BAREFOOT WALKING

Also by Michael Sandler and Jessica Lee

Barefoot Running

BAREFOOT WALKING

Free Your Feet to Minimize Impact,
Maximize Efficiency, and Discover the Pleasure
of Getting in Touch with the Earth

MICHAEL SANDLER
and
JESSICA LEE

Cofounders, RunBare Company

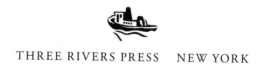

THREE RIVERS PRESS   NEW YORK

Library of Congress Cataloging-in-Publication data is available upon request.

ISBN 978-0-307-98591-0
eISBN 978-0-307-98592-7

PRINTED IN THE UNITED STATES OF AMERICA

For information about RunBare clinics, visit www.RunBare.com.

Editor: Sandra Wendel, Write On, Inc.
Cover design by Laura Palese

1 3 5 7 9 10 8 6 4 2

First Edition

Thank you, Pumpkin and Sawa, for blessing us with your lives, your spirits, and your lessons.

Life is good!

Contents

Preface

by The Sakyong,
author of *Running with the Mind of Meditation*

Walking is the most basic of human activities. It is also one of the most healthy forms of exercise. Not only is it beneficial for our bodies but also for our minds. It helps us connect with nature and the outdoors. It provides a natural basis for meditation and contemplation—a time of the day when we come in contact with our inner feelings, thoughts, and emotions.

As humans, it is essential that we have a moment in our day when we can self-reflect, release the busyness and stress, and for a moment, contact how we feel. These very brief moments of switching our allegiance from being extroverted to contacting an inner and deeper aspect of who we are is the cornerstone of living a meaningful life. It helps us prioritize. It allows us to reflect on the meaning of life itself—to come in contact with our inner purpose and motivation.

Walking is not simply how we get from one place to another. Rather, it can be a great mixture of mind and body—exercise and spirit. Therefore, walking is in itself a totality of human existence.

I am delighted that Michael and Jessica have highlighted many of these key points, especially encouraging how we, as humans, can contact the earth. We can do this as a personal form of health and well-being, or as humans, naturally within the ecosystem of our planet. By walking, we begin to re-contact that natural balance between humanity and our earth.

The Sandlers encourage us to remove our shoes and feel the earth beneath our feet, to walk on fresh green grass, to make contact with the sand along the beach, and even to venture out into mountain trails. All this is to reconnect with our own humanity. This is what I appreciate about the Sandlers' message—they utilize running, and now walking, not only as a way to exercise but as a way to connect with our own goodness and strength.

As humans, we have this basic goodness as the innate quality of who we are. However, through the challenges of life, we often lose contact with this intrinsic strength. When we lose contact with this, the fear and anxiety of life begin to overwhelm us. The natural harmony between mind and body gets disturbed and we begin to lose life-force energy. In order to restore a sense of vitality, meditation is helpful for the mind and exercise is helpful for the body.

In this light, walking is an excellent antidote to disharmony. It provides a perfect balance between movement and stillness. It slows our mind down in order to gain insight, while the increase of movement benefits circulation. Walking also naturally involves the breath. With the simple act of being aware of our breathing process, we are able to be present, which relieves anxiety and stress regarding the past and the future. This simple use of mindfulness is a natural component of walking. Placing one foot in front of the other, there is a natural inhalation and exhalation. As undramatic and simple as this may seem, it has a profound effect on our mental health and physical well-being.

We are living in a time when we are constantly being separated from the earth. Most of us live in heated buildings, drive cars, and walk on asphalt in our new shoes, rarely thinking about the earth that supports us. Even though these technologies serve humanity well, they have begun to create an unhealthy buffer between our environment and ourselves. Therefore, it is very much up to each one of us to reconnect with the earth.

In this wonderful guide, the Sandlers help us with the challenges we may encounter when we try to enjoy barefoot walking—from changes in posture and physiological differences to how we regard ourselves in the world. It offers a very thorough understanding of how barefoot walking can become an essential aspect of our natural health and well-being. It also communicates Michael and Jessica's spirit and joy in simply being alive. Based on personal experience, it presents walking not simply as a perfunctory form of transportation but as a symbol of life itself.

I hope this book inspires all of us to touch the earth and connect with our humanity.

The Sakyong

Foreword

by Dr. Mercola

If you are reading this book, health is a goal you are probably aspiring to achieve. It has been one of my primary goals for the last forty years.

In medical school I was surprised to find most education focused on treating disease rather than preventing it. After treating thousands of people it became abundantly clear the conventional approach to chronic disease fails to address the underlying cause, so it rarely resolves the problem.

The RAP Principle

I sought another model I now define as RAP (Replication of Ancestral Practices), based on the understanding that our genes and biochemistry take many centuries to adapt to environmental changes. If we follow similar patterns of our ancient ancestors, we will very likely optimize health.

Crucial Strategies to Improve Your Health

One big difference between modern society and our ancestors is they did not have access to refined food. So an important strategy is to avoid processed foods as much as possible.

If you drink soda it would be best to stop and drink pure filtered water instead, as sugar (especially corn syrup) and artificial sweeteners are particularly pernicious villains that will rob you of your health.

The Sun and the Earth

Most people ignore the numerous benefits of regular, safe exposure to the sun. Today the vast majority stay indoors when the sun peaks and do not receive vitamin D as our ancestors did. Though science is catching up, most people still take a supplement rather than the superior way from sunshine on their skin.

The Benefits of Grounding or Earthing

There are wide-ranging benefits of walking barefoot. For the few who walk and exercise outdoors, they typically wear shoes, which prevent contact with the earth. This is a major violation of RAP, as for millennia your ancestors had regular contact with the earth. While you could make a fairly solid argument for grounding based on ancestral practices, there is an emerging level of research to support the benefits. Much of this science is relatively recent and only fully appreciated in the twenty-first century.

It appears the earth carries a net negative charge and has a surplus of electrons it can donate if you are in contact with it. Not only does grounding appear to reduce inflammation, one of the primary influences of disease but also increases the Zeta potential of red blood cells, helping thin your blood and preventing clots from forming. While this may not seem important, there are many millions who take blood thinners or aspirin in the hope they will reduce the risk of heart attack and stroke.

Your Twenty-First-Century Bio Hacking

You most likely wear insulated shoes and live in an insulated home. So it is probable you regularly go days or months without being grounded for significant periods of time.

That is where *Barefoot Walking* comes into play. It provides practical strategies to implement earthing or grounding. It also does a wonderful job expanding on the theory and benefits of grounding.

So I strongly encourage you to aggressively apply the RAP principles and reap the benefits of your body's powerful healing mechanisms.

Dr. Mercola

Founder, Mercola.com

Most visited natural health site on the web

BAREFOOT WALKING

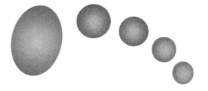

Introduction

People say that walking on water is a miracle, but to me, walking
peacefully on the Earth is the real miracle. The Earth is a miracle.
Each step is a miracle. Taking steps on our beautiful planet
can bring real happiness.
—Thich Nhat Hanh

Have you ever had a bad day, taken off your shoes, felt the ground with your bare feet, and suddenly everything felt right with the world?

There's something special—almost spiritual, even—about touching the earth.

Let's say you've had a challenging day at work. You come home. What's the first thing you do? Take off your shoes, right?

When you're barefoot, something special happens. You're connected and interconnected; you receive a flood of new information, yet everything's quiet. You feel the ground and suddenly all your anxiety dissipates.

A HEALTHY DOSE OF VITAMIN G

We were hiking through the jungle in Kauai, near the site of the filming of *Jurassic Park*, in the fall of 2010 when we started chatting about the main themes of this book. Admittedly, Michael was really sore when we started the hike. He'd gotten the flu on our travels, and though he didn't want it to affect our trip, he had full-body aches and chills. Not only that, but in a hurry to prepare for the Singapore Marathon (where he was to lead a team of runners and hold clinics), he'd rushed his training because we'd been stuck in a car all summer touring the United States, holding more than 130 clinics in 150 days. So he was far from being marathon-ready for Singapore.

So why in the world were we out hiking barefoot? Because we needed a healthy dose of vitamin G. Vitamin G is "vitamin ground," or the energy we get from the earth, which reduces inflammation, boosts our immune systems, calms our minds, and helps us to heal. We'll delve deeper into this topic in chapter 4.

In the jungle we walked over tree roots and lava stones, pine needles, seeds, small fruits, flowers, leaves, and much more. Each one of these has elements our bodies need to thrive and survive, and we absorb these nutrients through the skin of our bare feet.

As Michael walked along that day, he began to feel better and better. He started with a limp, and though he finished slowly, he finished tall and strong. His chills went away too, and his head began to clear. Only a week later he finished the Singapore Marathon, helping a forty-person team in the process.

MICHAEL'S STORY

I first discovered vitamin G after a nearly fatal accident in 2006. I was training for a cross-country skate, a world-record attempt to help students with learning disabilities. On a Sunday afternoon in April, I'd soaked my aching feet in a cool mountain creek, meditating for safety and guidance, then laced up my skates and pushed off, with the words of Dr. Wayne Dyer going through my head: "Everything in life happens for a reason." Going slowly, I rounded the first bend, and there before me, a tourist with a small toddler inadvertently stepped out onto the bike path. I threw myself down to avoid the baby. I lay broken and hurt but thankful I hadn't hit the child. I almost lost my life, and nearly lost my left leg. Months of rehabilitation followed. However, the accident put me on a new path in life, and over time, this turned out to be for the best.

With a titanium femur, a titanium hip, ten knee operations, nearly a one-inch leg length discrepancy, and little left of my lateral or medial meniscus, not to mention no ACL to anchor my knee, I was told I'd never be able to run again, and barely be able to walk.

Add to this my chronic plantar fasciitis (I had to wear hard-plastic custom orthotics in motion control shoes just to get across my living room floor), and there seemed to be almost no chance I'd be fully mobile again.

But little did I know I had nature on my side. And so do you.

We believe there's natural abundance all around us. The ability to heal is not limited to pharmaceuticals; instead, healing can be found in everything we see, hear, eat, breathe, and, in this case, touch or feel with our feet.

Being limited to life in a wheelchair wasn't acceptable to me, so I picked up a pair of crutches and headed out into nature, determined to heal. I felt a healing power there, as if something was drawing me to the trails—as if something healing was out there that I couldn't get on the sidewalks or bike paths.

And beyond that, something was drawing me to take off my shoes.

Now, I was literally a tenderfoot. My podiatrists had told me I was never, ever allowed to go barefoot. A grain of sand in my shoes or a pebble underfoot would nearly give me an anxiety attack. But as I worked my way off crutches and into shoes, something didn't feel right.

As my energy grew stronger, my body remained weak. How could I walk again, run again, or simply take a step and be pain-free?

On June 14, 2007, I began to find the answer.

I'd exhausted the road I was on and knew I had to find a different way. I'd been through shoe after shoe, orthotic after orthotic, I'd made my own, designed my own, yet nothing had worked. All I kept thinking to myself was that I needed a dynamic supercomputer on the fly, something that was smarter than I am, that could help me feel or sense the ground, accommodate for my challenges (such as having one leg an inch shorter than the other), overcome my numerous overuse injuries, and heal.

And then for some reason it came to me. Maybe it was the healing I was experiencing by being out in nature.

Whatever it was, I felt the pull to take off my shoes. Now, there were intellectual reasons for sure—as I said, nothing I was trying was working, and my

Japanese elite athlete friends mocked me for sporting bulky shoes—but this was something deeper, more visceral, like a voice in my head saying, "You've tried everything else, why don't you try taking off your shoes?"

And so I did. I told myself, "Let the grand experiment begin."

I was both scared and excited, feeling like I was standing at the start of a race waiting for the gun to go off. I reasoned, "What's the worst that can happen? I'm already broken." Ultimately, that's what gave me the courage and confidence to dive off the deep end.

So I prepared myself as best I could (I got the ice packs ready), snuck out the door, and ever so gently began my grand adventure.

I must say, the ground felt good. Even though I began on cement, it didn't feel as hard as I'd expected, but instead a bit light and springy. Now I could feel *everything*, and in particular the grain-sized pebbles beneath my feet. They didn't feel great, but they didn't scare me away either. I figured they were a temporary nuisance and would soon fade away.

The long and short of it is that it worked, and worked tremendously well. I went from walking 100 yards to running a 10K, and eventually running up to 30 miles a day barefoot. This from the guy who was barely expected to walk!

But something more precious came out of this: the healing power of nature. That's why we call it vitamin G—there's a healing power in getting grounded.

We'll go more into the science behind this in an upcoming chapter, but in brief, getting grounded, or getting vitamin G, can be one of the most healing experiences of all. It boosts your immune system, reduces inflammation, reduces levels of a stress hormone called cortisol, helps lower blood pressure, and provides our bodies with vital nutrients through the skin on the bottom of our feet. In essence, it's more powerful than any vitamin supplement you could ever buy.

PRESCRIPTION EARTH

Of course, Michael wasn't the only one of us who healed from an injury by going bare. Jessica injured her foot as we were coming off our whirlwind national tour for our first barefoot book, and the earth helped her heal.

In the spring of 2011 we moved to an Earthship—a self-contained off-the-grid home—in Taos, New Mexico. We were moving from the front range of the

Rockies in Colorado, with lush growth, good amounts of rain, and lots of snow, to a desert experiencing the start of what's been described as a "five-hundred-year drought." Our new house was built *out* of earth and built *into* the earth: the entire north side of the house was underground, the south part above ground with huge windows to take advantage of the sunlight all day long.

Living in and on the earth may still be the norm in many third-world countries, but we're very disconnected from that here in the United States. What we found was that though humble living situations certainly have their inconveniences, the experience at its core feels wonderful, almost indescribable.

Stepping into an Earthship feels and smells like going outside after a fresh rain that purifies the air. The entire length of the adobe home had a giant planter filled with garden growth. This added subtle scents of fruits, flowers, and vegetables while humidifying the air as well. We felt we were walking into our own Garden of Eden.

Walking on the property, or anywhere around the desert, we could feel the energy radiating from the ground—the same energy that has drawn Native Americans to this area for thousands of years. It's palpable and tingly underfoot.

On one of those walks, Jessica found a labyrinth buried under tumbleweeds in the desert behind our house. It was a circular path several hundred feet long, mapped out with desert stones and over fifty feet in diameter. Walking the labyrinth is a meditative form of reflective contemplation—and healing.

Clearing and walking the labyrinth was almost the first thing Jessica did, and when we had to move because of a nearby fire that clogged the air with smoke, walking the labyrinth was last thing she did as well. It was her way to connect, to wish a beautiful thanks and goodbye to our earthen home.

Michael's foot had healed too, and we know Mother Earth had more than a little something to do with that.

GREAT HEALERS DIDN'T WEAR SHOES

We are not saying vitamin G is the cure-all for everything, but certainly we know vitamin D, a product of the sun working in cahoots with our bodies, can help us, so surely vitamin G, a product of the ground, can help us as well.

Out on the trails of Kauai, our trail guide, Harold, was talking about the healing power of the earth and the great kahunas who have healed Hawaiians for countless centuries. He spoke of other great peoples too, such as the Maori of New Zealand, and their healing connection with the earth.

It seems you can find stories about the spiritual and medicinal benefits of going barefoot almost anywhere—if you ask. You will hear of great healers or spiritual people who do their best work, blessings, and prayers while being barefoot. There are great spiritual leaders of the past who went barefoot, such as the Buddha, who walked from town to town barefoot. Jesus had his apostles go barefoot. Even Gandhi is said to have meditated while walking barefoot. You hear stories about Muhammad going barefoot. There are stories in the *Bhagavad Gita*, in the Bible, in Hindu texts, in Buddhist texts, in the Torah, and in the Koran—story after story about connecting with God by taking off your shoes.

Think of the fire walkers of the island nations from around the world. Or of the African messengers who went barefoot or in straw sandals, traveling hundreds of miles at a time.

And there are modern Buddhists, both Eastern and Western alike, who practice walking meditations as part of their daily and weekly rituals. A wise monk, whom we quote in this book because of his marvelous insight, is Thich Nhat Hanh, who often practices his walking meditations barefoot.

One of the most inspiring stories is of the "marathon monks" of Mount Hiei in Japan. It turns out they walk the equivalent of two marathons a day—more than fifty miles—for seven years while on a quest for enlightenment and salvation in this modern world. They do it through snowstorms, thunderstorms, vicious summer heat, and the cold of winter. In dramatic fashion, they've vowed to take their own lives if they can't complete a day's journey during their seven-year quest.

Nearly as dramatic as the distance they travel is the fact that they do it nearly barefoot. For all seven years, they only wear a weak, unsupportive, handmade straw slipper. It's so fragile they may go through a pair or two a day.

By being nearly barefoot in thin footwear made of all-natural materials, they can absorb the healing energy beneath them. Along with their meditation, going shoeless helps them gain strength to make the journey. In fact, we would say it's *because* they don't wear shoes, not in spite of it, that they become stronger through the journey, survive, and, according to all accounts, reach a degree of enlightenment.

Jessica's father, a tai chi master, practices barefoot each day. He too talks about the healing power of the earth. The Lung-gom-pa runners, yogis of Tibetan tradition, train their breathing for up to seven years, sitting on the earth in solitude, before they begin walking and running vast distances of up to several hundred miles in only a couple of days.

When you're touching the ground, it's as if you've plugged yourself into an electrical outlet, one both of healing and of quieting the mind. In essence, once you've walked barefoot, it's hard to view the world in quite the same way again.

You're quieter, more peaceful, more compassionate and kind. You're more connected to the world, meaning more eco-friendly, and less likely to do harm to your neighbors. And your mind unclutters as well.

You gain new perspective with each barefoot footfall, and you'll find you are better able to separate what's important from what's not, and to know what you should and shouldn't do.

Have a tough decision to make? Go barefoot before you decide. Need a brilliant answer to an important question? Go barefoot and just listen. Feeling overwhelmed at home or work? Go barefoot and watch troubles fade away. Mind cluttered with so much information you can't sort it out? Simply go barefoot and see what you find.

To us, there's almost no difference between a great mindful walk barefoot, prayer in a place of worship, and meditation in a shrine. In each of these experiences, you're thinking of something greater than yourself and connecting with something deeply spiritual on the inside.

When you go barefoot, you're plugging into the source of everything. After all, as it says in the Bible, we go from dust to dust, or from the earth back to the earth. Therefore it only makes sense that we're touching what we came from when we're walking barefoot by plugging back into Source.

LIFE-ALTERING BENEFITS OF BAREFOOT WALKING

In this book we share what we've learned with you, so that you too can reap the life-altering benefits of barefoot walking:

- If you've never walked for leisure or exercise before, this book will be your guide to taking off your shoes with minimal risk of injury and maximum health and joy.
- If you're looking for a new twist on a tired old exercise program, you'll find immense success with barefoot walking, especially if you want to get off the treadmill of life (and off the treadmill at the gym) and try something refreshingly fun.
- If you're already a dedicated walker, this book will show you a much more aware way of getting into the zone and improving your stride, form, and performance.
- If you're overcoming an injury—as both of us were—this book will explain how barefoot walking can strengthen your feet and arches in ways you never dreamed possible.
- If weight loss is your goal, walking is a proven way to shed pounds—and you don't need any fancy equipment, rigorous diets, or scales to measure results. In fact, you just need to take off your shoes and step out the front door.
- If you think you're too old to start something new, we are here to tell you that you can teach your old "dogs" new tricks and why, as you age, you owe it to yourself to go barefoot.
- For the very young whose parents may be reading this book, we examine how going shoeless (or nearly shoeless) in childhood keeps those darling little baby feet fat and strong.

And for everyone, no matter your age, shape, or goal, if you're craving a more spiritual connection to the world, walking sans shoes will give you that as well. It will help you quiet your mind and begin a fantastic journey on the inside. Perhaps instead of "walking barefoot," this practice should be called "walking yoga" for its mind-body-spirit (or mind-body-earth) connection.

Even if you aren't ready to plunge fully into the barefoot scene, this book can still give you handy tips for exercise, diet, and strengthening your feet, until you're ready to slip off those shoes.

In 2010 we wrote a highly successful book called *Barefoot Running: How to Run Light and Free by Getting in Touch with the Earth*. We toured the United States and the world, holding clinics and retreats (for more on retreats and talks near you, visit our RunBare website). At every stop, we were asked about walking barefoot. We know not everyone is a runner—and some never will be. This book is for all nonrunners and for runners who are rehabbing from an injury or just need some be-kind-to-your-body cross training and connection with the earth.

This book has grown out of our nationwide and international quest to bring the message of going bare—whether you run or walk or just feel the earth beneath your feet—to millions of people the world over.

So kick your shoes off and let the journey of a million steps (in bare feet) begin right now.

YOUR STEP-BY-STEP WALKING GUIDE

Have you ever traveled to a new city and wanted to see the sights? The best way is to grab a guidebook, usually called a "walking guide." Think of this book as your walking guide to—ta-da!—walking without shoes. You'll see familiar terrain with new eyes and new awareness underfoot.

You won't have to tear off your shoes until chapter 7. First we present a brief introduction to walking barefoot and why it's so darned good for you—even if you are among those who still think it's a preposterous idea but were just curious enough to pick up this book. These first few chapters discuss why barefoot walking is a safe alternative and even more satisfying than wearing shoes while you walk.

Of course, if you're new to walking for exercise or just new to walking without your shoes, you'll need some of the basics, and that's in chapter 7 as we help you start by walking on a broad expanse of green grass. Then we'll stride right into the warm-up exercises in preparation for a real walking tour in chapters 8 and 9.

In chapter 10 we'll learn how to strengthen and condition our feet, revealing the marvel of nature's perfect design. Moving on up the kinetic chain brings us to chapter 11, in which we'll review proper technique and guidelines for drills, strengthening exercises, weight training, and cross training, for a total body makeover. Once our muscles are warmed up, in chapter 12 we'll keep them loose, supple, and injury-free by stretching.

Two special populations that are often overlooked in books on walking are children and seniors. Their particular issues with being barefoot are discussed in chapters 14 and 15.

Not every sidewalk or road is smooth and easy, so we'll show you in chapters 16 and 17 how to turn your feet into "all-terrain vehicles" and anticipate the roads less traveled and unpredictable weather conditions.

This comprehensive guide would not be complete without a serious discussion of nutrition, in chapter 13. And, unfortunately, injuries come with just about any activity—mostly while wearing shoes—but they don't have to be surprises, and surely you will need to know how to overcome any injuries or foot problems that sideline you, because you will want to be back out there quickly. Chapter 18 discusses the proven ways to stay healthy.

It seems odd to discuss footwear in a book about walking without shoes, but chapter 19 introduces you to minimalist footwear you might want to try—that is, *after* you've let your feet feel the ground.

Once you've mastered the basics and discovered the joy in walking and truly feeling the earth beneath your feet, you may remain barefoot for life. In chapter 20, we discuss going beyond barefoot walking, both in terms of activities such as running barefoot and in terms of stewardship of our planet. For when your feet meet the dirt, you'll never walk with a big footprint again.

You're about to embark on an exciting journey, one that we've been on and which continues to amaze us. Countless others have found pure joy, health, and emotional and spiritual well-being by stripping off their shoes and going barefoot. Now you can too. We'll be cheering you on, giving you advice, and helping you through the tough times. On that note, you can post your questions, find helpful tips, and follow our adventures on our Facebook page, www.facebook.com/RunBare. You can subscribe to our individual pages too, where we each share our own barefoot journeys and photos: www.facebook.com/RunsWith Spirit and www.facebook.com/JessicaLeeSandler.

You're about to step into a brave new world, so let's begin!

PART I

Why on Earth Would You Want to Walk Barefoot?

The miracle is not to walk on water.
The miracle is to walk on the green earth,
Dwelling deeply in the present moment,
And feeling truly alive.

—Thich Nhat Hanh

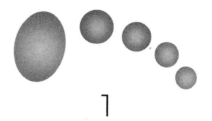

1
Walk Your Way to Health and Happiness

I only went out for a walk and finally concluded to stay out till
sundown, for going out, I found, was really going in.
—John Muir

No matter what, we always return to barefoot walking.

At our barefoot running clinics, people often ask, "What do I do if I'm not ready to start running?" or "What if I hate running?" Or they would tell us they were too weak, too old, or too heavy. For them, who were the vast majority, we would prescribe barefoot walking. It's an activity nearly everyone can do, and a kind and gentle way to exercise.

It's something kids can do to grow their feet and limbs strong. It's something seniors can do to roll back the clock, gaining balance, strength, flexibility, and even greater bone density. And it's something all of us can do, even with the most hectic of schedules, to get or stay in shape and quiet our minds in the process.

Walking barefoot each sunrise and sunset is where we do our best brainstorming for our books. It's where we swap ideas, feel things out, and have our greatest aha moments. You could call our barefoot walking time our "lab time" or our "creative time."

It's like a substitute for antianxiety medication without the side effects. Even today, if we start to get wound up, we head outside for a few minutes of barefoot walking or sitting on the ground. Both calm us and refresh us creatively.

Walking barefoot could be the deep breath we all need during stressful times. And for those seeking a spiritual experience, barefoot walking truly is the greatest exercise on earth.

It's hard to focus on your spiritual growth when your house (your body) is falling apart and your mind is wrapped up in thought. Barefoot walking helps your spiritual path, no matter what your religion, by helping you build a stronger foundation for your home and quiet the chatter. When you walk barefoot, you can't help but clear your mind and focus merely on your footsteps, or on the ground beneath your feet.

In essence, though designed to get us from point A to point B, barefoot walking is a powerful form of meditation or prayer, whether we intend it to be that way or not.

You'll gain a greater connection to your beliefs, to the earth, and to your higher power, whatever or whoever that is for you, with each and every step. You'll clear your mind and have time to breathe, to think, and to pray.

Quite simply, barefoot walking is our birthright. It's something each of us was born to do and can do, and it has some dramatic health benefits. And for us personally, it was our path to healing—Michael from an accident in 2006, Jessica from a foot injury in 2010, and both of us from a book tour that left us exhausted in every sense.

It was only by going barefoot and going back to basics, back to walking, that we began to heal.

ONE FOOT IN FRONT OF THE OTHER

You aren't likely to set any records for long-distance walking or to push your body into being a superstar athlete with barefoot walking. Though we will set modest goals together, when they are combined these small, incremental changes will be life-changing.

Our goal is to help you turn yourself into a healthy, happy human being. It's about helping you overcome your own challenges and grow, both physically and mentally.

"Ah, but isn't barefoot walking a strange way to grow?" you ask. "After all, you're just putting one foot in front of the other, right?"

Well, actually, that's the point. For when you put one foot in front of the other and can *feel* what's going on beneath your feet, something special happens. It's as if you've flipped the on switch for your body, which begins to wake up and sense what's going on.

When you go barefoot and commit to a practice, you can't help but get better. Your joints heal, your muscles grow stronger, you stand taller and with better posture, your blood sugar seems to be better regulated, your body's inflammation subsides, and overall you feel much younger. And that's just a few of the physical aspects.

Changes on the metaphysical level are even more dramatic. Your mind begins to quiet. In a world where we're going 24/7, being bombarded with texts, tweets, emails, and advertisements from all directions, and have more stressors and commitments than ever before, the toll on our minds is catastrophic. So if we can quiet the mind, we've gone a long way toward returning to health. For you can't have a healthy body without a healthy mind.

It all begins with the mind. Your inside journey begins with a single step. When you go barefoot and feel the ground, you begin to expand your inner awareness. And that's where the real fun begins.

Perhaps you've come to this book with a desire to heal, overcome injury, or cope with a long-lasting condition that's left you with poor health. Barefoot walking is a holistic, gentle way to turn your body, and therefore your health, back on. If you think of humans as being like giant trees, our health begins with our roots. For us, our "roots" are our feet.

Start to strengthen and heal the feet, and you strengthen your roots. It's a very simple process too. We start with short exercises and even shorter strolls. The great news is that it can be done anywhere, especially at your favorite places. For instance, head to your neighborhood park or a local arboretum or botanical garden. Who knew you could heal and get in shape just by looking at the beauty all around you?

As you get into barefoot walking, you will feel a revitalized sense of connection with nature. You may have heard the term *nature-deficit disorder*. Whether you live in the cities, the suburbs, or even the country, unless you're working on a farm, chances are you've become disconnected from your natural environment.

This disconnect is harmful because it can leave you lost, confused, and unsure of who you are, because since the beginning of time we came from the earth, lived on the earth, and worked as one with the earth.

Now that we're driving cars, living in multistory buildings, and walking on linoleum floors, we're completely disconnected from where we came. But as you begin to feel the earth beneath your feet, you begin to reestablish that connection, to plug back into the ground, and to renew your birthright of perfect health and joy.

We really were meant to dance with nature, play outdoors, and wander in the woods. It's what's healed us and sustained us for millions of years, and it's still there, beckoning us, calling us.

BUILD A NEW BODY

When Michael got into barefoot walking, he was broken, healing from a near-death accident and living with a new titanium femur and hip. He went from one overuse injury to the next. Only by feeling the ground was he able to heal.

Others of you have similar broken bodies. Maybe you're overweight or obese, or struggling with an autoimmune disease or diabetes. Maybe your joints ache. Your back hurts. You suffer from migraines. Perhaps that pain in your side is a broken relationship, an ailing parent for whom you provide daily care, a cruel boss, or a devastating loss of a friend or partner—an unfulfilled life, or broken dreams.

No matter what baggage you are carrying mentally and physically, barefoot walking may help you cope and recover.

The most important point is that we are not our bodies. Our bodies are merely the shells that house the soul. No matter what your body is like, it's yours just for this lifetime. Then your body passes on, eventually returning to the earth (hmm, there's that earth theme again).

If you believe in your mind that you can change your body, you can. Your body is a gift. Cherish it and treat it as best you can.

Think of your body like an expensive car—perhaps a true collector's item, or maybe the car you've dreamed about your whole life. Chances are you wouldn't buy the car and suddenly pack it with trash, dent the heck out of it, or fill it with bad gasoline.

On the contrary, you'd likely do your best to treat it well, give it the high-octane fuel it needs and the maintenance it deserves, and keep it sparkly clean.

Well, that's what we need to do with our bodies too. Treat your body well, and it'll treat you well. Where the analogy with the car stops is that we can regenerate our bodies. Nearly every cell in our bodies is replaced every three to five years. You don't have the same skin cells you had even yesterday, or the same bone cells you had just a few years ago. This means you can truly transform your body into whatever you desire it to be.

You can decide what type of new body you would like. When we first started our journeys, we wanted bodies that no longer felt cramped from being stuffed in a car or seated in front of a computer for too long. What are you looking for?

Start building your new body by putting your two bare feet on the ground. It's as if you're plugging into a computer and downloading instructions for perfect health. For when you feel the ground, you gain awareness, and with each step you are working toward a new and improved you.

Love your body, and it will love you. It's so simple.

Consider the discipline or practice of barefoot walking to be like a daily dose of love. You get up, you go for a walk, and you send love to your body. Each day as you walk, you're filling it with more love and more love—and reshaping it in more ways than one.

When you commit to a daily routine, either walking or stretching (to promote your walk), you're giving yourself permission to heal, permission to become healthy again.

No matter how far gone your health is, no matter how weak or tired you are feeling, you can make this change. All it takes is believing you can change and focusing on one gentle barefoot step at a time.

As you prepare to make this change, don't focus on any negatives. Instead, see yourself walking daily. Feel the joy of connecting with the earth. Imagine the stillness and peace of mind of focusing on your breath and on the beauty all around you. And watch it come into being. The path will clear ahead.

FEEL THE EARTH, FREE YOUR SPIRIT

When you're plugged into the earth, you're connecting with something greater than yourself. You go from a single soul of one to a community of everyone (the community of humanity). You go from an uprooted tree to one plugged into the soil with far-reaching roots connecting with a community of other trees. When you go barefoot, you're plugging back into the soil, back into the earth, and back into our global community. As Henry David Thoreau said, "Heaven is under our feet as well as over our heads."

When you feel the earth, you can't help but see the world in a more spiritual way, because even little things such as leaves, bark, pebbles, or clouds become so much bigger and clearer. In essence, by going barefoot, it's as if you're plugging back into Source—whatever that spiritual connection means to you—because you're going back to the ground from which we came.

How can it not be spiritual when we're feeling the beauty beneath our feet and suddenly we're looking in childlike awe and joy at the world around us? We see the beauty of a flower again, the grandeur of the tree, the amazing wonder of the feeling of the dirt beneath our feet. We begin to see the grand design of things and how we are part of that design.

To us, there's nothing more spiritual than plugging back into where we came from. Physically, that begins by going barefoot. Mentally, that begins with quieting our minds. And spiritually, that begins with the practice of letting go, surrendering, and just being.

For, as the expression goes, we are human *be*-ings. Our job is to let go, to be, to learn, to grow, and to see what happens. We can have this fully human existence, be spiritual beings having a human experience, only when we let go and be in the moment. And when you are fully barefoot, when your naked feet meet the earth (our shrine, our temple), in an instant you are present.

And what a beautiful instant that is!

Awareness begins with your first barefoot steps, awareness of the ground, awareness of your mind, and awareness of that still, small, yet growing voice inside calling you forward. That's your soul, your higher self, reawakened by the ground beneath your feet. By going barefoot, you step through the doorway and into the temple of the great outdoors.

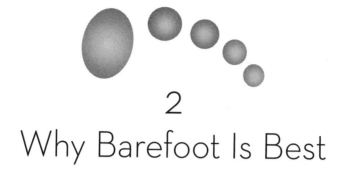

2
Why Barefoot Is Best

Speak to the earth, and it shall teach thee.

—Job 12:8

Monday, June 6, 2011, is a day we'll never forget. After holding a weekend retreat at the Kripalu Center for Yoga and Health in the Berkshires, I rushed to New York City for a whirlwind day of meetings with the top publishers in the world.

Our literary agent, Stephanie, had miraculously planned ten back-to-back meetings in one day. To make each meeting on time, we'd have to walk at top speed from one corporate office to the next. But she'd mapped it out well and clocked each leg, so we were well prepared for the challenge.

Tromping through Manhattan to our first meeting, however, Stephanie's feet began to ache. She wasn't wearing anything overstated or terribly disfiguring on her feet, no stilettos or pointy-toed shoes. Instead, she'd donned a tasteful open-toed dress sandal, quite appropriate for late spring meetings with execs, though perhaps a tiny bit too narrow in the toe box.

But as we walked briskly down the city streets and Stephanie watched me going barefoot, she proudly declared, "Oh, what the heck!" and stripped off her shoes.

And her feet came back to life.

First her feet took to springing, then bouncing, and finally even bounding at times. Fortunately, Stephanie had read our first book, *Barefoot Running*, and she is also a burgeoning yogi, so she was already well practiced in barefoot movement. Even so, she was astounded by how much better her feet were feeling walking barefoot. We felt like kids, playing along the streets of New York. She was giddy with delight.

Into meeting after meeting, both Stephanie and I made our entrance barefoot. It became the topic of conversation among department VPs and senior editors, some of the nicest yet toughest individuals in the city. These were often no-nonsense New Yorkers with strong ideas, traditionally not quick to change. And yet when Stephanie showed up barefoot, they soon found themselves following suit and delightfully stripped off their shoes. It was contagious.

This book is the result of that day. And so are some extra-happy feet. On a day when her feet should have been killing her, Stephanie was delighted to report, her feet survived the streets of New York and felt better than ever. "Why didn't I think of this sooner?" she asked.

FREE SHOES FOR EVERYONE

How could something we have for free—our bare feet—be better than shoes that cost money? After all, shoes are designed to protect our feet—aren't they?

The truth about walking in shoes, especially high heels and rocker-style aerobic shoes, is that they can be downright dangerous to your feet and your overall health.

An Iowa State University study evaluated women wearing flats, two-inch heels, and three-and-a-half-inch heels. You don't need to be a researcher to figure out how this went. The higher the heel, the greater the forces on the inside of the knee. These forces, over time, can contribute to osteoarthritis of the knee, leading to a lifetime of pain and a need for knee replacements. And if that isn't painful enough, high heels force women to bend forward at the pelvic bone, causing undue stress on the lower back and the spine.

While previous studies have examined the effect of high heels on joints, the ISU researchers found that the higher the heel, the slower women walked, the shorter their strides became, and the more compression they experienced on the inside—or medial side—of the knee.

That's the dirty little secret the shoe manufacturers don't want you to know.

Perhaps the safest, most comfortable shoe in your closet is your bedroom slipper. Think about it. What shoes do you put on when your feet hurt? When you're just hanging out at home?

A LIGHTER STEP

Our feet have the most concentrated group of nerves in our body. So when we walk, our feet have a natural desire to feel what's going on. It allows them to adjust to different surface conditions on a moment-by-moment basis.

When we wear cushioned shoes, though, it reduces the ability of our feet to sense what's happening beneath them. We'll therefore automatically hit the ground extra hard with each step just to compensate for not feeling the ground directly.

Here's how the problem was explained by orthopedic surgeon Joseph Froncioni in the pivotal article that confirmed to Michael that taking his shoes off would speed his injury recovery:

> [When barefoot,] the ball of the foot strikes the ground first and immediately starts sending signals to the spinal cord and brain about the magnitude of impact and shear, getting most of its clues about this from the skin contact with the surface irregularities of the ground. Take away this contact by adding a cushioned substance [a shoe] and you immediately fool the system into underestimating the impact. Add a raised heel and the shod runner [and walker] is forced to land on it. Strap the cushioning on tightly with the aid of a sophisticated lacing system and you block out shear as well, throwing the shock-absorption system even further into the dark. The system responds by landing harder in an attempt to compress the cushion and "feel" the ground.

The repeated high impact from walking in shoes creates terrible stress on our ankles, knees, legs, and hips. The cumulative effect of these micro traumas to which we subject our bodies leads to stress fractures, plantar fasciitis, bunions, and a variety of other ailments of the knees and back that can sideline casual and avid walkers alike.

Discover Your Springs

The calcaneus, or heel bone, is magnificently designed for standing and walking, helping us balance over any kind of terrain. When we walk barefoot and with proper form, we land very lightly on our forefoot, or may even roll off the heel. The twenty-eight bones in each of our feet work in harmony with our muscles to absorb shock and bounce back. This giant "spring" is one of the greatest marvels of the human body.

Landing hard on your heel, whether barefoot or shod, is harmful to the body, but a cushioned shoe gives you a false sense of security. Those cushy shoes lead your brain to the false conclusion that it's okay to land on your heel first—you're protected. But that heel strike sends a shock wave straight through to your ankles, knees, hips, back, and neck. It's as if you're striking bone on bone; once the impact travels past the shoe, there's no stopping it.

Get Low, Feel High

Barefoot walking begins from the ground on up. But in order to meet the ground correctly, you first need to unlearn a bad habit we all learned in a shoe.

You see, a typical shoe—almost any shoe, whether for walking, for running, or for dress—isn't just a shoe, it's a high heel. Take a look at your shoes. In fact, look down right now at what's on your feet.

Note the size and shape of the heel. Chances are it's between one and two inches in height. That may not seem like much, but it has a dramatic effect on how you stand and walk and puts pressure on your legs, feet, and joints.

If you think about walking in true high heels (if you're a guy, you'll have to use your imagination), you know that if you don't adjust how you stand, you'll fall forward, flat on your face. That's because high heels lean you forward. Just watch little kids playing dress-up in high heels. They lean forward (and often fall).

To stay upright in high heels, you need to lean back. The way your body adapts to this lean is to hinge at the waist and kick your butt back. In anatomical terms, you're rotating your pelvis forward. This shifts your center of gravity

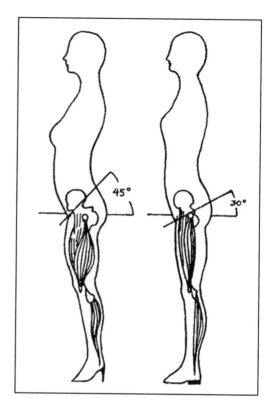

Wearing heels creates stress and strain on the hamstrings, knees, shoulders, neck, and back by forcing the pelvis to dip forward and the butt to rotate back.

back and keeps you from falling forward. It's also why some people think high heels make women look more shapely, because they have to adjust with their derrieres.

Now, whether it's a true high heel or a running or walking shoe doesn't make a difference: when your heel is higher than your forefoot, you need to adjust how you stand so you don't fall forward on your face. It's another telling argument for getting rid of all those high-heeled shoes.

For every inch your heels are up off the ground, you're tilting your pelvis forward at least 10 to 15 degrees. Stand up and try it. See what we mean?

This kind of change in our anatomy, how we stand, is highly significant in terms of the body. And it's unnatural.

Your body works as a kinetic chain, or a series of movements, each one affecting the next. If you think of the body as a series of interconnected links in a chain, you must move one link before the next, and if one of them is out of position, it can disrupt the smoothness of the chain. When you rotate the pelvis forward to compensate for a high heel, for example, you cause several detrimental

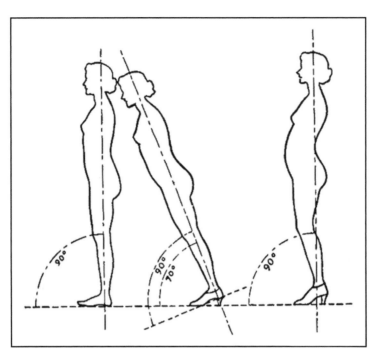

If you want to stay upright in high heels, you must rotate your pelvis, swinging your butt backward while painfully exaggerating the arch in your lower back.

changes to how you stand and walk (just look at the arched back and pooched belly on the woman on the far right in the diagram above).

First, your pelvis pulls on your back and hamstrings. If you've ever gotten tight hamstrings (the muscles on the upper back of your thighs) while you walk, it's because of the tilt in your pelvis. More often than not, it pulls on your knees and lower back muscles, making them sore as you walk, stand, or move throughout the day.

Believe it or not, this also affects your upper back, shoulders, and neck, because as you lean forward, your back, shoulders, and neck are forced to do the work of holding you up. They become fatigued and strained.

In a sense, it's as if you've attached a weight to your neck by a string. As you lean forward it pulls on your neck, straining your entire neck, back, and shoulders throughout the day. If you could stand truly upright, the strain would go away. Unfortunately, so would your balance in a typical shoe.

It also causes you to lean forward, putting more pressure on your thighs,

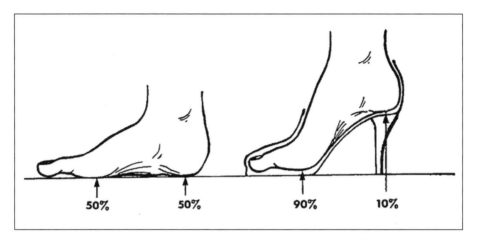

Note the even weight distribution throughout your foot while standing barefoot versus wearing a shoe with a heel. The greater the difference in weight distribution, the greater the chance of injury and deformity.

knees, and even feet. This awkward posture is sure to fatigue you. It will make you sorer as you walk. It also makes you less stable and more likely to fall. No wonder you want to intuitively kick off your shoes when you come home from work.

One final point on posture: when you lean forward, you're squashing your poor feet in shoes. Leaning forward puts extra pressure on your feet, which are trapped in shoes. Even in a well-fitting shoe, if you're leaning forward, you're pushing your feet forward, smashing your toes right into the toe box of your shoes.

Chances are, unless you've been in sandals or barefoot your whole life, your feet are telling a tale. Take off your shoes now and look at your toes.

Injuries and misshapen toes have two main sources: a shoe that's too tight and small for the foot (more on this shortly) and leaning forward and jamming your foot into the front of a shoe. Foot problems aren't caused by genetics, as some people think. You don't have to have bunions or squished toes. Over time, you can positively change the shape of your foot. The only thing you can blame on Mom and Dad is what they made you wear as an infant and how they influenced the type of shoes you wore as a child and perhaps even as an adult. Mom and Dad likely put you in the same type of shoes they wore.

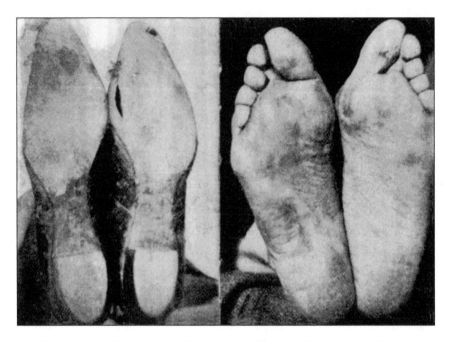

Note how the feet take the shape of the shoes and how the big toes are cocked inward.

How far your feet can go toward returning to normal depends on the amount of time and dedication you want to put into it, but you can get your feet looking and working better. And they will feel better too.

DONALD DUCK KNEW BEST

Perhaps you've heard this analogy: Place a frog in hot water, and it'll jump right out. But place the frog in cool water and then gradually bring the water up to a boil, and the frog will stay right in the pot up until the end and boil to death. (Don't worry—no frogs were harmed in the making of this analogy.)

Think of your feet as the frog.

More than a hundred years ago, doctors were already talking about the incredibly harmful effects of footwear, and they hadn't even come out with modern high-heeled walking or running shoes yet. Back then, doctors recognized and documented the differences between the feet of those who spent their lives barefoot and those who habitually wore shoes. Shoes can quickly yet quietly deform our feet and cripple our bodies.

Because feet are very plastic or malleable, they'll conform to or take the

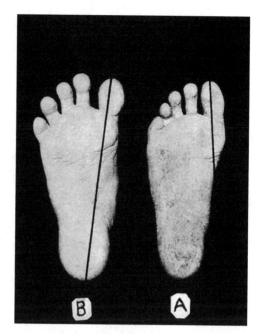

The person with the foot on the left probably never wore shoes and has a natural, wide triangle to stand on. The person on the right has been wearing shoes, and the foot has taken on the shape of the shoes.

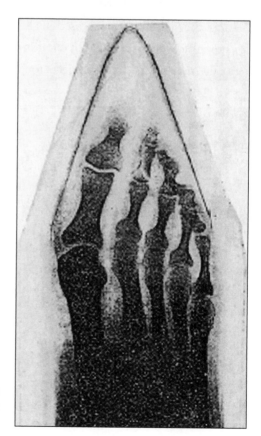

Note how the bones of the foot are squashed together in a shoe that's not shaped like a natural foot.

shape of anything we put them in. Like shoes. You can see your foot shape by simply stepping into a puddle with bare feet and parading down your driveway or sidewalk.

In nature, our feet develop to a natural, wide triangle, an incredibly stable platform on which to stand. That platform may have a high arch or a low arch, a high instep or a flat foot. Studies show that the height of the arch has absolutely nothing to do with the foot's performance, the walking gait, or injuries. Unfortunately, that's a long-standing myth about arches. Instead, it's all about foot strength.

The average natural foot—though it comes in all shapes and sizes—more often than not is as flat as a pancake. Why? It's likely that muscle and fat padding have filled in around that great strong arch. But again, there's no one ideal shape, size, or height of the arch.

Natural, unencumbered feet are triangular, or almost paddle-shaped, like Donald Duck's. These feet have far greater stability, resilience, and strength. The toes of the lifelong barefooter are also stronger and often tend to be longer, because they haven't been encased in shoes. And they work better too, not only for propulsion but also to aid in climbing, dancing, and picking up things (yes, feet can grab and hold on to objects too).

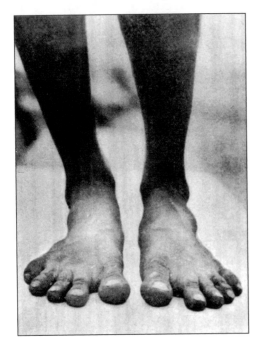

When unshod, toes spread and feet naturally develop to a wide triangle, an incredibly stable platform on which to stand.

This may sound strange, but look at how a baby uses her toes. In the beginning she's using her toes and feet as fingers and hands. She doesn't know that's not what she's supposed to do. In fact, it's exactly what she's supposed to do for good, strong, healthy feet.

We're all born with these amazing feet. And then we stuff them into narrow shoes.

Modern Chinese Foot Binding

As we've noted, our feet are quite malleable or plastic. They can take on almost any shape. That's where Chinese foot binding comes in. This practice was designed to compress or deform a girl's foot so that it would grow to no more than four and a half inches long—basically just a stub. The woman would never be able to stand still when upright: she would have to constantly move back and forth to keep her balance, or she would need to be assisted when walking. Her feet were completely deformed by her footwear.

Our feet are also misshapen from our shoes—although not quite as dramatically as with foot binding. Like the frog in the pot, adapting to an ever-warmer environment, our feet change without us even knowing it. From those cute little baby booties to tiny sneakers, Mary Janes for dress-up, clunky work boots

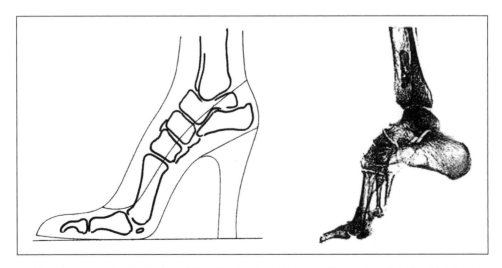

We deform our feet for fashion. Note the similarity between the modern foot in a high heel and a foot subjected to Chinese foot binding.

with superheavy soles, ever-higher heels, and narrow, pointy-toed dress shoes for work, each takes its toll.

We may think it's normal for the foot to get tired or even sore at the end of the day or after a shopping trip to the mall. But we don't associate that with our shoes. Our toes may hurt or get sore, but we don't associate that with our shoes. Or we may get bunions (something our doctor may have told us we inherited from our parents, which is not true), but we may not realize that these problems are caused by our shoes.

⦿°°₀ FOOT NOTE

"Our feet have not changed since pre-shod times; foot pathology is not hereditary, but directly caused by being placed in shoes. Foot pathologies are also not tied/linked to arch height or size, but to being placed in shoes." This conclusion was drawn from a study published in the *Journal of Bone and Joint Surgery* more than a hundred years ago.

And here's the kicker: we all have narrow feet compared to the unshod, and we never realize, think, or even care about the fact that this narrowness came from our shoes.

And why should we? What's wrong with a foot that's rectangular or tube-shaped instead of one that's a triangle?

Well, actually, everything.

Perhaps a good analogy is to look at the difference between a tricycle and a bicycle. Our feet were meant to be trikes. They have three wheels or landing points (behind the big toe, behind the little toe, and the heel), which make the foot an incredibly stable surface. That's the natural foot.

Today, our feet are something different. They're more like bicycles. They have two very narrow points of contact, one under the center of the front of the foot, and one at the center of the heel.

No wonder more and more people are getting plantar fasciitis, which is a pulling of the rope-tight connective tissue that runs from front to back, right under the center of our foot. This tissue takes all of the pressure because of how we've mangled and weakened our feet.

And it goes far beyond this.

A triangle-shaped foot is good for stability. It helps you balance and keeps you from rolling an ankle, twisting or straining your knees, or falling and abusing your hips.

The triangle-shaped foot is also great for propulsion. If you ever get a chance, rent a canoe. First put the paddle in the water with the wider, almost triangular shape down. Scoop the water—feel the resistance and see how far and how fast you go. Now flip the paddle around and put the narrow end in the water. Scoop at the water and notice the difference. You can't go anywhere with the narrow end, and you have almost no control. That's what's going on with our feet.

If you're trying to stand upright or erect with triangular feet, you stand tall, like a great oak. But if you're trying to stand tall on bicycle-like feet, it's in essence as if you're on ice skates, and you're in trouble. Just the act of standing is straining your feet, which are digging into the ground trying to get stability. Your feet are wobbly and unstable. It's easy to roll an ankle, easy to twist or strain a knee, and easy to fall.

Our bodies are amazing compensatory machines if we give them even half a chance. However, when our feet are stuck in shoes, it's as if we're blindfolded. We've deadened the senses of the foot and cut off the entire nervous system's ability to feel the ground. In essence, the nerve endings in our feet are supposed to communicate with our brain. Even when your feet are in shoes, your mind and feet still try to find a way to get balanced.

So what do they do?

If you've ever skied, you'll know exactly what to do if you're stuck with two narrow skis underfoot. You'll move the heels of your feet to the outside, forming the shape of a *V*, to get stability. You did this when you first skied. If your feet are the shape of skis instead of stable triangles, you'll do the same thing—you'll turn your feet to the outside and try to mash them down in order to gain stability.

We call it *pronation*, and we say it's bad, but turning our feet outward is the most natural way our feet and body deal with a completely unnatural circumstance. By turning our feet outward and then trying to drop our arches through the floor, we're trying to regain our stability and the natural triangle we once had.

And it's killing us. Or as the analogy goes, the frog is now being boiled.

We've reshaped the foot, taken away its ability to hold us upright, forced it to rotate outward (straining our ankles, knees, hips, and even backs) to try to regain stability, and forced it to crush the arch into the ground to try to make a stable surface.

We've completely deformed the foot and ruined its ability to propel us forward, hold us upright, and allow us to stand tall, stable, and strong without pain. Instead, in order to stay upright, we hunch forward to get low. Why? Because we're now like a tree with its roots lassoed and tied together. If the slightest wind blows, we're knocked over.

Our feet are not naturally weak; they are naturally strong when they're allowed to work, allowed to do their jobs, and allowed to have their natural shape.

Okay, now that your blood is boiling (as well as the frog's), what do we do about it?

SAVE YOUR CHILDREN'S FEET!

First, whenever possible, keep your kids out of shoes. It's not a safety issue if they're not wearing shoes—it's a safety issue if they *are* wearing shoes. Keeping them barefoot helps them grow a healthy, happy, and strong body, from the roots on up.

The longer children are barefoot, the greater their chances of developing powerful, healthy feet with strong arches and of their mastering balance, enduring impact, and achieving great posture. A 1992 study of 2,300 children found that the chances of developing flat feet were more than three times greater for the kids wearing shoes than for those going barefoot.

Putting shoes on our children as soon as they can stand may cause more harm than good. When it comes to shaping the foot, consider the findings of Dr. Bernhard Zipfel and Professor Lee Berger: "Studies of Asian populations whose feet were habitually either unshod, in thong-type sandals, or encased in non-constrictive coverings have shown increased forefoot widths when compared to those of shod populations."

So shoes not only weaken feet but increase the chances of deforming them. A healthy foot, as described later, grows wider to accommodate the forces of

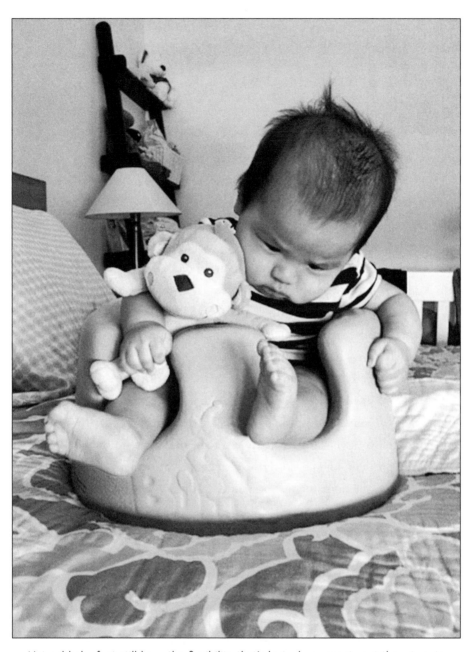

Natural baby feet still have the flexibility that's lost when parents put them in cute little shoes.

running and walking. There's much more on the benefits of barefoot living for children in chapter 14.

Grow Tall like the Oak

But you're not a kid anymore. Can your feet get back to their natural state?

It all begins with our shoes. As a species, we're like oak trees planted in flower pots. How are we supposed to thrive and survive in such a tiny pot? And if we miraculously do gain some height, how do we stay upright without tipping over? How are we supposed to grow roots to nourish our leaves and stay healthy? How are we supposed to spread our branches and gain energy from the sun? And how in the world are we supposed to dance with the wind or a breeze?

We're in constant danger of tipping over or falling down, and our roots must be killing us, tangled all over each other and trapped in such a tiny pot.

That's what we've done to our feet. Studies show that 88 to 90 percent of women are trapped in shoes too small for them. Why? Because the feet can conform, and do so willingly, with bearable discomfort, at least in the beginning.

Instead, let your feet feel the ground. Let them grow naturally strong. Let your body tell you what it needs. All you have to do is take the blindfolds off your feet, be patient, and go slowly. These changes won't happen overnight, but given a chance, the human body, no matter its age, will begin to change, adapt, and grow stronger.

It's as if there's a message or a code in the ground just waiting to wake up our feet and wake up our health. To reprogram the body, to unlock the doors to health, all we need to do is interact with the ground and let it reprogram us for perfect health.

Our feet contain almost 25 percent of all the bones in our body. This isn't by accident; it's because our feet developed as intricate propulsion devices over millions of years. Feet are designed to be sensitive enough to feel minute changes in surface conditions and to make moment-by-moment adjustments to keep us continuously balanced and safe—like the suspension system in a car. Yet we continue to encase our feet in devices that have little bearing in terms of shape, size, scope, or mobility to the very thing they're encasing. With shoes on, you can't feel the ground, so your feet are deprived of the detailed moment-by-moment information they crave. Instead they're sliding around in your shoes, which interferes with balance, and hitting the ground extra hard in an attempt to gather the information they're blocked from directly obtaining through touch. Furthermore, your feet can't grab or move freely within shoes and so are substantially limited in the adjustments they can make to provide you with optimal balance and stride.

There's a reason our feet are so supersensitive: it's to read the ground and make changes on the fly. Turn on your own incredible, built-in supercomputer by simply taking off your shoes.

SAVE GRANDMA'S HIPS!

Even if you're convinced that going shoeless is good for kids and adults, you may wonder whether it makes sense for older people. By this point, though, you can probably guess the answer. When we grow old, we often lose our sense of balance. In fact, one of the major sources of injury and death among the elderly is falls. It's not the fall itself that's so problematic, but the broken hip, hospitalization, and lack of mobility, which create a downhill spiral.

Going without shoes—an idea that many older people find insane—just might give them a new sense of their natural balance and allay any fears of falling. Barefoot walking will help reactivate the senses in an elderly person's feet and restore the natural balance with which we're born—and which shoes disrupt. Feeling the ground will also strengthen the feet, eventually resulting in greater bone density (an ongoing issue for old bones ravaged by osteoporosis), leg strength, core strength, and stability.

In addition, the stimulation of going barefoot will increase an older person's desire to exercise. And there's no better medicine for old age than regular exercise, as it helps bones avoid becoming brittle and risking fractures, and it staves off such killers as heart disease and countless other maladies. The path to going barefoot must be a slow and gradual process, especially for the elderly, and convincing Grandma may be tough. But with patience, going barefoot can add additional quality years to an already long life.

HELP OUR RETURNING TROOPS

We also think people with head injuries may do better rehabilitating without shoes, including our soldiers returning home. We especially salute the injured troops who struggle to regain their ability to walk after suffering head trauma while valiantly serving our nation.

Going barefoot helps people with head injuries develop a connection between the feet and the mind. This begins the rewiring or remapping process in the brain for proper balance and awareness of time and space. It helps people figure out where their bodies are, helps them determine whether they are landing or standing erect, and helps prevent a sensation of spinning and vertigo. With proper supervision, this can be an excellent tool to help rehab, rebuild, and return to mobility and health.

BENEFITS OF BAREFOOT WALKING

The difference between walking in and out of a shoe is as dramatic as the difference between playing a sport as a video game and actually participating in the sport. In both you see the action, but in only one are you a part of the action, feeling what's going on and producing chemical and physiological changes to the body.

While any walking is quite beneficial to your health, it's as different as night and day without shoes for a number of key reasons.

- **Awareness.** When you're walking barefoot, you're walking awarefoot. You're in touch with your surroundings, as if reading Braille with your feet, and the trails are the words. Find a good path or trail, and you're reading a great book. Unfortunately, in the vast majority of shoes, you can't feel the ground beneath your feet. When you're walking awarefoot, you can feel the ground, which gives you the feedback necessary to walk light.

- **Walk lighter.** When you go barefoot, you receive immediate feedback from the ground. Gone are the days of the heel strike or the heavily extended foot smacking into the ground. Instead you become light, because the alternative is painful. You start to relate to stories of Native Americans who moved through the forest without a sound. You begin to understand why barefoot walking is so much kinder and gentler on the body. And you may begin to startle others, walking up to them without making a sound. You'll notice you're walking through the house with a lighter step too.

- **Lower injury risk.** In a shoe we send shockwaves up through our bodies. Out of a shoe, we're letting the feet and legs work as the natural springs they were intended to be. Therefore, out of a shoe there's far less wear and tear on the body. Additionally, in a shoe our feet and legs are forced to go where the shoe wants them to go (via motion control or abnormal curvatures in the design of the shoe sole), rather than where we want them to go, increasing the chance of overuse injuries.

- **Balance.** The nerve endings on the bottom of your feet aid in your response to the ground and to each imperfection in your path. There's an incredible mind-body connection that occurs as you go barefoot. Your feet are in instant communication with your brain. As neuroscientist Dr. Michael Merzenich describes, your brain literally creates new neural connections, developing a mind map, or mental image, of the terrain and your body in relation to it. As your mind map grows with new information from your bare feet, your balance improves, as do your reaction time and your ability to recover. When you're wearing shoes, this mind map is fuzzy or blurry at best. It's hard for the brain to take the necessary steps to keep you from falling, improve your balance, and improve your reaction time. We've heard from Dr. Merzenich and other doctors, along with hundreds of people at our various clinics, about how their balance was improved or restored by going barefoot and feeling the ground. In essence, just feeling the earth began to wake up the nerve endings on the bottom of their feet. Even for people with vestibular challenges such as vertigo, feeling the ground helped them reprogram their minds and find better balance.

Walking Yoga

Think of barefoot walking as walking yoga. You would never think of doing yoga with shoes on. That's because you need the connection with the ground to stay balanced, to help you get in position, and to help keep you strong. In essence, all of your poses or asanas come from the ground up, which is why you need your toes to be free, to grab the ground, give you support, and give you stability. If you've heard the term "yoga feet," then you know dedicated yoga practitioners develop strong toes and strong feet. Whether you engage in barefoot walking or yoga, no matter how weak your feet are to begin with, they always grow strong once they're asked to serve a purpose. For yoga, they must grow strong to assist with your poses, to help you get and stay in position, and to stabilize your entire body. The same thing happens with barefoot walking. As barefoot walkers, we need strong feet—in essence, yoga feet—for all of the same reasons.

Both barefoot walking and yoga require a heightened sense of awareness, of both the body and the ground. In yoga you start all of your poses barefoot, focusing on the connection between your feet and the floor. And in walking barefoot, you must focus on the connection between your feet and the earth. Both disciplines ask you to concentrate on quieting the mind, listening on the inside, and perhaps even going on a spiritual journey. Yoga and barefoot walking help develop the mind-body-earth connection that aids our health, our spirit, and our mental well-being. They also give us greater strength, mobility, and control over our bodies. These complementary practices are empowering, giving us a sense of freedom, clarity, and peace.

- **Strength.** As you stand more erect, engage your core, and let your body move naturally, your entire body begins to strengthen. It's now getting signals from the ground to grow strong, to hold you erect, and to properly move you forward. This strengthening begins with your feet. Like the roots of a tree, the energy begins to move upward, from your feet, to your legs, hips, buttocks, back, arms, even shoulders and neck. Holding yourself in position takes work for the body, work that pays big dividends in terms of better tone and strength throughout the body.

- **Bone density.** There's often a question of which came first, the broken hip or the fall that broke the hip. Either way, the answer is clear: strengthen your hips as much as you can, along with all of your bones and joints along the way. The entire body, including the bones, works on the "use it or lose it" principle. If you work your bones by doing weight-bearing exercises, you get to maintain strong bones. If not, those bones weaken and break. That's because the bones receive more stimulus from muscles that are working harder to keep us erect. For example, studies show walking or running is better for our bones than cycling or swimming. Barefoot walking takes this to an entirely different level by forcing us to rely more on our stabilizing muscles. Since our muscles pull on our bones (through tendons), the very act of contracting our muscles stimulates bone growth and increases bone density. Working on the muscles around the hips for stability not only helps keep us from falling, but builds the hips stronger to protect us in case of a fall.

- **Foot strength and stability.** When you're in a shoe, the footwear is doing the work of stabilizing and supporting your foot, rather than your foot muscles. This causes your foot to atrophy over time. As it atrophies, you may find your foot sliding around in the shoe. In other words, you have no support. Therefore you tend to get an even more supportive and narrower shoe to support the foot and keep it from sliding. Unfortunately, feet adapt to their environment and now weaken further because the muscles don't need to work in the more supportive and narrower shoe. Conversely, if you spend time out of a shoe, your foot strengthens and begins to grow wider, your toes begin to spread naturally, and you start to gain stability back. Additionally, the more time you spend barefoot, the more your big toe separates from the other four. A gap appears between your first (big) toe and your second as your first stretches inward, acting as an anchor and giving you a stable platform. One excellent device we recommend to help promote toe spread (and reduce bunions) is Dr. Ray

McClanahan's Correct Toes (www.nwfootankle.com). It's similar to another product you may have heard of, Yoga Toes, but fits inside shoes with wide toe boxes. If you wear these toe separators for a few hours a day, you'll see your foot returning to a more natural shape in only a few short weeks.

- **Core strength and stability.** Want abs of steel along with a stronger back, arms, shoulders, and neck? When you're in a shoe, your footwear does the job of stabilizing you. Out of a shoe, you do that job. That means you need to tighten your core (abs and back) and use your arms to stabilize your entire body. This helps you grow incredibly strong and resilient abdominal and back muscles, helping you in all of your day-to-day activities, not just in walking.

- **Cardio.** When you begin going barefoot, your heart rate is elevated as you work to pump blood to muscles that didn't need it before. Later on, as you gain efficiency, you'll likely find yourself moving more freely and easier than ever before. It's as if you're flying, and the miles are moving effortlessly by. When walking becomes easier and more enjoyable, you're far more likely to get a great workout. The formula for fitness is really quite simple, and it has nothing to do with discipline. Focus on the fun. If something's fun, you're more likely to do it, and the quality of your activity will increase. Have fun walking barefoot, and you'll likely go farther and faster than ever before and thereby greatly increase your cardiovascular benefits. Walking barefoot is a perfect cardiovascular activity because it raises your heart rate, but without overstraining your body. This promotes a stronger heart and lungs, and can reduce blood pressure and LDL and overall cholesterol levels; it can even help thin your blood. It can also aid with circulation, producing more flexible arteries, and returning blood to the heart more efficiently. A stronger cardiovascular system also stimulates the production of mitochondria within the cells. These mitochondria are responsible for giving you more energy and help regulate body temperature.

All of this means you'll feel better, be less winded in everything you do (such as that flight of stairs that always gets you), and have better stamina throughout the day. Oh, and did we mention the "runner's high"—or in this case, "walker's high"? It's real. You get a dose of some fantastic neurotransmitters (such as serotonin, the "happy chemical") while walking. When Michael used to coach learning-disabled and ADHD students, he always recommended they *exercise* aerobically for at least twenty to thirty minutes daily. Why? Because the neurotransmitters released during cardiovascular exercise helped students stay calm and focused throughout the day, and helped them fall asleep and stay asleep each night. Stay connected to the ground, work that cardio with a smile, and you too will reap these benefits.

According to Dr. Merzenich, barefoot walking may help the cardiovascular system in a new way: when we walk over uneven surfaces, the minute changes (flexing and bending) the foot makes to keep us balanced require nearly instant changes in local blood pressure through the smallest blood vessels and capillaries. This ability to quickly adjust blood pressure and heart rate helps build a more robust and resilient cardiovascular system. In essence, the cardiovascular system must try to compensate between heartbeats to adapt to new terrain, thus strengthening the heart and reducing blood pressure.

As an aside, all of these benefits can occur without initial weight loss. Don't be scared off if you don't see pounds being shed instantly. We often replace initial fat loss with muscle gain, and that's a great thing, as muscle burns more calories than fat!

- **Blood pressure.** According to studies, reflexology—stimulating the nerve endings on the bottom of the feet—can reduce blood pressure, lower anxiety levels, boost the immune system, and more. Similar results have been found in subjects walking barefoot on cobblestone mats (it stimulates the bottom of the foot much like walking on an uneven surface outside). Scientists have noted a significant drop in blood pressure in subjects who walked on the mats compared to subjects who didn't walk on the mats. It's hard to get the stimulating benefits of reflexology when you're walking on a flat, unchanging surface, as you are when your foot is encased in a shoe and cushioned with a sock.

- **Instant stress reduction.** This may be the best bonus of all. Going barefoot isn't good just for the body, it's great for the mind and spirit as well. We've all had the experience of coming home from work and wanting to take off our shoes and walk through the grass, or wanting to feel the sand between our toes as we walk barefoot on the beach. It's a universal feeling, and perhaps it's why kids fight us so much when we want to put them in shoes. Not only does being barefoot feel good, it helps us empty our minds. Barefoot really is awarefoot. It's an exercise in mindfulness. Suddenly everything that's not important in the moment fades into the background as we focus on the task and sensation at hand.

  Even a simple barefoot walk midday can reduce stress. An evening walk may help you sleep like a baby. And that morning walk may stimulate incredible creativity while decreasing the likelihood of anxieties and worries in your upcoming day. It's instant meditation, clearing out all the junk of the day and leaving us blissfully in the now.

- **Immune system.** You may be aware that light-to-moderate aerobic exercise boosts your immune system, but did you know going barefoot gives you an additional boost? Here are five key ways.

  1. Connecting with the earth's negative charge decreases inflammation and cortisol levels in the body, allowing your immune system to work better. (More on this in chapter 4.)
  2. Being connected to the dirt helps draw toxins out of the body, and exposure to microbes in the dirt helps train and strengthen your immune system. (More in chapter 4.)
  3. By stimulating all of the nerve endings on the bottom of the feet, the way acupuncture and acupressure do, you directly stimulate the immune and lymphatic systems.
  4. Your lymphatic system relies on movement, such as the movement of your foot (something you can't do in a shoe), to draw out excess fluid, waste, and toxins from the feet while delivering nutrients, oxygen, and hormones. (For instance, the lack of movement is why your feet and legs swell on an airplane or in

a shoe.) When you increase movement in your feet, you help circulate fluid and support this vital system.

5. In winter months, sensing the cold through your feet helps turn on the immune system and regulate your internal temperature. It's ironic, but the cold sensation helps you stay warm—a key to staying healthy.

- **Gratitude.** When you're connected to the earth and feeling the ground underfoot, it's hard not to be walking in a state of gratitude. It's as if you're instantly thankful for the day and for the opportunity to take this walk, no matter how stressful the day or the challenges ahead. It seems that walking barefoot naturally puts you in a state of "ahhh," the way a great massage does. You can experience this state of gratitude by simply taking off your shoes and feeling the ground.
- **Spirituality.** The spiritual benefits of vitamin G are spelled out in the introduction. Many barefoot walkers think this benefit is the best. The rest are just nice bonuses.

CHALLENGES OF BAREFOOT WALKING

Of course, there are some challenges with barefoot walking. Most of these challenges are health-promoting.

- **You slow down.** You may walk slower in the beginning, particularly on more challenging surfaces. This isn't a bad thing; it's your body's way of adapting. The feet need to grow stronger and to adapt to the challenges. Your body needs to grow stronger and carry you more erect. And everything from your muscles and ligaments to your tendons and bones needs to adapt for greater strength and endurance. You may feel slower in the beginning, but even at a snail's pace, you are likely challenging your body more than you've ever done before. It's as if you're learning to walk all over again. So don't worry about starting slowly or taking it slow. You've just stepped into the greatest exercise on earth.

- **Your dog may be confused.** Michael couldn't walk our dogs, Pumpkin and Sawa, as fast as they wanted to go in the beginning, and it was a big challenge to keep his eyes focused on the trail *and* walk them without tripping over the leashes at the same time. He needed to focus 100 percent on putting one foot before the other. Sometimes he simply had to leave the dogs at home. Other times he had to work on their patience skills. But over time he grew faster, he and the dogs grew more patient, and it became a fantastic bonding experience.

- **Your shoe collection will take a hit.** Try as you might, over time you just won't want to wear your old shoes anymore. Who wants to wear something that not only hurts the foot but mangles it? The great news here, unless you plan on walking barefoot full-time, is that you're going to need new shoes. There goes the shoe budget. But it means it's time to go shopping!

- **People will look at you funny.** And they'll say stuff to you. At first this may be the people in your neighborhood or on the trails, wondering why you're going barefoot (or, more likely, how they can get into it too). They'll wonder if you're in a weight loss program or a gym training program, or if you've discovered a new therapy or found a new lover. In short, they'll wonder where the new you came from, the one who stands taller, has greater confidence, is less anxious and stressed, is thinking more clearly, and is fitter than ever.

- **Up may become down.** You may find that paths you once enjoyed are too challenging to begin with and others that were once boring now hold the greatest charm. Either way, once you've entered the three-dimensional world of going bare, where you'll want to walk will change based on the stimulus each place provides to your feet. Just remember to go slowly and listen to your body.

- **Look out, James Dean.** You may become a bit of a rebel, desiring freedom for your feet at all times. Why can't you go shopping barefoot? Why can't you take off your shoes at the office? And who says you can't walk down the street sans shoes? As you grow your own shoes and your confidence increases, you'll find yourself wanting to go bare (or out of your old shoes) as much as you can.

- **You'll establish a new rule.** We have a rule at our home: if we're walking in the city, we must wash our feet before climbing into bed, and ideally upon entering the house. Yes, there'll be more work involved in washing your feet, but you'll get to know your feet better as well, watching them change, adapt, and transform into strong, healthy propulsion, support, and cushioning devices before your eyes.
- **You won't allow shoes in the house.** Once you've gone bare, you'll realize everything people *walk through* in shoes without knowing it. With this newfound knowledge you'll think twice about bringing your shoes into the house or having others wear theirs indoors. You'll soon understand why many Asian cultures do not allow shoes in the house.

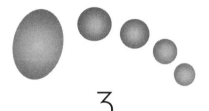

3
Barefoot Walking: The New Fountain of Youth

Walking is the exercise that needs no gym. It is the prescription
without medicine, the weight control without diet, the cosmetic that is
sold in no drugstore. It is the tranquilizer without a pill, the therapy
without a psychoanalyst, and the fountain of youth that is no legend.
A walk is the vacation that does not cost a cent.
—Aaron Sussman and Ruth Goode, *The Magic of Walking*

Jessica says, "Michael and I stood beside each other before the bath-room mirror in our new ohana, or cottage, on Maui. We had just spent nearly thirty-six hours traveling from my parents' home in New Jersey to Maui via Monterey, California, where we paid a quick visit to our wayward storage unit. We had in total eleven pieces of luggage, including books, camera equip-ment, two iMac computers, hiking and camping gear, the bare essentials of clothing, and two large cardboard bicycle boxes. Considering the ordeal of transporting our lives five thousand miles, one might assume it'd be natural to look as gaunt and worn out as the two of us did.

"Approximately eleven months after the day I met Michael, we hit the road for five months straight on a cross-country book tour. We packed up our entire lives, our two dogs, and our new business into my little Suzuki SX4 hatchback and miniature four-by-six-foot trailer. All told, we hit more than 130 cities and drove more than 40,000 miles in 2010. With so many hours spent behind the wheel, a poor diet from living on the road, and an irregular schedule, we were not kind to our bodies, and the wear and tear showed.

"On Maui we were determined to turn back the clock. We reinstated mandatory morning meditations; we added to our diet fresh fruit smoothies, more local foods, sprouts, and leafy greens, eventually even going "raw" (more on this in chapter 13); we got eight hours of sleep each night and improved our stress management skills; and of course we spent more time out walking the trails. We set our intentions and started paying attention to our bodies *all* the time, not just some of the time.

"After just a month of living a reformed life, we stood before the mirror again. 'You look younger today,' I told Michael.

" 'Thanks. So do you. *Much* younger,' he said."

It's never too late to roll back the days, months, or years. There are simple small changes you can make in your life. One of them is simply committing yourself to walk. As Auntie Puanani Mahoe, a *kapuna* or wise Hawaiian elder, explained to us, "I walk. Therefore, I live."

Although it's unlikely you'll become immortal by going barefoot, this humble exercise can roll back the years and make you feel, act, and look younger. Greater circulation does wonders for the skin, as does toning and healing your whole body.

Barefoot walking, or going bare, is a true paradigm shifter. Any activity that is difficult or challenging can become pure joy. Have fun with your barefoot walking experience and watch yourself slowly transform as you roll back the years. You'll be amazed at the results, as will those around you.

ANTIAGING BENEFITS OF WALKING BAREFOOT

Going barefoot isn't just a new experience; it's an old experience, one you likely had as a child. Letting your feet feel the ground taps into the muscle memories and pleasant recollections of your youth. You find yourself smiling, giddy, and filled with the laughter we all had as children. As your body changes, you grow stronger, and as your aches and pains subside, you'll find yourself feeling younger. By all methods of physical measurement, you'll become younger.

A smile (and perhaps unexpected laughter) will come with every one of these happy experiences. Here are other ways in which the simple act of freeing your feet restores your youthfulness.

- **Grow taller.** You will stand taller and with better posture. When you feel the ground, you gain awareness of your body and your posture. You feel all of your muscles firing. You can feel if you're hunched, if you're pooching out your belly, or if you're sagging at the knees. This immediate feedback helps you tighten your core and stand tall. You stand more erect, you eliminate your slouch, your shoulders stop rolling forward, you tuck your pelvis underneath you, and you stand more like a ballet dancer. It won't be just you who notices this; those around you, and your chiropractor if you see one, will notice as well. Who said you have to start shrinking as you age?
- **Get abs of steel.** Your core, from your abdominal muscles to your back, begins to tighten and strengthen to hold you in position. You'll feel it in your clothes (they'll drape better) and in how you feel. Now you can reach things above you without as much stress, wobble, or strain. You can carry things more easily, you feel stronger overall, and you feel more powerful too, as your inner power comes from your core.
- **Say goodbye to foot pain.** In the beginning your feet may fatigue as you go barefoot. But that's not a bad thing; it's like lifting weights at the gym. Your muscles get tired and then grow back stronger. As your feet begin to strengthen and adapt, you'll notice many of the daily aches and pains of your feet and lower legs going away. Soon standing on your feet will be a more enjoyable activity.
- **Gain greater circulation.** You'll quickly begin to notice your feet don't feel as cold. Over time you'll see an increase in warmth or blood flow to your feet and lower legs, and a decrease in your varicose veins—all without laser therapy. You'll feel warmer on the cooler days, and cooler on the warmer days.
- **Grow baby feet again.** Those cute, chubby little feet you had as a child just might return. The fat on the bottom of your feet went away because you've spent too many years in your shoes. Great news here: once you go barefoot, the ground stimulates your feet and the fat

you've lost since you were a child begins to return. The skin starts to thicken, but not as unsightly calluses caused by high-friction areas in an ill-fitting shoe; rather, it occurs as an even thickening over the entire bottom of the foot where your sole meets the ground. This fat pad will make challenging surfaces much easier to negotiate.

- **Gain confidence.** There's something empowering about knowing you can go anywhere you want with just your two feet, and without even needing shoes. With confidence comes grace and poise as well.

- **See the world with new eyes.** Your feet have eyes (or maybe your eyes have feet). You begin to look at the path, at the hillside, even at the trees in a different way. You are no longer a spectator in the world around you but an active participant. Even that boring park you've been through a thousand times seems to transform once you take off your shoes. It's as if you have a child's newfound excitement and enthusiasm for the world around you. Though you've been there a hundred times before, you may wonder what's around that next corner.

- **Quiet your mind.** You may find yourself taking out your iPod earbuds, shutting off the cell phone, and just listening to your steps. Not only will you find that the external world becomes quiet, but the internal chatter of your mind settles down too.

- **Simplify your life.** Once you go barefoot you'll find yourself seeing the world and your daily life with clarity. You suddenly have new opinions on what's important and what's not. This leads to better decisions and also means you begin to let go of the things that aren't important in your life, that don't bring great happiness and joy, or that have been a burden on you.

BAREFOOT BRAINPOWER

Want to be smarter and have a better working brain? Then go barefoot. So says Dr. Michael Merzenich, professor emeritus of neuroscience at the University of California at San Francisco. His premise, and ours, is that going barefoot helps wake up the mind in many ways.

Without our realizing it, the modern human brain has become quite dysfunctional. Not only have we disconnected from a major source of stimuli—what's beneath our feet—but our minds have been compartmentalized, each part separated from the next. Our human brain was meant to be fully integrated. Out in nature we would hear, see, smell, feel, and often even taste things, all at the same time. This integrated way of thinking led to a more effective or efficient brain, something people often call a sixth sense.

Unfortunately, today that's no longer the case. In the digital world, we focus on one or perhaps two senses at a time, completely ignoring the rest. As evidence of this change, we needn't look further than the epidemic of attention deficit disorder in children. Our attention spans are down, our anxiety levels are up, and our minds seem more overburdened, overtaxed, and overwhelmed than ever before.

But what does that have to do with going barefoot, and how can going barefoot help our minds?

Going barefoot can help in three key ways:

1. It helps us rewire our minds and reintegrate all of our senses.
2. It helps us train our bodies and minds to better handle "surprises," which are in essence learning experiences.
3. It helps our minds grow sharp, for a lifetime of greater intelligence and a longer useful life.

Going barefoot may be one part of the elixir that makes up the fountain of youth, not just for our bodies but for our minds as well. Nowhere else in our daily lives are we integrating all aspects of our brains better than when we're barefoot on the trails or in the city, because all of our senses are heightened and we're no longer going through the world on autopilot. You can't go on autopilot when you're barefoot in the woods or in the concrete jungle, no matter how much you try (and you wouldn't want to anyway).

Now let's look at how going barefoot can help our brains.

Brainercise

First point: when you're barefoot, you're exercising your brain. When you step out of your shoes and begin to feel the ground, you begin to rewire your mind. You're sending signals to the brain about texture, temperature, pressure, hardness, and much more. All of these sensations work on the mind in much the same way as reading a great new book does.

More than that, the mind has to kick into high gear to analyze everything beneath your feet and put it into perspective. For instance, if you're walking, your brain has to know if it's safe to put your foot down, if you might trip, if you need to shift your weight slightly because of a pebble, or if there's a slope your mind needs to take into account.

Not only are you sensing the ground, but when you take the earbuds out of your ears, then you're giving your brain context as well. Now, in addition to seeing what's all around you, you're hearing it too, instead of Bruce Springsteen. And of course you're feeling it beneath your feet. You're smelling the world around you, and if something in the air is strong enough, you may even be tasting it too.

Taking in everything at once is something we rarely do in our modern world. We typically have our cell phones glued to our ears, or our thumbs are flying while we text. Maybe music is blaring, or we're watching TV (the latter is a truly unnatural act, as we're watching things in motion but aren't actually in motion ourselves), or we're hypnotized by the computer screen. The point is, we're rarely focused on all of our senses at once—something Dr. Merzenich calls *integration*.

What's so important about integration? When you integrate, you strengthen the mind, increasing its efficiency, its effectiveness, and, in essence, your intelligence.

That's right, you heard it here first: you can get more intelligent by going barefoot. Dr. Merzenich says it can increase your brainpower by a factor of two. How'd you like to be twice as smart?

Your Brain on Nature

We've established that going barefoot makes us smarter, but add nature to the mix and we've catapulted our intelligence to the moon. Everything in nature, from the dirt under our feet, the microbes in the air, the amazing scenery, the tactile stimuli, and the fascinating scenery before us, has been shown to improve our focus and concentration, heighten our awareness, and increase our intelligence.

Though a walk down a city street may be just as stimulating as a walk in nature, your brain processes them quite differently. Studies show that when we're in nature, we integrate all of the sights, sounds, and smells around us into one pleasing picture. Going barefoot and feeling the details of the ground adds another information-rich layer. Meanwhile, in the city, the brain perceives everything around us, such as cars, traffic lights, and billboards, as signals for us to take action. In other words, nature scenes induce peace of mind, while city scenes induce a stressed-out mind.

Contrary to the city walks, the relaxing experiences in nature help quiet the mind, leading to less stress and fatigue, along with more efficient memorization, information processing, and attention. In a day and age when we are constantly bombarded with information overload, a reprieve in nature is invaluable, especially for children. This has been particularly important for Michael, someone who struggled with ADHD for nearly thirty years and went on to author *College Confidence with ADD*. He attributes his focus and success to his required daily dose of nature, which can be as simple as a walk in the park.

The richness of the experience has been shown to boost our creativity too. If you want a great idea or inspiration, head out into nature. It appears to be cumulative as well: the more time in nature, the better. Perhaps that's why many of our greatest minds, including Einstein, Thoreau, Emerson, and Godel, all religiously took daily walks in nature. It just so happens that's where our best ideas come from too.

The next logical questions are why and how. It happens because you're linking all parts of your brain, including your left and right hemispheres, something that occurred naturally in humans until recent times. This helps you put together all of the information you're getting with thoughts, ideas, and emotions.

It means you're recording information better too, for with every surprise on the trail, you're triggering the recording mechanism of the brain. This mechanism kicks into high gear when it thinks there may be something important to remember. With each step there's the potential for a surprise or a fall, so the recorder is always going. We have our recorder off in our day-to-day lives, allowing us to drive across town or even across the country virtually on autopilot. The more we turn off the autopilot by drinking in and feeling the world around us, the more we engage the recorder of our minds and begin to strengthen it.

What kind of impact can this have? In adulthood we seldom challenge our minds, so they get sleepy or go on autopilot. They become less well integrated, because we rarely use multiple senses at the same time, and they become hardened and slower, struggling to process new information. We assume this is natural, but it's far from that.

Something that's normal is not necessarily natural. In a shoe it's normal to come down hard on your heel when you're walking. But take your foot out of the shoe and you see that it's anything but natural. It's just an accepted norm. Similarly, in modern society it's normal for our brains to slow down and become less flexible or less plastic as we age, but as Dr. Merzenich points out, that's anything but natural. The separation of the various parts of the brain may be normal too in our modern age, but it's anything but natural. It's just that we've switched over to cruise control.

A good example of this is our daily exercise. When you're wearing shoes, the activities of walking, hiking, and even running are just pounding movements you do for your health. It's a repetitive, mindless stride. Maybe you stick in the earbuds, crank up high-energy tunes, and just get it over with. And even if you're enjoying the activity, you're still blocking out most of the world around you. It's just a repetitive motion, stride after stride. There's little information here the brain needs to record or even think about.

But when you're out of a shoe, there's the potential for surprise with every step. This puts your mind's recorder into high gear, exercising and stimulating your mind.

EXERCISE

Engage Your Recorder

The next time you head out for a walk or a hike, turn your mental recorder on. Try to take in all of the information around you—everything you hear, see, smell, taste, touch, and feel beneath your feet. When you get home, sit for five minutes and try to replay the walk in your mind. What did you sense? Additionally, what are the feelings you got with each sense? What did it feel like inside your body and inside your mind? Do this later in the day for a second time and recall what you can. During the replay, jot down notes or start a walking journal.

In the beginning you'll remember very little, but each time you do this exercise, you're rewiring your mind, strengthening your recorder, and re-integrating your senses, so they're more like they were when you were a child (this is one reason it's so beneficial to let your children play in the woods or in city parks).

Keep practicing, and you'll find yourself remembering more and more, and not just on the trails or your walks but throughout your day. You'll find you're processing information better, making sharper decisions, and feeling that your mind is clearer, as if you're more on top of your game.

As Dr. Merzenich says, "Doing this stimulates the heck out of the hippocampus, the part of your brain responsible for formation of new memories and navigation." You're strengthening your entire mind and creating new pathways for thoughts to flow along. Especially as you age, this can be a powerful tool for reawakening your mind.

Forget crossword puzzles and Sudoku—head outside without shoes on.

Historically, men and women were always active and always on the go. Human brains were designed to do their best thinking while moving, according to Dr. Merzenich. It's very unnatural for us to sit at a desk in a classroom, at a workstation, or before a computer and try to focus on something.

Our minds, just like the rest of our bodies, operate on a use-it-or-lose-it principle. Keep thinking about the details, taking in and truly examining information, and you continue to learn, continue to rewire your mind, continue to keep it strong, healthy, resilient, efficient, and effective.

Studies show we can start to rewire our minds at any age. Dr. Merzenich has repeatedly told us about an interesting rat study by Dr. Hubert Dinse. Lab rats live a very predictable life, which lasts about three years. Researchers did an experiment in which they started enriching the rats' lives, offering them challenges and giving them more to think about. Suddenly the rats were living 15 to 20 percent longer or more! Other preliminary studies show rats exposed to more challenging surfaces and terrain may live even longer.

Why is this? Because their minds are getting stimulated and have to work again. It's as if the lights are turned back on.

Footloose and Fancy Free

Barefoot walking is like being a kid again. Children are wide-eyed toward the world (at least if we keep their thumbs from texting and playing video games). They're constantly exploring, discovering, and learning about the world around them. They aren't deadened to the world or moving through the abstract, but are swimming through the details of the world.

As Dr. Merzenich suggests, get off the path, walk through the woods, drink in the unpredictability of everything, and be a kid again. Barefoot, the whole world becomes new to us again, flipping on the light switch of our minds. The biggest danger is a world without surprises.

Ever notice how you get your best thoughts when you're out of the house or the office, walking to work or home or the subway, or through the park? Movement stimulates our minds. It's where our species was meant to think. We may stop for a moment to examine something on the trail, but we always keep moving and keep thinking.

You're stimulating so much of your brain when you're out barefoot that if we did a brain scan, we'd see your brain light up like a Christmas tree. Why? Because details are coming in from every direction, warming up the mind and creating new neural pathways.

Mental Sticky Notes

From Michael: "I almost always get my best ideas when I'm out on the trails. I'm trying to focus on the trail, giving thanks for being out there, and trying to be both mindless and mindful at the same time. I focus on everything around me, but without letting my mind go wandering or walkabout with a particular idea, thought, concern, or worry.

"As I do this, suddenly ideas pop into my head. Lately they're about my writing, since that's what I'm focused on. While the ideas are great, I try not to write the chapters in my head as I go along. Instead, I make a mental sticky note so I can remember the ideas for later."

Try this the next time you're out on a walk. Quiet your mind and let go of all of your thoughts. Just exist in the awareness of the world all around you. If a bright idea comes to you, make a mental sticky note and associate it with a letter of the alphabet as a way of helping yourself remember it, such as A is for apple, as in pick up apples at the store. Then let it go. You can even make an acronym, such as AOK, apples, oranges, kale. Once you get back to your desk, go back through your letters, write down the associated ideas, and watch your creativity flow.

EXERCISE

Waking Up the Mind

As we get older, we start to go on autopilot, viewing things only in the abstract and sleepwalking our way through life. Not only can we drive down the highway this way, but we can live through weeks and months without being fully aware of the time passing, and then all of a sudden we wonder where the years have gone.

To truly be alive again, we need to wake up our minds and be filled with wonderment at the world all around us. This means becoming surprised again, awake again, and aware again. As we say, going barefoot is becoming awarefoot.

This is a very simple exercise. For this, head out for a barefoot walk along your favorite trail, path through the park, or city sidewalk. Walk with one specific purpose in mind: see how many times you can be surprised by something.

For this, you'll have to start examining the world more closely. Maybe it means looking behind the bushes, or up into the trees, or really studying what the people, plants, or animals are doing all around you. But open your ears, widen your eyes, and feel what you can feel. What do you see, hear, smell, touch, taste, or notice beneath your feet that you've never noticed before? What were your emotions like when you touched a tree or felt a pine cone beneath your feet?

Once you're back home, see what you can remember and write it down. Try this exercise at least twice a week and, after a month, notice how differently you're now viewing the world. It feels exciting to be engaged again, doesn't it? Not only will you be sharper and more engaged, but notice how much calmer you feel, more empowered, and how many new ideas you're coming up with! Do this for a month and you'll never sleepwalk through life again.

NATURE'S VIAGRA

It's natural that as men and women grow older, we often experience decreased sex drive. This can be caused by psychological conditions such as stress, anxiety, or depression, to name a few, or physical conditions, such as heart disease, diabetes, or high blood pressure, among others.

But your sex drive also has to do with how active and physically fit you are. The better shape you're in, the better things work, and the better you feel about yourself, making for a continuous cycle.

Barefoot walking can be a natural Viagra for many key reasons: First, you feel better about yourself. You start to get more physically fit, more active (sex after all is an exercise), more energetic, and more confident. Numerous studies now show that after you begin to exercise, your sex drive starts to go up. They claim it's a combination of increased blood flow, increased hormones, and increased endorphins. Plus, of course, you just feel better about yourself.

You also get the blood flowing more, which helps with arousal and erection. And you get gobs of vitamin D, a natural sex drive stimulant. That's one reason why people are more stimulated to have fun in the summer months. When it comes to libido, the most common bits of advice are to exercise and get outdoors more.

Getting outdoors gives you more vitamin D, but going barefoot also gives you loads of vitamin G. That's important in everything from mitigating psychological conditions (including stress, anxiety, and depression) to helping relieve inflammatory conditions that, if left unmanaged, contribute to decreased libido.

Who can argue with the sensual stimulation you feel on the bottom of your feet? That just might transfer to the bedroom.

So get outside and feel the earth, and then you may want to do what those birds and bees keep doing.

A final thought about the life-transforming benefits of barefoot walking from our expert, Dr. Michael Merzenich: "Do you want to be smarter? Do you want to be more understanding of the nuances of what you're seeing, of what you're feeling, of what you're hearing? That's what barefoot walking is all about. Do you want to be more alive? Then walk barefoot."

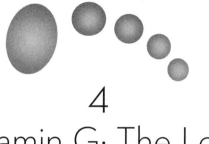

4
Vitamin G: The Lost Supplement

The foot feels the foot when it feels the ground.
—Buddha

In August 2010 we pulled off the road early from our *Barefoot Running* book tour. We'd been on tour for over five months, covering over thirty states and conducting clinics with barefoot fans from coast to coast.

During that time we were traveling with our two dogs: Sawa, our wunder-kind service dog, and Pumpkin, our wise-elder coyote mix.

At the time, Pumpkin was struggling with cancer. She'd been battling it on and off for nine years, and she never let herself get down. But giving her chemo and keeping her healthy on the road was too much, and so we ended our tour early.

We think she wanted a chance to rest, to have peace, and to bring us to a safe place so that she could feel comfortable letting us go and moving on.

Once we got back to Boulder and settled in our apartment, she started a fast decline. It was as if she hit the off switch and was ready for departure. But it wasn't overnight, and she struggled a bunch. Her cancer had moved from just beneath her skin into her GI tract.

We could have put her down; however, we'd promised a wise Tibetan woman we'd keep her comfortable and let her go naturally. For Pumpkin still had lessons she wanted to teach us, up to her very last moment.

She smiled the entire time, even when clearly in discomfort. She'd wake up each morning, even if she was too weak to eat or almost too weak to stand, start smiling, and with her beaming eyes declare, "Life is good." Even on the last day of her life.

But there was something else she taught us in her final days. In the house she would whimper, clearly in major discomfort. But outside, lying on the ground, she would smile. If we brought her in, she'd whimper. Take her out, and she'd smile.

Now, this was a dog who preferred to be inside, by our side, at all times. She loved the trails, but lived for the indoors too. And here she was, wanting to be outside every moment she could.

It took us a while, but we figured out why. It was the same reason Sawa, before she passed away a year later at age fifteen after battling pancreatitis, would stay outside for hours, either walking the yard (she put in miles a day) or lying in the dirt.

Both dogs knew that the earth felt better than lying indoors. They were soaking up the medicine of the earth; it calmed them, soothed them, and made them feel better than any medicine could.

This was a powerful lesson both Pumpkin and Sawa taught us: if you're not feeling well, spend some time walking, sitting, or lying on the earth. Now whenever we don't feel well, or we've gotten sick, or our heads are just spinning, we do like Pumpkin and Sawa did, head outside and plug back in.

We call it vitamin G for "ground," but maybe we should call it vitamin G for "good."

AN INCH OF RUBBER AWAY FROM NIRVANA

Michael says, "Before going barefoot I struggled with overuse injury after overuse injury, swelling after swelling. As part of my healing, I began going barefoot outdoors, first every other day, and then every day. As I did, the swelling in my body began to melt away. It wasn't just the physical act of moving. It was the near-miraculous anti-inflammatory benefits of being connected with the earth."

What's missing today is a physical connection to the earth. We're spending too much time indoors, and even when we're outside for a walk, we're separated by an inch of rubber, which is a fantastic resistor to electricity.

This brings us to the physics of getting grounded—how we're truly connected to the earth and vibrate at the same frequency as the earth, what that means for our health, and how barefoot walking can help.

On a spiritual level, we're no longer connected to the ground from where we evolved. On a physical level, we're no longer connected to the earth's magnetic field and particle charges. On a mental level, we see ourselves as distinctly separate from nature and other living beings.

Since the beginning, we've been in nature, not just foraging for food, not just to survive, but for our enjoyment and spiritual experiences as well. Organized religions know this: sacred texts give us scenes of Jesus in nature and images of the Buddha on his travels and meditating while sitting under a tree on his path toward enlightenment.

Though in many ways we're more advanced than at any other time, we're also the most unplugged. We all feel a desire to connect, to feel the earth and get grounded again. We just have a hard time finding the way or letting ourselves do it.

Perhaps what's missing is that we're literally no longer touching the ground. We're told that in advanced societies people no longer touch the earth in that way; it's considered dirty, taboo, or even dangerous. So we've developed devices (shoes) to keep us above the ground.

However, as a species, we evolved to hunt, farm, gather, and be outdoors. We didn't evolve to be indoors sitting at a desk all day or to wear shoes. We have beautiful strong feet and an incredible means for connecting with nature.

At our barefoot clinics, it's nothing but ear-to-ear grins once participants

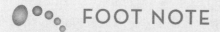 FOOT NOTE

The Most Dangerous Job in the World

A BBC interviewer once asked Michael, "Don't you think barefoot [walking and] running is dangerous?"

Michael responded, "The most dangerous thing in the world is working at a desk job nine to five. Sure, I might get scratched up if I go barefoot in the beginning, but it's nothing like the risk of being sedentary to guarantee harm to my cardiovascular system, heart, lungs, blood pressure, insulin response (as a risk for diabetes), and so much more."

If you work at a desk, it's best to take frequent breaks, get up and stretch, sit on the ground and get your vitamin G, get out for a barefoot walk whenever possible (not to mention slip those shoes off under the desk if you can), and consider a grounding pad (more on this later).

shed their shoes and frolic in the grass. It's not just physical; it's soothing on an emotional and spiritual level.

NATURE'S DRUGSTORE

Disease—think of it as *dis*-ease—comes from an unsettled mind. Connecting with the earth, plugging back in, quiets our minds. Spiritual author Deepak Chopra often describes disease as coming from stress and harmful chemicals (such as cortisol or stress hormones) ravaging our bodies.

Walking barefoot is connecting with the greatest drugstore on earth, our minds. We often don't know how a drug works, but we do know that it triggers the release of chemicals from the brain. Dr. Maureen Traub, a medical doctor on Maui who believes in the power of self-healing, hasn't written a prescription in five years. She likes to say, "There goes another forty thousand dollars!" every time you smile, laugh, or simply take a deep breath. In other words, you just produced another $40,000 worth of amazing, healing drugs for the mind. When we're grounded and having fun, a simple smile can produce more powerful cancer-fighting and health-generating drugs than anything else in the world. Perhaps this is a great benefit of being barefoot—connecting with the earth and taking those deep breaths help heal and center us from deep within.

GETTING IN SYNC

Our dogs Pumpkin and Sawa (and our new wonder cat, Bam Bam) always wanted their food at exactly the same time every day. But how did they know it was time to eat? They weren't wearing puppy or kitty watches, but their internal clocks told them when to wake, sleep, and even salivate for food. All animals except for humans, with our artificial light, computer screens, and TVs, have synchronized their body clocks with that of the earth. But by exercising regularly, particularly barefoot and feeling the ground, we can reconnect with and reset our internal clocks.

Once you're ready and prepped to go barefoot, we recommend walking outside on a regular basis, particularly at sunrise and sunset, which tends to synchronize our bodies to the twenty-four-hour cycle of the sun. Whatever hour of day you choose, try to go out every day at that same time. The body will learn when to rise and when to sleep, when to think, and when to go quiet. This body knowledge helps us let go, relax, and get in sync with the earth.

THE PHYSICS OF GETTING GROUNDED

Getting grounded isn't merely a spiritual feeling; it has its roots in physics. (Extensive documentation to support the science introduced in this discussion is cited in the notes at the back of the book.)

Since the beginning of time, we humans have walked, slept, and spent most of our time with our bare feet on the ground, unaware that this physical contact transfers natural healing electrical energy to our bodies.

For the first time in history, our modern lifestyle has disconnected us from the earth's energy, making us more vulnerable to stress and illness. We wear insulating rubber- or synthetic-soled shoes, travel around in metal boxes with rubber wheels, and eat, sleep, and work in structures raised above the ground. New research, spearheaded by Clint Ober, is showing that when we reconnect to the earth by way of our bare feet, or by using a grounding device, a myriad of things happen to support health and vitality.

Clint Ober, the Father of Earthing

Clint Ober is a true pioneer in the field of grounding, or what he termed "Earthing." A former cable television network expert, he lost his health and nearly his life after an infection from a root canal compromised 80 percent of his liver. The infection spread throughout his entire body and he was given just months to live. However, after experimental surgery his liver grew back to its original size. During the healing process, he experienced a paradigm shift. In his book *Earthing: The Most Important Health Discovery Ever?*, he wrote, "A stark realization came over me that I didn't really own my home and the mountain of possessions I had. Rather, they owned me." He sold his possessions and business, bought an RV, and spent four years driving around the country in search of his purpose in life. In meditation, he thought, "I want to do something different. Whatever time I have left I want to dedicate it to something worthwhile and with purpose."

One day he sat on the bay in Key Largo, Florida, and asked for guidance. When he returned to the RV, he heard these words: "Become an opposite charge." Years later, thinking about static electricity (which caused "snow" and white lines on TV) he wondered if being insulated from the ground in footwear would have an effect on people's health. He realized that electronic and electrical equipment had to be grounded, and thought perhaps humans do too.

And thus began his quest. First he developed a grounding pad that could connect someone with the earth when indoors (he simply calls it an "extension cord" for the earth). He performed a humble study showing that of the people who used the grounding pad, 85 percent went to sleep more quickly, 93 percent reported sleeping better throughout the night, 82 percent experienced a significant reduction in muscle stiffness, 74 percent experienced elimination or reduction of chronic back and joint pain, 100 percent reported feeling more rested when they woke up, and 78 percent reported improved general health. This was just the beginning of a long career in research on the effects of grounding.

Clint Ober's research is a major reason we now have science starting to catch up with what we intuitively know: that getting grounded is good for us.

When you touch the ground, something special, almost magical happens. Or perhaps we should say that something *electrical* happens. Because when you touch the ground, you're connected electrically with the earth.

Look at it this way: the earth is a giant negatively charged electrical battery. That's why our electronic equipment is grounded and why electrical plugs have a third, grounding prong.

Anything disconnected from the earth tends to hold a positive charge (which is why there are electrical storms or why your hair stands on end, particularly in the winter). How many times have you shuffled across the carpet and then zapped someone? Shocking!

That static charge is harmful. For example, computer chip makers avoid static electricity because it can fry a circuit board. Anyone who works around gunpowder or fills up at gas stations knows the danger of stray sparks causing an explosion.

Those charges build up in our bodies. The earth was always there to take the hit, so to speak. But along the way, we became disconnected from Mother Earth. Our ancestors walked barefoot or in leather-soled sandals. They slept on the earth, tilled the earth, and, in a very real sense, were one with the earth.

Not so today. Because we're insulated from the ground, that static electricity charge builds up—with no place to go.

When you slip off your shoes at the end of the day, walk barefoot through the grass, or squish your toes on a sandy beach, you're not just draining tension away, you're off-loading the excess positive charge clinging onto and in your body. You're plugging back into the earth, getting grounded, and getting your dose of vitamin G.

Here's some more good stuff. When it comes to injuries and disease, the number one word you'll hear doctors use is *inflammation*. It's linked to high blood pressure, heart disease, various cancers, diabetes, autoimmune diseases, and plenty more of our modern ills.

And where does this inflammation come from? One major source of inflammation is free radicals, those pesky little electrically charged buggers we're all trying to get rid of by taking antioxidants such as vitamins A, C, and E.

Think of free radicals as electrically imbalanced or electrically unstable charged particles in your body. They are a by-product of metabolism and are also produced by your immune system (specifically by white blood cells) to go hunting for problems. Trouble is, when they don't find something unhealthy to latch onto and clean up, or a way to be drained from the body, they build up, creating inflammation and latching onto healthy tissue, causing damage.

Studies reported in the book *Earthing: The Most Important Health Discovery Ever?* and in the *Journal of Alternative and Complementary Medicine* show that going barefoot reduces your excess charge, and voilà—bye-bye free radicals, hello reduced inflammation, blood pressure, cortisol levels, stress, pain, and muscle tension.

Earthing: A Natural Blood Thinner?

As the expression goes, blood is thicker than water. But thick, inflammatory, clumpy blood, typical in patients with cardiovascular disease and diabetes, isn't a good thing. That's why there are some very expensive drugs on the market to help us thin our blood.

Here's the good news. In a 2009 pilot study by cardiologist Dr. Stephen Sinatra and Dr. Gaeten Chevalier (to be published in the peer-reviewed *Journal of Alternative and Complementary Medicine* in the spring of 2013), it was found that grounding, even for a very short period of time (two hours), dramatically altered the zeta potential of a cell by an average of 270 percent. The zeta potential relates to the degree of negative charge on the surface of a red blood cell. The higher the zeta potential the more likely the blood is to be thin and flow freely, which means a much lower risk of clotting.

While more studies are needed, this study suggests what we've seen time and again: you literally get healthier by plugging into the earth, even for brief periods of time such as your barefoot walks. In this case, your blood gets thinner and healthier, helping it flow better. And it means, in Dr. Chevalier's words, "if Earthing affects blood as we have seen in this pilot investigation, that means Earthing really affects the metabolism of the entire body at the cellular level. This further supports our hypothesis that grounded people have a different physiology than people who are ungrounded. As more research rolls out, we may find that we need to rewrite physiology books!"

In Michael's case, with barefoot walking he was on the world's largest dose of anti-inflammatory and healing drugs, all in one, just by plugging into the ground.

It turns out that planet Earth has a frequency, or a heartbeat, called the Schumann resonance, of approximately 7.83 hertz. This number is important because it's approximately the same frequency our brains use. In other words, we evolved to vibrate at the same frequency or heartbeat as our planet does.

We vibrate in sync with the world around us. When our environment is out of sync, we're out of sync too, which can have significant harmful effects on our bodies and minds. Studies are showing that when our environment is not vibrating at approximately 7.83 hertz—for instance, in an environment bombarded by cell phone signals and electromagnetic waves from all sorts of other devices (which some call "electro-pollution"), brain wave function can be disturbed, causing ADD-like symptoms, depression, and other psychological conditions along with a number of medical conditions. Unfortunately, as cell phone use becomes more ubiquitous, electro-pollution continues to rise, as do corresponding health risks. We're not even safe in our beds at home; we're still bombarded by electrical radiation as we sleep, from cell phone signals, household appliances, the wiring in the walls behind our beds, and even microwave towers miles away.

While the earth's frequency averages 7.83 hertz, it cycles throughout the day, peaking twice, around 8:00 a.m. and 5:00 p.m wherever you are in the world. These peaks help keep our bodies in tune with the twenty-four-hour cycle of the planet. Since our bodies and minds are in tune with the earth, these cycles give

◐°°₀ FOOT NOTE

Ever wonder why you experience jet lag or feel so out of sync after a long flight? It's not just the time zone change or lack of hydration—it's because you are literally out of sync with the earth. If we go barefoot after we travel, or spend thirty to sixty minutes sitting or lying on the ground, we start to vibrate in harmony with our new environment, and feel much better. It's why we're both barefoot the minute we get off a plane.

us our circadian rhythm or internal twenty-four-hour clock, helping us naturally know when to rise and when to sleep. However, when our environment's overloaded with artificially created electromagnetic radiation, we're thrown out of sync with the natural circadian rhythm.

Being barefoot for just a few minutes a day may not be enough to bring you back in sync. It's not just a matter of dissipating the charges, but of resynchronizing ourselves with the cycles and vibration of the earth. This takes time, such as long barefoot walks, runs, or hikes daily (or even twice daily, following the cycles of the earth).

Additionally, being barefoot for a few minutes each day doesn't protect us from the harmful electromagnetic frequencies we're virtually swimming in. To protect ourselves, we must be grounded. When we connect to the earth, we become part of the earth's circuit. We not only begin vibrating with the planet, but the earth helps protect us and keep charges from entering our bodies.

If you've ever heard of lightning striking a car, the reason the people inside the car aren't killed isn't because of the thin rubber tires. It's because the electricity travels around the car instead of into it, and then exits through the ground. This is similar to a Faraday effect. Our skin works the same when we're connected to the ground. Electrical waves with much lower charges than a lightning strike hit our skin and go around our bodies to the ground when we're barefoot. In this way grounding protects us from the incredibly harmful electromagnetic pollution. The more time you spend being grounded each day, the better.

Grounding sheets and pads have a silver or carbon mesh and plug directly into the ground via a wire and grounding rod or into a properly grounded electrical outlet. You can sleep on them, lay them on your office chair, or even place them on your favorite couch. There are also stick-on patches, which Jessica used to heal her foot. Personally, we have grounding sheets on our bed, which help us sleep better, and we work with grounding pads at our desks, which seems to help calm the mind and give us greater creativity. Others who use these pads swear by them for increased productivity, improved health (greater resistance to colds, for example), and far less stress at work, even while being bombarded with high levels of electromagnetic radiation. Though we feel they make a big difference, whenever possible we prefer the greater benefits of being grounded by sitting, standing, or walking directly on the earth.

Flower Power and Vitamin G

A recent proof-of-concept experiment by Dr. Gary E. Schwartz at the University of Arizona illustrates the importance of being grounded, at least for flowers. A team took sunflowers and put them in vases, grounding half and leaving the other half ungrounded. Then they observed the sunflowers and took photos for two weeks. The results? The grounded sunflowers remained strong and vibrant, while the ungrounded flowers began to wilt and die within days. Just think, if grounding does that for sunflowers, what will it do for us?

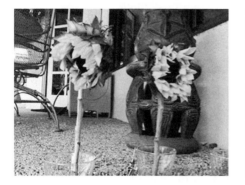

Ungrounded Sunflower

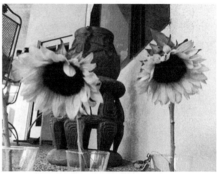

Electrically Grounded Sunflower

SPIRITUAL GROUNDING

That is why the old Indian still sits upon the earth instead of propping himself up and away from its life-giving forces. For him, to sit or lie upon the ground is to be able to think more deeply and to feel more keenly; he can see more clearly into the mysteries of life and come closer in kinship to other lives about him.

—Standing Bear, Oglala Nation

Although you don't need to be religious or spiritual to enjoy barefoot activities, you may find the act of shedding your shoes and touching the ground to be a spiritual experience.

We call it "the big G," as in God. However, the nomenclature of spirituality isn't what's important. Call it God, the Divine, Mother Nature, Universe, *chi*, love, Source, or whatever term best fits your belief system, but the universal power is all around us and supports us with life-giving energy. To us, touching the earth helps us plug back into Source. It's as if while wearing shoes or being indoors all day we become unplugged from an energy source, and when we're touching the earth barefoot, we're plugged back in.

Here's the extra bonus: barefoot time and vitamin G are cumulative. The more time you spend barefoot, the better you feel. So go barefoot today, connect with the earth, and feel your stresses drain away, your blood pressure drop, your health increase, and your mind quiet . . . all by plugging in.

EXERCISE

Greeting Mother Earth

Dr. Warren Grossman, author of *To Be Healed by the Earth*, believes the greater the awareness we have of the energy in the earth, the more it helps us. This exercise helps you grow your sensitivity to vitamin G.

Lie down with your back flat on the ground, with your arms spread outward and your palms facing down. If possible, lie directly on the ground,

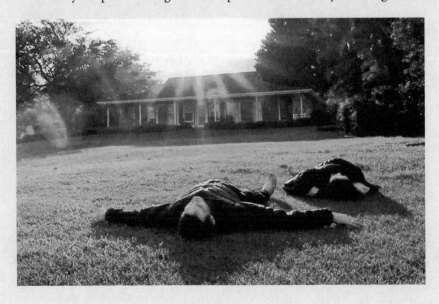

but if needed use a thin blanket made of natural material such as wool or cotton. To begin, start with your knees bent and your feet flat on the ground. Focus on your breathing as you try to sense the earth. It's typically a tingly or ticklish sensation.

1. Focus on your feet and their connection to the earth. What do you feel, or sense?
2. Next put your legs down and feel your calves connecting to the earth. What do they feel?
3. Move up your body and feel the earth. Next are hamstrings (back of your upper thighs).
4. Glutes (gluteus maximus)
5. Hands
6. Arms
7. Entire back
8. Shoulders
9. Neck
10. Head

EXERCISE

Plugging into Source

This meditation will help you recharge your mind, body, and spirit. When you actively focus on plugging into the energy of the earth, you're teaching your body to plug in automatically. In this seated meditation, we'll focus on feeling the earth's energy entering through your fingertips.

Sit directly on the ground. (Direct contact with the ground is preferred, but it's okay to sit on a towel or blanket made of natural materials.) Cross your legs and sit as tall as you can. As if you are playing the piano, place

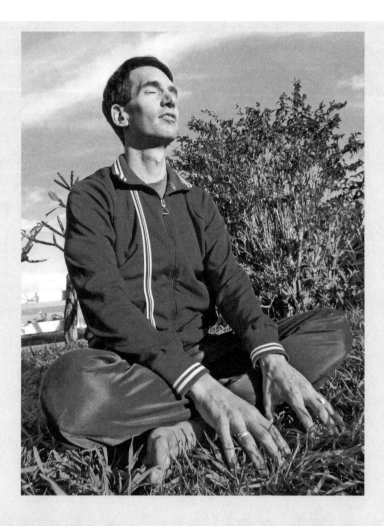

your hands in front of you with each of your fingertips independently touching the ground.

Concentrate on slow, deep, controlled breaths as you bring your awareness to your hands. Feel the tingling of the earth in each finger, and in particular your thumbs. Note any sensations in your hands, such as changes in temperature. It's not uncommon to feel your hands or palms become warm. Then begin to sense that energy traveling up through your fingers to your head and then as a gentle wave down your spine and back into the ground. In a very real sense, you're completing an electrical circuit!

The more you circulate this energy, the more awake, vibrant, and alive you will become. Plug into the earth and turn your light on!

DIRT—IT DOES A BODY GOOD

As we walk through the landscape, not only are the birds aware, and
the bears, and all the other animals of this forest, but all the
microbes of the soil are aware of our presence.

—Paul Stamets, *Dirt! The Movie*

Dirt is the living, breathing skin of the planet. A random handful of dirt likely contains all of the five kingdoms of life, from the one-celled monerans to the protists, plants, animals, and fungi. As Gary Vaynerchuk, host of *Wine TV*, puts it in *Dirt! The Movie*, "I think it's very obvious dirt might be more alive than we are."

Without dirt we wouldn't exist or be alive. From dirt come all of the vitamins, minerals, and building blocks of our existence.

Nearly every indigenous people tells a story of being inextricably tied to the land. Without one, there is no other. Hawaiian people are called *kama'aina*, which literally means "children of the land" or "children of the earth." There's a similar expression in Navajo too: the original term for the Navajo people before the Spaniards arrived was *nihokáá' dine'é'*, meaning "people of the earth" or "holy earth people." Countless other such expressions are found all over the globe.

For that matter, we are all children of the earth, children of the dirt. We are all made up of the same basic elements that make up the earth.

Ancient texts, including the Bible, tell how mankind was fashioned, molded, or given life by God or some force, directly from the earth. In Genesis 3:19, for example, it says, "For out of [the ground] you were taken. For dust you are and to dust you will return." In Hebrew, the very name *Adam* means "dirt" or "clay."

From *Dirt! The Movie:* "In our earliest stories we celebrated dirt as the source of who we are and where we come from. In the Amazon jungle it's said that one day Sun hurled a stick rattle into Mother Earth and out we came. Ancient Egyptians believed that the gods shaped clay into humans and put them in an earthly paradise. Jewish, Christian, and Muslim traditions share the story that God scooped up dirt and blew in the breath of life."

In this society we may not treasure dirt, but dirt is the most sacred substance on the planet. Without good dirt, we wouldn't exist. Period. It's not that we wouldn't have the same quality of life; we wouldn't have any life. For good soil is required for everything we eat, for the water we drink, and for the trees that produce the oxygen we breathe.

And yet we forget that. We think dirt is, well, dirty.

We have it backward. Without dirt we wouldn't exist. Dirt is life.

Every vitamin, every mineral, everything that we need as a building block for our existence comes from the soil. Look outside. We're made of that very thing beneath the grass and concrete.

A Dirty Little Secret

> *The people who make the greatest wines in the world love their dirt.*
> *They pick it up, they coddle it, they kiss it, they put it in a jar, and it*
> *sits on their mantle in the living room because they know, they know.*
> —Gary Vaynerchuk, *Dirt! The Movie*

How much would you pay for something that would boost your immune system, reduce or prevent allergies, strengthen your mind, reduce anxiety, alleviate depression, lower the chance you'll ever develop dementia, and tame inflammation to boot?

How about if it'd also make you happy?

Sounds like a miracle cure, doesn't it? Well, it's much simpler than that. It's dirt.

There's a dirty little secret out there, one that's been around for thousands of years, one that every kid knows and that many parents abhor.

Dirt is good for us. (So is mud, but we're getting ahead of ourselves.) It turns out dirt may be the secret ingredient for great health and a great mind. And that's according to researchers!

Dirt has been shown to do all of these things and more. Which is impressive, particularly since we live in a society that treats dirt like dirt.

Our society abhors getting dirty. There's been a campaign for years to eradicate dirt from the home. The theory is that the cleaner our homes and cities, the less communicable disease there'll be. To a large extent, it's worked. We don't have outbreaks of typhoid, tuberculosis, the plague, or other major challenges.

However, we may have gone too far.

There's a new hypothesis in town, and it's called the hygiene hypothesis. According to this theory, we've gone too far to eradicate dirt, and we're paying the price with autoimmune disorders, allergies, and weakened immune systems.

It's true that at no point has our society been on more of a cleaning rampage (just look at the number of antibacterial products out there today), and at no point have we had more allergic and asthmatic kids or people with autoimmune disorders.

Thinking about it a different way, there are more than 90 trillion organisms living on and in your body at any time. Every few square inches of your body has a unique ecosystem of bacteria that is unlike any other surface on your body, let alone anyone else's. In general, we live in harmony with these microorganisms, working together to exist and thrive. If we start killing them off because we think they're harmful, then we can throw the whole thing out of whack. For instance, we wouldn't want to kill off all our stomach flora, because those bacteria are essential for the digestion and absorption of food and nutrition. By the way, when you see yogurt or kefir labels that tout "probiotics," that's just a fancy word for the bacteria that protect your stomach and aid in digestion. Today, the majority of yogurts are pasteurized, a process that kills off living probiotics. Make sure you look for yogurt with "active cultures." The vast majority of bacteria are actually good for us, working with us or helping us build a strong immune system.

In other words, we need to live in symbiosis or harmony with the wee beasties that are in us, on us, and in our environment. We evolved together on this planet, and most of these little microorganisms help us to survive.

Proof positive? In third-world countries where they have a different perception of "clean" and use antibacterial soaps sparingly, they don't have nearly the frequency of allergies or autoimmune disorders that we have. That doesn't mean such societies don't have their health issues or that we should stop being clean; we just need to know that a little dirt may go a long way toward bringing our bodies back into balance.

So, realistically, how can you get the great benefits of dirt? Well, we're biased, but the simplest way may be to walk, run, or play barefoot in the dirt. Of course, gardening is another effective way to get our hands in the dirt and be exposed to its positive benefits. There are also mudbaths, mudpacks, and eating dirt, but more on that later. In short, we reap the benefits of dirt through our permeable skin, the air we breathe, and the dust we ingest.

International Mud Day

Imagine a day when kids can get muddy, *really* muddy. When there's a giant mud pit at the local park and hundreds if not thousands of kids are slipping, sliding, playing, or generally just covering themselves in mud.

There's just such an event taking place each year on International Mud Day, and it's growing. The event started in Nepal and since then has spread even to the United States.

One of the biggest events in the States takes place in Michigan, where they combine 20,000 gallons of water with 200 tons of topsoil to make a giant mud lake. Here kids and grown-ups get together to play in the mud, rejoice in the mud, and even hold organized games and races in the mud. It's a chance to get down and dirty without getting in any trouble!

And yes, there are showers—*many* showers—to get the mud off the kids before going home.

Playing in the mud sounds like fun, doesn't it? Do you really need a special day to celebrate mud?

Dirt, the New Prozac

Researchers have been discovering what all children intuitively know: that playing in the dirt makes you feel better and smile. As researchers were looking into the hygiene hypothesis, they stumbled across another benefit of dirt, specifically from the soil bacterium *Mycobacterium vaccae,* which they believe helps alleviate depression. After researchers injected lung cancer patients with the bacteria, patients reported improved mood and a better quality of life. Other benefits also included alleviation of nausea and pain. In a separate experiment, the bacteria were injected into mice. Researchers found their brains had increased levels of serotonin, the "happy chemical," just as would happen in mice given Prozac. According to the lead researcher at Bristol University, Dr. Chris Lowry, the dirt studies "leave us wondering if we shouldn't all spend more time playing in the dirt."

Dirt for Wound Care?

Michael says, "During our film shoot on Maui I spent a day running on the road along a dry, windblown coast. It was a desert, the last scene you'd expect to find on a tropical island, receiving perhaps a fraction of an inch of rain a month.

"At one point, the director asked me to jump off the paved road and down a dry old jeep road pointed toward the ocean. I stepped off the road and landed in a giant poof of dust. As my foot hit the ground, plumes of dirt exploded from beneath me. This dirt was so soft and powdery, I could only imagine it's what moon dust would feel like. And it felt great, as if any and all life on the planet could grow in it, if only there was any water.

"That dirt was some of the most amazing soil I have ever run on. It, along with some of the soil I've felt in corn mazes, resonates strongly with me.

"At the time I had a cut on my toe—not on the bottom, as you might expect from walking barefoot (getting cuts is actually quite rare), but on the top of my toe, from running wildly through a bamboo forest trying to keep up with Jessica for our film shoot. I'd accidentally caught a broken branch with the top of my foot.

"The cut was fairly fresh when I did this road photo shoot. But something strange happened: I had the desire to cover my foot, including the cut, with this newly discovered soft dirt.

"I think the dirt bound to my wound, thereby protecting it from further harm, and promoted formation of a thick scab. I also believe it gave it minerals needed for healing. Because dirt is negatively charged, it helps draw toxins from the body and aids in reducing inflammation. A quick search online found that indigenous people have used dirt to cover, protect, and heal wounds for thousands of years. Now, we're not recommending throwing dirt on an open wound, but it does make you wonder."

Get Down and Dirty

There are likely as many types of dirt as there are species of life on the planet. Next time you're walking on a dirt path, stop and pick up some dirt in your hand and spend some time examining it. Look closely at its texture and composition. Feel it. Smell it. And if you're daring enough, take a little taste. You'll discover that some kinds of dirt will resonate with you more than others. And you'll know if it resonates by how good it feels to you. Our bodies know best. If you really fall in love, you won't want to put it down—and it's probably good for you too.

Mud, the New Anti-inflammatory

Struggling with swollen joints, a nagging injury, or troubled skin? Try mud.

Mud, also known as healing clay, has been used for thousands of years to help draw out toxins and reduce inflammation. We swear by it when it comes to overuse injuries, and for Jessica's skin. (We've been using Aztec Secret Indian Healing Clay with Bragg Organic Raw Unfiltered Apple Cider Vinegar.) For injuries, mix powdered clay with apple cider vinegar plus sea salt, and apply the mixture to the swollen area. You'll experience nearly instant relief. We attribute mud's power to the negative ions in its composition and its ability to draw out toxins. For younger-looking skin, allow the mud mixture (without salt) to dry for twenty to thirty minutes (ten to fifteen minutes if you have sensitive skin); then wash it away. Watch your skin glow! Go mud and go primal!

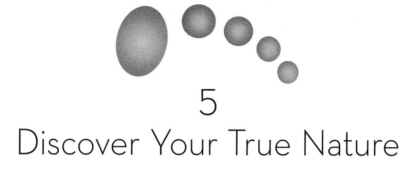

5
Discover Your True Nature

You can't know who you are until you know where you are.
—Wendell Berry

One of our first missions on Maui was to find an eco-friendly means of travel. Michael had always imagined us zipping around in a Mazda Miata convertible, sun in our faces, wind in our hair, and best of all awesome mileage. So we scoured Craigslist and found a promising 1997 Miata. Though we didn't know if this would be the one, we knew we would make a friend. So we headed down to Kihei, a beachcomber's paradise along the sunny southwest shore.

As we stood in the driveway talking to the owner of the car, a rusty white pickup truck, a true "Maui cruiser" held together with bungee cord and twine, pulled in behind us. The bungee cord held the grille to the car, while the twine kept the passenger door on its hinges. The truck gently growled at us before the engine cut off. In the driver's seat was David, jack of all trades, king of passion fruit pies, eco-home remodeler, and founder of Maui Mystical Tours. He was here to remodel a bathroom.

David hopped out of his truck barefoot, and it was immediately obvious that his were not virgin feet. No sock or shoe tan line. Muscular. A wide forefoot with space between the toes. After quick introductions, we knew instantly he got "it" even more than we did.

"The earth speaks to me," he said. "She tells me where to go." He began to share his discoveries on the island, and we understood we would have much to learn from him. He would be our guide. We all hugged and became instant lifelong friends.

Before each of our trips, David would sit in meditation and ask Mother Earth and the ancestors where to take us. This first trip would be our introduction to Maui, much like saying, "Maui, meet Michael and Jessica, your new students," and "Michael and Jessica, meet Maui, your new teacher." In his meditation, David heard he needed to introduce us to a sacred ancient burial ground where Hawaiian warriors once interred the remains of royalty. They would gather the bones and bury them in holes in the ground and in the rock walls. This wasn't exactly a place you'd take tourists or your friends and family if they came to visit you on Maui.

David explained, "This is truly sacred land, which no one should set foot upon unless guided to do so." (Hence in this book we have left this place unnamed and without location.)

We were crammed together in the passenger seat of David's truck. As we pulled off the paved road onto a rutted dirt track, Jessica pushed herself forward and peered up at a steep hill jutting up from the sea. From our point of view, it appeared to have an awfully jagged top. With the gray morning mist still hanging low, this hill looked ominous and dangerous.

Secretly Jessica thought, "We're going to hike up *that* thing?" It had been a long road to recovery for her left foot, and she hadn't tested it with something this strenuous yet. She wondered if her foot was up for the challenge.

As we approached the hill, it seemed to grow in size. Meanwhile, a drizzle changed to fat drops and came at us sideways. We had to keep our heads down to keep the water out of our eyes and see the path before us. Michael jokingly called it a "shower" and asked for shampoo. But David called it purification: "You guys need to be cleaned of any negativity before climbing her."

At the base of the hill, we realized this was much more than a hike. This was rock climbing. With the combination of cold rainwater dripping into her eyes and mouth, Jessica felt off her game. We were facing chunks of porous igneous rock held together by clay, typical for Hawaii but unfamiliar to her. Would it be slippery in the rain? Would it hold her weight or would a chunk of the rock wall come off in her hand?

David later explained, "Everybody thinks clay is slippery when it's wet, but they don't actually go out and feel it. It's the opposite—sticky!" Jessica had to trust David and trust that she was *supposed* to climb this hill and reach the top.

As she reached for each handhold, she had to trust that her fingers would grip the rock. With each foothold, she had to trust that her toes would grip the rock. David bounded ahead a few yards but turned around to guide her hands and feet. "Be the mountain goat . . . be the mountain goat," he gleefully yelled back.

As ridiculous as it may sound, being the mountain goat helped. Jessica felt springs loading in her legs and felt her legs and arms working together to propel her forward. She didn't just feel like a mountain goat anymore; in fact, she felt extraordinarily human as her body began remembering what it was designed to do. The fear that had caused her muscles to tighten was more tiring than simply allowing her body to move freely.

If you've ever tried rock climbing, you know that if you stay in one spot for too long, contemplating whether or not you should go for the next hold, you waste precious energy, diminishing your chances of making it to the top. Once you know your body can do it, you just have to go for it. Once Jessica let go of fear and relaxed into her body, she started having fun.

Eventually the terrain began to level out. The harsh rock was now covered by soil and tall grass, and soon we found ourselves mounting the crest of the hill. The rain cleared and the sun emerged. Looking down at the waves crashing about the seemingly tiny rocks, we realized what dizzying heights we had just come up. It was like a rite of passage. We had walked, scrambled, and climbed our way into the next stage of discovering what it means to be human.

We're not suggesting you jump into barefoot climbing just yet. This is simply where we were in our journey and a demonstration of learning to trust. We hope that you learn to trust your own personal knowing about what you can do now and what you may have to wait for in the future. You may be simply mustering up the courage to walk barefoot ten feet down your driveway. That's okay. You're just beginning your own personal journey to discovering your true nature. Allow this exciting new world to unfold before you.

BAREFOOT IS HUMAN

Humans are bipedal, meaning we walk upright on two feet. This distinguishes us from all other animals on the planet. If we were born with weak, meek feet, we wouldn't be standing upright and we wouldn't be the most dominant species on the planet. Nothing else in the animal kingdom has anything like our feet. In other words, our successful evolution as a species stems in large part from our two feet.

Children know what it means to be human, to run, play, and stand on their own two feet. Do they want to be in shoes? No. Do they kick them off every chance they can? You bet. And do they run and play in the dirt and mud out in nature? Heck yeah.

It's human to play in the dirt, to run barefoot in nature, to explore, and to put one bare foot in front of the other.

The nerve endings on the bottom of our feet give us the information we need to step lightly and safely. We also get the information we need to move efficiently, which was important when we had to walk (as nomads once did) hundreds of miles for survival and food. It gave us the ability to feel the ground to stay out of danger or to avoid missteps. And sensitive feet helped us find the swiftest, most economical stride to help us chase, catch, and bring home dinner.

We were given these smart, sensitive feet to guide us along our way. Ever feel you're supposed to go right instead of left? Or ever heard the expression "She got cold feet"? Or how about "happy feet"? These are examples of emotions, information, and warnings coming to us from our feet. Animals flee before earthquakes, floods, and tsunamis, because they feel something's not quite right. A few remaining indigenous tribes haven't forgotten how to use their bare feet either.

||||||||||||||||||||||||||||||||||||||||||||||||||||||||||||||||||||||||||||||||||||||||||||||||||||||||||||||||||||||||||||||||||||||||||||

Awaken Your Sixth Sense

People think of the mind as being located in the head, but the latest findings in physiology suggest that the mind doesn't really dwell in the brain but travels the whole body on caravans of hormone and enzyme, busily making sense of

the compound wonders we catalogue as touch, taste, smell, hearing, vision.

—Diane Ackerman, *A Natural History of the Senses*

The latest studies suggest thought isn't limited to the mind, or to the five senses we thought it was. According to Richard Louv, author of *The Nature Principle*, scientists have discovered conservatively ten and possibly as many as thirty senses (such as the ability to sense time without a watch), senses that awaken once we spend time in nature. To us, it's all about awareness, what you perceive, sense, and feel in new ways.

When the giant 2004 Indian Ocean tsunami struck the Andaman and Nicobar Islands, most villagers were oblivious to the oncoming danger. The barefoot Jarawa tribe, however, safely evacuated to higher ground, deep into the forest. According to the Jarawa, they sensed danger and fled. In other words, they used the sixth sense they had developed in nature as an early tsunami warning system.

Walking in nature, particularly barefoot, helps us develop our own sixth sense, an enhanced awareness of our environment. According to brain researchers at Washington University in St. Louis, the brain's early warning system is centered in the anterior cingulate cortex, which is designed to pick up subtle signs and cues. This ability to sense is what vision researcher Ron Rensink at the University of British Columbia calls "mindsight." In essence, mindsight is the ability to take in information from the senses unconsciously and know what's going on, even before you've had time to process the data. It'd be like successfully avoiding an accident by turning the car before you've even heard the bus or seen it coming toward you.

This mindsight, or sixth sense, is important in nature, in cities, and even on the battlefield. A large military study found that people who grew up playing or hunting in nature are better able to spot anomalies or a roadside bomb before it's too late. According to researcher Army Sergeant Major Todd Burnett, "They just seemed to pick up things much better.... They know how to look at the entire environment." For us, it means nurturing an intuition that is just as valuable as intellect. It means that instead of asking, "What do you think?" we ask, "How does it feel?"

When you develop your sixth sense in nature, the world doesn't just grow richer, but clearer too. We only need to listen, or turn on our mindsight.

DANCE IN THE WOODS

We all yearn to reconnect with nature. This is visible in our art, entertainment, language, and prayers. In almost all that we do, on some level, we yearn to plug back in.

Throughout the history of mankind, for as long as there've been paintings, drawings, and petroglyphs, humans have been fascinated with nature. We desire to live in the mountains or down by the sea. We put lakes and parks in our cities and bring nature into our homes with aquariums and plants. We use flowers to express love. We paint landscapes and photograph panoramas. And baseball, our national pastime, takes place on a "field of dreams."

As kids, we yearned to be outdoors. Sadly, there's an epidemic of kids disconnected from nature. Richard Louv, author of *Last Child in the Woods*, says today's children have what he calls nature-deficit disorder. They've been cut off from nature and lost their chance to play outdoors and to connect or plug into the world around them. It's why we're found at the beach on weekends, or in the country, or skiing on the slopes, or craving almost any other outdoor activity you can think of.

In fact, even when we're indoors watching a movie, chances are nature or a beautiful backdrop is featured prominently throughout the film. For many, connecting with nature is what draws them to walking—and to this book. We yearn to breathe fresh air, quiet the mind, and be outside—laughing, playing, and enjoying nature, as we once did as children. On the beach, we let our feet squish through the sand and feel the water lap our toes. In the park, if we're lucky, we take off our shoes and also dance through the grass. These sensual experiences harken back to simpler times.

NATURE PLAY

Nature play—playing in and with nature—is the easiest way to feel connected to the earth, to feel like a human being. What better way to get to know a place than by playing in it? And what better way to know yourself than by experimenting with your body outdoors? The instructions are simple—because there are none. It's about following your instincts and listening closely to your body to know what your body is capable of and what it still needs time for.

As children, we felt invincible. There are some practical reasons for that: our bones were far more flexible and healed much faster, and we had a lower center of gravity, so when we fell, we didn't fall as far. In a sense, nature play is a gradual process of regaining some of that feeling of invincibility. Your body will tell you when it's had enough or if it's not ready for the next step.

When you feel ready, try walking along a log on the ground or hopping from one flat stone to the next flat stone. With time and practice, you'll be able to take on more difficult obstacles, just like a kid again.

Like on our rock-climbing expedition with David, it's always amazing what our bodies are capable of and surprising the conditioning our bodies naturally undergo just by walking barefoot. When you explore nature like this, you turn exercise into joyful play. Playing is a part of being a human being. If you listen to your heart, it'll tell you how.

On Bare Faith

One morning Jessica was cooking eggs after a morning meditation, thinking about how to help Michael with his ADD coaching, when out of the blue she had the idea to start a barefoot running school. Jessica hadn't even been barefoot running for a month yet, nor did she have any idea that the barefoot movement would become so popular. At the time, not many people were considering taking off their shoes. In fact, we were sometimes ridiculed or scoffed at. All she knew for certain was that a lot of people could benefit, and if our mission was to help people, we couldn't fail.

This was in 2009, less than three months after we met. Two months later, we had both quit our jobs and with little savings started writing *Barefoot Running*. It just felt like the right thing to do. Many of our friends and family thought we were crazy. It was difficult to explain where our knowing came from, so we attempted to explain by creating a business plan. Still, they couldn't understand the risk.

Sometimes there's no sense in waiting around for the science to back something up that you already know to be true. If you believe in the existence of

God or a divine energy that is greater than yourself, it's like waiting for science to prove that God exists. Why wait to believe when you can feel it's true?

It was both exciting and incredibly scary taking these leaps of faith, but we took each one because we felt we were being guided. It helped to know that it wasn't *our* plan but a *divine* plan, and therefore it must be a much better plan than either one of us could ever devise.

We went nearly broke three times in our first few years together. Each time we had just enough to get by. Once we were left with just one dime in our bank account after paying for a parking meter in front of the post office, where we were mailing a certified check to free our first five thousand books from the printer. Each time we saw what was left as a miracle, a symbolic gesture that we'd always make it.

Each time you feel as if you're going out on a limb based on your knowing and you see that you're still okay, the next time it's a little less scary. You grow braver and braver until one day you realize, wow, you're really living for the first time in your life. Trust that there is a divine plan conspiring for your best interests, no matter how daunting the mountain is that stands before you. There's a good reason for that mountain to be there—to steer you in the right direction.

So check in. Shut off the mind chatter. Feel your heart, feel your body, feel the earth, and listen. If it feels right, try a little barefoot play.

Tree Huggers, Unite!

In 2010 we held our first RunBare clinic at Kripalu, a yoga and wellness center in the Berkshires. There, after several days of barefoot walking and connecting with the earth, we walked the group out into the woods with the specific purpose of hugging some trees, though we didn't tell them that yet.

We went out silently, focused on the ground beneath our feet, and doing an exercise in which we focus entirely on each of our senses, one at a time, to wake things up, gain awareness, and grow fully into the moment. And then we stopped at a large grove of trees, some hundreds of years old.

It was supposed to be a five-minute exercise, but everyone in the group lingered for at least another ten minutes. People were captivated by what they felt, dumbfounded even.

"I never expected to hug a tree," said a physical therapist.

"I can't believe it—my hands were tingling," said a doctor.

Another person said, "It felt so alive!"

Whenever we are out on the trails, we're constantly touching the trees around us. It's as if we're giving them handshakes, or perhaps it's the other way around. But we're connecting with the woods and the forest as we go along.

If we find a special tree, we may stop and lean up against it or hug it and see what we feel or even what we hear. Trees are all expressions of the earth—think of trees as standing dirt. My favorites right now are the strong, incredibly solid eucalyptus trees soaring over 150 feet high, and the banyan, a tree that has roots going up and down in an intricate weave and can cover an entire city block with roots, branches, and more roots. Both of these trees have their own unique feel, and each is incredibly special.

The Tree Marks the Spot

Jessica says, "Have you ever stopped to wonder if a tree is conscious? I love to stop at an old-growth tree, put my hands on it, and wonder about what it's seen, heard, and felt over the course of its long life. Though trees can't rationalize or problem-solve quite like humans, it doesn't mean they're not aware of being alive. I say hello. I apologize for the state of the environment, say thank you for producing the oxygen we breathe, listen, and send it love. I get the sense that the tree appreciates my gratitude."

Adds Michael: "I started hugging trees after my 2006 accident. I go back to the spot where it happened each year and give thanks for the accident and all that's occurred since then. And how do I give thanks? By hugging a tree just next to the spot and thanking it. On my last visit in 2012, I was astonished to see a handprint in the bark, exactly where I place my hand each year. Every one of our actions makes an imprint of some kind.

"For the tree is an expression of nature, and of the earth. It's still fully plugged in, and just a manifestation of the ground. It's like standing earth.

"I especially remember a morning when I was strolling past ivy leaves just as the sun began peeking out from behind some trees. One leaf held a tiny dewdrop, and the first rays of the sun sliced through it and brought out all the colors of the rainbow. It was such a beautiful sight. I cried.

"From that day on, I began looking at the world in a new way and started taking a camera with me on my barefoot adventures. My photos have had gallery showings and have been purchased by art lovers around the world. They never would have happened if I hadn't slowed down long enough to see and appreciate the beauty all around me."

BARE YOUR SOLES

We are not trying to be rebels or nonconformists when we travel around barefoot. But after years of going barefoot, we're no longer comfortable in traditional shoes.

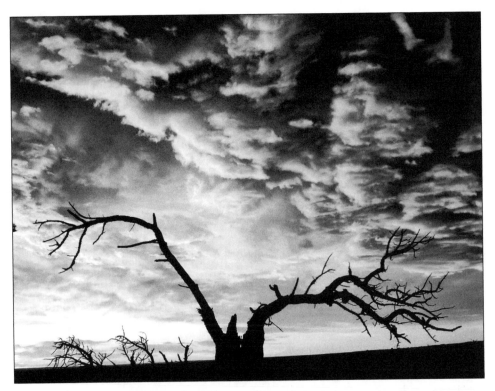

One of Michael's early photos, *Embracing Nature's Energy*. Connected to the earth, you begin to see the world in a new light.

Reach Out and Hug a Tree Today

Next time you go for a walk, pick out a tree that calls to you. It could just be a tree that you find beautiful, intriguing, happy, or sad. Walk up and place your fingertips on the bark. Note how your hand feels.

Then wrap both your arms around the trunk. Use all of your senses to experience what you can. Focus on these sensations. Press your ear to the tree and listen as well. And listen too, with your heart. At minimum, try to feel the energy that the tree is drawing up from the ground. The process by which a tree or any plant drains water and minerals out of the soil is ionic, or electrical, in nature. Each cell in a plant or tree has a tiny charge that pulls up water from the deepest soil to the highest leaf. So what you're feeling is real. For instance, an oak tree can bring more than a hundred gallons of water from its roots up into its leaves each day. Just imagine the energy that process requires.

After you've spent at least five minutes hugging the tree, give it thanks.

If we see a sign at a retail store or food establishment that reads "Shoes Required," we may slip on some footwear before entering. We're not trying to push the rules or make employees uneasy, so in these situations we wear minimalist shoes, sandals, or flip-flops.

Although it's not illegal to be barefoot in any American establishment, a store has the right to enforce its own dress code. For instance, a suit or tie may be necessary in one restaurant, or no jeans allowed at another. So an establishment has the right to tell you to wear shoes.

The laws about going barefoot—or the social norms and myths—have everything to do with socioeconomic status rather than health codes. Michael was escorted out of a Whole Foods market one day when he'd forgotten to bring shoes. Why can't you go barefoot in a store? Likely because at some point in the past, store owners believed that if you didn't have shoes, you didn't have money and might be out to steal from them. The same thought pattern may occur on public transportation. While we'd like to believe they're making us wear shoes for our own good (even the security guard may believe he's keeping you safe), it likely goes back to keeping the riffraff off the bus.

When you first begin going barefoot in public, you might walk tentatively. Yes, some people will stare at your feet and then study your face. However, overall, most people are quite absorbed in their own worlds and will hardly notice, and those who do could benefit from a little barefoot time themselves.

Where should you go barefoot? Well, anywhere you feel comfortable. It's up to you. Just go with your gut. If it feels good, go for it. If not, don't. Over time

⚫°°•。 FOOT NOTE

Our Right to Bare Feet

Despite what you may have heard, it's not a crime to go barefoot. Not in a food establishment, not driving your car, nor just about anywhere. Now, that doesn't mean if a shop owner asks you to put on your shoes, you can claim some constitutional freedom to bare your feet. A shop owner has a right to ask, and a right to refuse to serve you (or ask you to leave) if you don't comply. Typically, they're concerned that allowing barefoot customers would get the store in trouble somehow, or that it would scare away other customers.

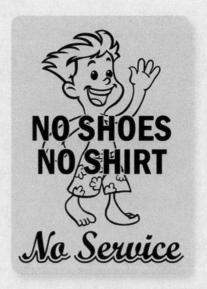

But despite the common claim that it's a "health code violation" or "against the law," that's really not the case. If it were required by the health code, then the signs you see saying "No Shirt, No Shoes, No Service" would be followed by a state statute. Instead, it's a discriminatory artifact from our past. There are no health code regulations requiring patrons to be barefoot because it does not affect the health of other patrons.

However, there may be health code restrictions against workers going barefoot, and Occupational Safety and Health Administration regulations to protect workers as well.

As for driving barefoot, it's another urban myth. We'd contend that going barefoot is a safer way to drive because you can feel the gas and brake pedals better, feel the road vibrations beneath your feet better, and are quicker to respond (plus there's no chance of catching your sticky-soled shoe on one pedal when you're trying to move your foot to the other). Race car drivers wear the thinnest shoes they can to have the best possible feel of the pedal. (Yes, their shoes are lined with Kevlar because of the heat buildup on the uninsulated floor of a race car, or the chance of a fire if a race car crashes.)

To dispel this myth, AAA used to state in its digest of motor vehicle laws that it was legal to drive barefoot. We contacted AAA about this and were told that it is still legal in all states except Oklahoma. We contacted the Oklahoma Department of Motor Vehicles, which passed us on to the state patrol, which said that (as of 2012) it is "absolutely legal to drive barefoot in Oklahoma."

At present there are no states where driving barefoot is against the law, and police officers are not regularly checking to see whether you're wearing your shoes or not. However, if a police officer deems that going barefoot made you a dangerous or reckless driver, then you can be cited for that, not for the actual act of going barefoot.

you'll grow more courageous about where you choose to go bare and about what feels right for you. As your feet change, you'll likely find the freedom, comfort, relaxation, and grounding too much to resist. And with practice, you'll find yourself barefoot, or nearly barefoot, in more and more situations.

Yet you needn't go fully bare. Although barefoot may be best, there are many shoes coming on the market that give your feet a much greater sense of freedom than shoes of the past. We discuss alternative footwear options in chapter 19.

Barefoot walking, or being barefoot in general, is only now becoming socially acceptable again. For centuries it was seen as unclean, uncouth, or socially unacceptable, something done only by the poor (those who couldn't afford shoes), hippies, rebels, or social nonconformists.

Before the interest in barefoot running, yoga, and other more natural activities, going barefoot was a big no-no in society. And many still look down upon it, although this is rapidly changing.

Being barefoot is more of a collective reawakening to the human body, human spirit, and mind. And once you feel the ground and wake up, there's no turning back.

In essence, we need to give ourselves permission to return to nature, to be more natural, and to experience humanity the way it was intended, with our two bare feet.

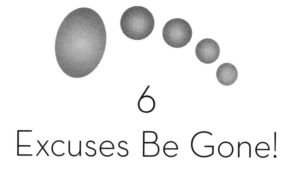

6

Excuses Be Gone!

Fear less, hope more; eat less, chew more; whine less, breathe
more; talk less, say more; hate less, love more; and all good things
are yours.
—Swedish proverb

While at a recent running industry conference, we were discussing this book with industry insiders. Even among the pros—people who work day in and day out in the athletic world—reason after reason came back to us as to why barefoot walking (and barefoot running) might work for *us*, but not for *them*.

A vice president of a major shoe manufacturer turned to Michael and said, "Well, you guys are still young, I couldn't go barefoot at my age, I'm forty-two." Michael didn't have the heart to tell him that he was forty.

Some objections have a rational basis. Others are based on misconceptions or preconceptions. Ultimately, they're all based on one thing: fear. It's scary to go barefoot. Ever since we were children, we've been told to make sure we have our shoes on or we're going to get hurt.

Fear is a powerful lion, but one often tamed by knowledge. Here are the top objections to going barefoot, and the knowledge you need to turn a growling lion into a purring pussycat.

LOVE OVER FEAR

Focus on the positives, on what you have to gain, not what you have to lose.

We recently made a post on our Facebook page about taking kids walking barefoot through corn mazes. The responses were surprising: there were people worried about chiggers (little insects that bite), burrs, and who knows what else—perhaps even attacks of killer corn.

There are always reasons *not* to do something. Heck, it's even a risk to get out of bed in the morning, let alone start your car or cross the street.

But if we focus on the negatives, where would that leave us? Hunkered down under the covers, hiding from the day?

So why not live life to the fullest? No more excuses. Give barefoot walking a try. What do you have to lose? Your fear. What do you have to gain? Stronger feet, grounding, plugging into nature, dancing with trees, and a host of health benefits.

In this chapter we'll cover all of your major worries or concerns and tell you how you can step on past them and give barefoot walking a try.

EXCUSE #1: THAT LOOKS PAINFUL

It's true that barefoot walking can be painful at times in the beginning. But thirty minutes in high heels is way more painful. When you commit to barefoot walking, your skin strengthens quickly and quite dramatically. For the first few weeks the skin is really tender and soft, and that's a good thing: it acts as your coach and keeps you from doing too much.

After only a few short weeks the skin grows strong and the fat pads on your feet, lost after you began to wear shoes as a kid, begin to return. In only a few short months, in addition to developing strong skin, your feet become spongy, cushioned, and springlike. They do not become callused and crusty, which is a common misconception, but rather strong and quite smooth. If you live in a warmer climate, this occurs even faster, no matter your age.

EXCUSE #2: I COULD STEP ON SOMETHING SHARP

Yes, you could. At least in the beginning, you could certainly step on something sharp and hurt yourself. But it's not nearly as big a concern as you think. Why? Because when you start walking barefoot, you're hypervigilant. You have two eyes and you are using them to look for anything in your path. Over the first few weeks you'll know the location of every stick, stone, seam, and crack on your path. When you're walking barefoot, you're walking awarefoot. You'll be in the moment, incredibly focused and mindful of each step and everything before you. Your eyes will keep you safe as you scour the ground.

Soon enough, glass will become no more than a sharp pebble, something that you'll feel underfoot but that won't cut your feet. Over time you'll find it's not the glass that gets you, but sometimes a tiny thorn, or if you're in cactus country a barb or goathead. All of these are minor, sometimes requiring you to stop for a minute or a bit more. But none of them is the type of catastrophic injury we think of when we think about going barefoot.

FOOT NOTE

Keep a Sharp Eye Out for Rock Salt

We're often asked about the worst injury we've sustained when walking or running barefoot. Both of us cut our feet while going barefoot on rock-salt-treated pavement in the winter. While salt is often applied to roads, sidewalks, and steps during the winter to melt ice and keep people from slipping, it wreaks havoc on bare feet.

Why? Well, when it's dry, rock salt is sharp and hurts like the dickens. If it's wet, it acts as a meat-tenderizer, softening the skin, thus making our feet susceptible to normally benign road hazards. A piece of glass that normally would never bother us now poses a potentially painful threat.

EXCUSE #3: I HAVE FLAT FEET
(OR HIGH ARCHES)

Your arch shape doesn't determine whether you can go barefoot. It's a myth. In fact, study after study says it has absolutely no bearing on whether you can go bare or not. Your arch, like your fingerprint, has its own unique shape.

We could find no correlation in the scientific studies between the shape of the arch and how it functions. However, what we did find is that the shape of the arch changes as you go barefoot. You start to strengthen the arch, and it grows taller. In essence, you're building a stronger spring. However, for many people, after the arch grows taller, the foot gets more muscular and better padded, and so, like the greatest African barefoot runners, the foot may fill out and appear to be flat again. But this time the muscle is hiding a beautiful strong arch on the inside.

Your feet are made up of muscles. Just as you can strengthen your arms, no matter how weak, you can strengthen your feet as well. Weak feet are only a starting point.

For some reason, countless people have been told by their doctors, shoe salespeople, or others that their high arches equal troubled feet. We don't understand this one at all. A tall arch is a great thing.

Why? Because it means you've already got a strong spring underfoot. If you wake up that spring and strengthen it some more, those high arches can become some of the greatest propulsion devices and shock absorbers in the world. A high arch is a sign of an incredibly strong walker or athlete in the making, no matter how old he is or what type of shoe her foot has been caged in.

Years ago, Michael was told by many a podiatrist that he had the flattest feet in the world. When he shares this with people at our clinics, they immediately stare at his feet, then shake their heads in disbelief. Surprise! He no longer has flat feet.

As podiatrists later told him, "We don't know how you did it, but you grew an arch." That's exactly what happens after going bare: your feet strengthen and become toned. Then voilà—you have an arch, the perfect spring to give you light and effortless steps.

EXCUSE #4: MY FEET ARE REALLY SENSITIVE

Often people look at our bare feet effortlessly stepping along and grimace with pain. They remark, "I could never do that; my feet are far too sensitive. I wince if I even have a grain of sand in my shoe. There's no way my sensitive feet could go barefoot."

First, sand or pebbles inside a shoe would bother anybody's feet, even ours. Our skin becomes moist and soft when it's trapped in a sweaty shoe. At that point anything that protrudes would bother us.

However, when you get out of a shoe and dry out your skin, pebbles and sand are hardly an issue.

Still, technically these naysayers are right. In the beginning your skin is thin and incredibly soft. But just like the muscles of your feet, your skin can be strengthened. Skin is a living, breathing, dynamic tissue, capable of great adaptations. With the exception of rare circumstances, all of us have skin that can regenerate when injured and strengthen when stimulated.

When you wear shoes, the skin has no need to grow. It's pampered and coddled in a damp, sensation-free environment. The trick to strong skin and less sensitive feet is to wake them up. By taking them out of a shoe, giving them oxygen, and letting them feel the ground, you send a message to the brain that stimulates new skin growth and stronger skin. You also order up more padding to handle the sharp stuff.

Consider barefoot time the body's opportunity to read a new how-to manual. With each step it's given instructions on what to do. In this case, the instructions are clear: grow stronger muscles, thicker skin, and padding for the feet. Give these instructions to your brain on a regular basis, and you'll go from supersensitive feet to superstrong feet.

The skin begins to grow stronger almost immediately after getting the message. In only two to three weeks, it starts to dramatically change, and in three short months you can be walking on almost any surface (granted, you still might not enjoy a gravel road barefoot after three months, or even three years for that matter). You'll find out more about strengthening skin later in this book.

EXCUSE #5: MY FEET WILL BECOME UGLY

This is one of Jessica's favorite questions to answer. At clinics and talks people always want to look at (and touch) our feet. They want to see if Michael's skin is rough like an elephant's (it's not) or if it looks like it's been through a war (it doesn't). They comment, "It's not fair—your feet look better than mine, and I keep my feet in shoes."

As for Jessica, they want to check out her feet and poke her pads. They can't believe how soft and supple her skin feels, how pink and rosy it appears. She tells them her feet used to have terrible circulation and were always cold, until she began to go bare. Now she has pliable skin, great pads, and warm feet that are rosier than ever.

People note in particular that our feet have not gotten ugly. There are no hard calluses or thickened abnormalities on our feet. Why? Because calluses like that form from hot spots or friction points in a shoe. If there's no tight shoe, there are no hot spots, and therefore no hard calluses.

They also think we'll have alligator skin or feet that look like a rhino's. We take care of our feet and use beeswax products such as Waxelene, Climb On!, or other natural salves (avoid petroleum products on your skin if at all possible) to make sure our skin doesn't crack, but overall the skin looks smoother and softer because it's been woken up and has a job to do.

As for bunions, see Excuse #15 for more details.

EXCUSE #6: IT HURTS WHEN
I LAND ON MY HEELS

We're getting ahead of ourselves here, because we'll cover this in the "technique" section, but you're right again—it does hurt when you strike down on your heels barefoot. Why? Because we were never meant to strike down on our heels. And we no longer do so once we go barefoot.

Our heels are for standing, balancing, or rolling off of, but never, ever were they designed to land on. That's why it hurts. We'll teach you new techniques to land on the front of the foot, or roll off the middle of the foot, but never to land on your heel. The heel is the third part of the tripod that helps balance us when we stand; it was never designed for repetitive slamming into the ground.

With the new technique in barefoot walking, you'll walk lighter than ever, like a Native American with a quiet step, and with almost no force resonating through your heels. With barefoot walking your heels will be happy, as will your feet, knees, hips, back, shoulders, neck, and other joints.

EXCUSE #7: THE GROUND IS TOO COLD

Depending on your local climate, ground temperature typically isn't a problem, unless you try to build up too quickly. Certainly if you're picking up this book in mid-December, it could be too cold outside. However, over time your feet adapt to the cold, and in surprising fashion.

Here's what happens when you wear footwear in cold temperatures. Since your footwear does the work of supporting your body weight instead of your feet, your body takes blood flow away from the feet to parts of the body that need it more. This is called "shunting," and it makes your feet feel cold.

Conversely, when you're barefoot or in minimalist footwear, your feet must do the work of supporting your body weight. The body therefore pumps additional blood to the feet, helping them become beet red and hot. This increased circulation serves an additional purpose: healing.

Both cold and warm weather walking (along with walking on uneven surfaces) help wake up the vasculature of the feet and bring greater perfusion, or delivery of oxygen and nutrients to the feet for fuel, heat, and healing. This blood flow's great for overcoming chronic injuries, such as plantar fasciitis that won't fully go away, or an ankle you've been told is permanently weak. When you wear ill-fitting shoes, your feet don't receive enough blood flow. But if you spend a moderate amount of time barefoot in the cold, you stand a much better chance for healing.

EXCUSE #8: IT'S TOO HOT OUTSIDE

This is a very common misconception. Certainly in the beginning, even walking across a parking lot in the summer can be too hot, particularly in southern climes such as Arizona, California (Death Valley, anyone?), Florida, or south of the border. But if we think of the evolution of humankind, there's hope.

If we did indeed evolve on the savannah in Africa, then we weren't just walking in soft mud. That mud would harden and become bone dry and hot in the summertime. We've all seen pictures of vast lakebed with cracked dry mud. Summertime on the savannah was hot, and our feet had to adapt. A good modern example is the Aborigines of Australia, who still walk barefoot through 100-degree-plus desert heat.

It turns out there's nothing better for stimulating strong pad development than walking on hot pavement or hot sand. The challenge is that you need to build up to this incredibly slowly, or you'll really hurt yourself. Yes, you could end up in the hospital with third-degree burns on the bottom of your feet if you don't start slowly.

How slowly? How about walking fifty feet or less (ten or twenty feet if it's really scorching) if you're starting in the summer? Better still, start in the morning, when the ground is still cool (it feels invigorating around dawn or pre-dawn in the summer), and then gradually go out a bit later and later in the day, until you're handling the midday heat.

Always let pain be your guide when it comes to heat or cold (more on this later in the book), and do not veto your body. Your pain receptors are there for a reason: to give you the feedback you need to stay healthy and safe. Respect this information. If it hurts, it's too hot. Immediately hop off a hot surface onto a cooler surface such as grass, and try again when it's cooler. If it's still too hot, put on your shoes and head for home.

Barefoot walking isn't about pain tolerance, being tough, or being a hero. It's about developing the discipline of listening to your body. Just be safe.

EXCUSE #9: I'M A HEAVY PRONATOR (OR NEED EXTRA SUPPORT)

This is a common fallacy. For some reason we've been taught that if our feet are weak and roll inward (which is called pronation), we need to give them crutches and prop them up rather than strengthen them.

Think of your feet as your home. Imagine you have a flimsy home that could blow over in heavy winds. Would you prop up some two-by-fours against the frame to keep it from tipping over, or would you build the walls (and foundation) stronger?

Our bodies aren't fixed and unchanging. They're incredibly adaptable. If something's weak, we can strengthen it. This means you can work to keep your feet from rolling in and give them the strength they need to function properly.

If your feet roll in too much when you walk, it stresses your ankles, knees, hips, back, and more. The rolling itself isn't bad, but when your ankles dive inward, it affects the entire chain of the body (think of the body as a series of interconnected links in a chain—if one link is out of alignment, it affects all the other links).

However, the answer to pronation isn't to panic and order overbuilt orthotics or highly supportive shoes. The answer is to slowly work on strengthening your bare feet.

EXCUSE #10: I'M TOO OLD TO TRY GOING BAREFOOT

On the surface, this one sounds like a logical objection, but dig beneath and you'll see that it hides an insidious assumption: that you can no longer heal or grow strong as you grow older in life. That assumption is not just wrong but downright dangerous. If you believe your body can no longer handle anything that comes your way, you're in for a gradual decline in health. The truth is, you don't need to give up your power to heal or grow strong.

The great news is that at any age, your mind and body can adapt and change. Just as your finger can heal from a cut or wound, your feet can grow stronger, your nerves can wake up, your body can adapt, your brain can learn better balance, and you can grow stronger.

Particularly as you age, you owe it to yourself to grow the strongest, most perceptive feet you can. And by perceptive, we mean feet that can feel the terrain and adapt and adjust to changes underfoot.

As you age, that crack in the sidewalk may seem as though it becomes the most dangerous hazard of all—but in fact it should be the greatest teacher of all. That crack should be welcomed, as uneven terrain helps wake up your body, teaches greater balance, and over the long run keeps you from falling.

Build up in small doses and in a controlled manner, and you can safely retrain the body for better balance and stability, and help prevent that dreaded fall—not by walking in the most cushioned shoe and avoiding uneven surfaces, but by feeling the ground, waking up the feet, and slowly challenging yourself on terrain you once avoided.

EXCUSE #11: I'M TOO HEAVY

Often the corollary to "I'm too old" is "I'm too heavy." Quite the opposite is true.

When you're overweight, you can't afford to be in traditional shoes, pounding your feet. Instead you need to learn how to walk lightly, to be as gentle on your body and joints as possible.

The heavier you are, the more important it is to include some daily barefoot time into your day. In the beginning, go extra slowly, because your feet will have to hold a lot more weight than is ideal. But as you gain strength in your feet, you gain mobility. And this mobility can go a long way toward helping you regain your health.

We've helped many overweight and obese people (even some defined as morbidly obese) regain their health by rebuilding their foundation and feet. As they began to walk more lightly, with greater stability and less effort, they became mobile and active again. And they discovered walking barefoot to be the greatest exercise in the world—the best way to burn fat, reduce weight, and regain the freedom, self-esteem, and positive self-image they'd been looking for. If you're overweight, you owe it to yourself to try barefoot walking.

Losing Weight with Barefoot Walking

Barefoot walking is one of the most efficient, yet kind and gentle, exercises for losing weight. You won't be headed to the gym for searing, sweaty workouts that'll cause you injuries or set you back. You can go consistently and naturally and let the body melt away the pounds.

Barefoot walking does a much better job than traditional walking or other exercises for shedding pounds because it's more of a total body workout. You have to engage all the muscles in your body to stay balanced, upright, and moving forward, particularly on uneven terrain.

With that said, you don't need to be completely out of breath and be experiencing searing pain in your leg muscles in order to be in the fat-burning zone. This zone is a state of metabolism in which activity burns fat without you working too hard—if you have a heart rate monitor, you're at about 60–65 percent of your maximum heart rate (which is calculated by subtracting your age from 220). In short, you can burn just as many fat calories at a heart rate within the fat-burning zone as at a higher heart rate. Just keep in mind you won't be burning as many total calories.

You don't have to go fast to burn fat. Think of it this way: if you're walking at a pace just above one that allows you to smell the flowers but not so fast that you're out of breath, then chances are you're in the fat-burning zone. You don't have to tax the heart much to burn fat; you just need to go at a decent walking pace.

We recommend that for the first month (if not longer), you hold off on purchasing your first heart rate monitor. However, after that, a good heart rate monitor may be a helpful portable motivator. Even so, stay more focused on the inside, on how your body is feeling, than on what a gadget is telling you.

Says Michael, "I've personally used a heart rate monitor since 1986, when they were just coming out with the first chest-strap monitors. I'm a strong believer in a heart rate monitor to learn about your body. However, it's very easy to get caught up in the readout of the watch, rather than in paying attention to where you're going, what you're doing, or your barefoot steps. As a game of awareness, any additional input can take your focus away. Since going barefoot I've given away my heart rate monitors."

A simple rule of thumb for staying in the fat-burning zone is this: walk at a good pace, one where you can comfortably talk but notice that you are breathing faster. If you're having trouble talking and feel short of breath, then you're going a bit too fast. What about going too slowly? Particularly early on, you're going to be slow; that's how you're going to build up to this safely. But over time, the big issue will be going too fast, not going too slow. Still in doubt? Get that monitor and get yourself in the zone.

If you're overweight, you need every advantage you can to get yourself fine-tuned and working well again. If you hurt when you walk, if your joints ache, if your hips or knees or back are killing you, or if your feet are uncomfortable, then it's going to be very hard to keep up any workout program for an extended period of time. We need you feeling light, feeling strong, and working with the ground (and your feet) rather than against it. That means getting you out of your shoes. The heavier you are, the more you owe it to yourself to grow the strongest feet you can.

Be kind to your body if you're overweight or obese: get out of those shoes and learn to land light. Yes, you've got to start extra slowly to give your muscles a chance to catch up with your frame. But in the long run it's a life changer and well worth the effort and patience.

EXCUSE #12: THERE'S NO PLACE I CAN GO BAREFOOT

When getting into barefoot walking, it's common to think there's no place to go. But that's just not the case. In all but the roughest environments, there are bike paths, parks, or even running tracks where you can begin. And if it's winter, you can head to your local mall before opening hours. There you can walk to your heart's content in the safest, most controlled environment possible (this is the best way to keep your feet in shape during the snowy season). Perhaps your local health club or gym has an indoor track, and certainly you can find a treadmill (we have some cautionary advice about treadmills in chapter 11).

For your first day, all you need is a short swath of grass (twenty or thirty feet in length or more). If that's not available, you can use a short stretch of debris-free pavement or asphalt. Your driveway may even suffice (you'll learn later in the book that the harder the surface, the easier it is in the beginning). If you start slowly, the feet are much more resilient than you think. That's why they worked as the ultimate all-terrain vehicles for several million years.

Just as with everything else, you'll want to baby-step your way in. Begin on either smooth or rough terrain (harder surfaces are preferred to softer ones, because they help you "feel" the ground better and land lighter, and they strengthen the feet) for a few short minutes or less, and then build your way up. Indoors, outdoors, on a track, on trails, in a park, or even at the mall, there's always a place you can begin.

EXCUSE #13: PEOPLE WILL LOOK AT ME FUNNY

Sure they will. But don't take it personally. Chances are they're confused, oblivious, or just very curious. Strange as it sounds, they may be scared too. Perhaps since the beginning of time, people have always criticized or looked down on what they don't understand or what they consider different, new, or threatening. Don't let other people's judgments prevent you from doing what it takes to regain your foot strength and overall health. After all, your health is most important, and it's your right to live a healthful lifestyle.

Until Christopher McDougall's story about barefoot running in *Born to Run* came out, people looked very strangely at anyone walking or running barefoot. But times are changing. People are no longer looking at barefooters as throwbacks to the 1960s; rather, they look instead inquisitively, as in "What are they doing?" or "How do I start?"

We're not the strange ones going barefoot anymore, but the hipsters and the trendsetters. Just look at all the movie stars, millionaires, and celebrities giving it a try now! So go barefoot and be proud. Your body will thank you for it, and as your friends start following your lead, they'll be thanking you too.

EXCUSE #14: I'LL STEP IN DOG POOP

In nearly five years of barefoot running and walking, Michael has stepped in dog poop only twice, and both of those times it was our own dogs' poop, as the dogs were rounding him up with their leashes. (Fortunately, feet are easier to clean than shoes.)

Walking barefoot is an exercise in awareness. You become more aware of your environment and of every step you take. While you're looking twenty feet before you, you're also scanning the ground just beneath your feet, always on the lookout for hazards coming your way. Dog poop, except in thick grass in the park, is almost always avoidable.

Don't sweat the poopy stuff; just walk aware and you'll be fine.

EXCUSE #15: I HAVE BUNIONS

Michael says, "Until I met Jessica, she was in denial about her bunions, but after meeting her and checking out her bare feet, it was one of the first things I mentioned. (Note to men: this is a really poor icebreaker!)

"But I was forgiven, and I was right. Her shoes, even her most comfortable pair, were pushing her toes inward, particularly squeezing her biggest and smallest toes."

This is not the natural shape of the foot, and bunions are not hereditary. Instead, it's our feet directly adapting to the shape of our environment.

But why the bunion? The bony callus on the side of your foot is a protective mechanism, trying to get the shoe off your toes to give them room to breathe and move properly. Over time that bunion can become quite painful if you don't heed its warning and give your feet the room they need.

Bunions, however, are reversible! Once you begin taking your feet out of their medieval torture devices, they begin to return to their natural shape. Walking barefoot can be corrective for bunions in helping wake up the foot.

As Dr. Ray McClanahan, a leading podiatrist in the Northwest, puts it, foot surgery, like that for bunions, typically isn't corrective surgery, but cosmetic surgery, done to help your feet fit into fashionable footwear. If you're willing to go barefoot, you can help correct your bunions naturally, for free.

EXCUSE #16: I HAVE WEAK ANKLES

This is not an objection at all. It's actually a reason to walk barefoot (though start slowly). Weak ankles are caused by too much support (and a lack of mobility) in a shoe and not enough blood flow to the ankles.

Consider this: our shoes are typically the cause of ankle sprains. In almost any athletic shoe, you're raised above the ground at least a half inch or more (and sometimes up to two inches), and they have super grippy tread. The higher you're off the ground, the more likely you are to catch this tread on a rock, a curb, a crack in the sidewalk, or almost anything, and roll an ankle. Moreover, grippy rubber is supposed to be good for traction, right? Well, yes . . . except if it causes your foot to stick or catch a surface while momentum continues to carry your body mass forward. When you want to go one way and your foot is stuck going another, you could end up with an ankle sprain.

Here's the good news. When you're fully barefoot, you're directly on the ground so it's much harder to roll an ankle. And if you're fully barefoot, you tend to skim over obstacles rather than stick to them and twist.

Sure, if you step on a ball or other obstacle accidentally underfoot, you can always roll anything, but when you're barefoot (or in very flat footwear) you're already almost on the ground. There is no place to roll.

Ankles can be strengthened over time by being barefoot. Unless you have pins and other hardware in your ankle that prevent mobility, even short distances barefoot can benefit your ankles. Just start slowly and listen to your ankles. If they start getting tired, stop.

If your ankles are weak, you just need to start slowly with barefoot walking and focus on the other exercises mentioned in this book. The ankle is a

FOOT NOTE

The average person engaging in nonstrenuous activity walks about 4 miles (10,000 steps) every day. That works out to about 115,000 miles in a lifetime—that's the equivalent of walking almost five times around the planet. That's also over half the distance to the moon!

system of interconnected muscles, ligaments, and tendons, and therefore can be strengthened. It just takes time and baby steps.

In nature we never had anything wrapped around our ankles. Even a tall Native American moccasin was no more than soft leather that covered the ankle. The ankle must be allowed to move unencumbered in order to stay flexible and strong.

You can bring that flexibility and strength back through barefoot walking, particularly on uneven surfaces.

EXCUSE #17: I'LL GET PARASITES OR DISEASES

Not true, unless you're walking in very unsanitary conditions, such as stagnant water or some third-world country areas without plumbing.

In general, parasites that enter through the skin are rare in the United States and found only in the hottest states in the South. Even there, as long as you're not walking or standing around in festering pools of water, there's little chance you'll pick something up, and it's extremely unlikely you'll pick up something that's life threatening (you have a much higher chance of winning the lottery). However, please do not walk around a dog park without shoes. There, we've said it.

The greater harm to your health is not getting out and exercising.

Last thought here: keep your tetanus immunization up to date. Boosters are given every ten years. If you can't remember when your last tetanus booster was given, check with your doctor. Although cuts when going barefoot are rare, particularly after your first few weeks, it's better to be safe than sorry here. And remember, if you've got a cut on your foot, do not go barefoot until it's healed.

Dirty Feet

If you don't want to get your feet dirty, then there is good news and bad news. First the bad: if you go barefoot, particularly in the city, your feet will get dirty. However, that dirt washes right off, particularly if you keep a wash basin or wet wipes by your front door.

So here's the good news. Your feet are likely cleaner going barefoot outside than they are in your shoes. Why? Because we almost never wash the insides of our shoes, and we sweat in them every day.

Shoes are known to harbor thousands if not millions of molds, fungi, and disease-causing bacteria in and on them before we finally succumb and throw them out in favor of a new pair. *Good Morning America* once tested eight people's pairs of shoes as well as two dogs' paws and found the shoes carried the most bacteria, up to 66 million organisms each. This compared to toilet seats, with only 1,000 organisms. And nine out of ten pairs contained coliform bacteria from human or animal feces. They can also carry pesticides, toxic chemicals, and pollen. Yet we rarely (if ever) wash our shoes, because we don't want to ruin them. So instead we slip our feet into germ traps, sweaty environments devoid of oxygen that are just perfect for wee beasties to fester in and on. And we track them around our houses.

The rule in our house is this: whether we've washed our feet when we've entered the home or not, we must wash our feet again before we go to bed.

And there's even more good news. Research shows that microbes in the dirt (not those in our shoes) are actually good for us, and exposure to them contributes to a stronger immune system. More on this fascinating topic in chapter 4.

Going Bare at the Gym

You would think the gym's a perfect place for going barefoot, with yoga classes and other fitness classes that would seem to be in natural alignment with barefoot activity.

But something funny happened on the way to the gym. People have gotten liability crazy. Out of concern that you may drop a weight on your foot (which would break your foot in or out of a shoe), trip (something you're more likely to do in a shoe), or catch your foot on a contraption, gyms are wary about having you go barefoot.

From Michael's experience: "At my favorite gym I had to write my own waiver after a lengthy discussion with management about being able to use a treadmill barefoot. In the waiver, I stated they were not responsible if I hurt myself. I also had to promise that I would scrub down the belt afterward so it wasn't dirty for the other patrons (who, oddly enough, would be in shoes that were never washed, even after walking in public bathrooms). Even then they were hesitant to let me use the treadmill."

Other strange oddities at gyms abound. There are fitness classes and even yoga classes (though this one is silly) where you have to at least wear socks, if not shoes, when working out. However, you're more likely to slip and fall, particularly in a pose, if you can't grab with your toes.

Working out barefoot at the gym is a great way to increase proprioception (your perception of movement and spatial orientation of your body and its parts), balance, strength, and overall health. However, if you find you just can't do it at your gym or the stares are too much, then simply get yourself the most minimal shoe you can. (There are even toe socks, with rubber nubs for traction, designed specifically for yoga classes.)

But, wait, you say. What about the gym locker rooms? If our feet are cleaner out of a shoe, what about getting athlete's foot at the local gym? That occurs because people take their sweaty feet with festering foot fungus out of their shoes and then walk around barefoot in the locker room and showers.

In these environments, if your foot is going back into a shoe, it's easy to pick up the fungus and spread it to your shoes. But if you're staying barefoot, the fungus can't survive in oxygen, so your feet should be just fine. When in doubt, wipe your feet, especially in between your toes, with tea tree oil, organic raw apple cider vinegar, or raw honey. Flip-flops will serve you well here too.

Absolutely wear shoes in public restrooms, on the streets in third-world countries, and anywhere else you see or smell unsanitary conditions or feel uncomfortable.

EXCUSE #18: I'M PREGNANT (OR PLANNING TO BE)

The good news is that going barefoot adds additional benefits for future mommies during pregnancy. Swollen feet are common during pregnancy, and many women find themselves shedding their shoes anyway. Consider these benefits of truly going barefoot:

- **Minimizes swollen feet.** One of the big considerations for pregnant women is circulation. It's known that women's feet get bigger during pregnancy, and a large part of this is fluid gain, often caused by not working our muscles. However, fluid gain goes down as you use muscles more. When you go barefoot, your feet have to work more. That's a great thing when pregnant, because a working foot is like a fluid pump, bringing fluid up out of the foot and the lower leg and delivering it back to the heart.

- **Improves overall circulation.** The increased circulation doesn't just end with the feet. Your lower legs also do more work when you're barefoot, particularly as you shift your weight toward your forefoot. This increased circulation acts as a fluid pump and helps keep your legs healthier, happier, and stronger.

- **Builds balance for less wobbling.** One of the greatest benefits of going barefoot is that your feet are closer to the ground, which brings more stability during a time when your center of gravity is shifting. You can also feel the ground beneath your feet, which helps you re-awaken and work the stabilizing muscle groups from your feet to your legs, hips, and up into your core, improving your balance for increased maneuverability and lower chances of falling.

- **Strengthens core muscles for delivery day.** If you think of the human body as a series of interconnected links of a chain, each one connected to the next, you start to get a real sense of the benefits of going barefoot when pregnant. After your legs, the next link in the chain is your core. Now, a stronger core isn't just about the stomach; it includes all the muscles from the pelvis on up. In essence, when you've fully engaged your core, you're doing somewhat of a Kegel exercise, just to hold yourself in place—muscles essential for an easier delivery day.

- **Develops a healthier back for a happier mommy.** Keeping the back healthy and happy during pregnancy is often a big challenge. After all, you're carrying a very heavy weight in front, and your back often arches forward. Having a stronger core helps greatly in protecting the back. And by working all of the muscles from your feet on up, you assist the circulation of your cerebrospinal fluid, in essence lubricating your spine and keeping it loose.

- **Stand with better posture for more comfort.** Since you're working right up the chain and have better body awareness, better circulation, and a stronger core, you also end up with better posture, because you can feel what's going on beneath you—especially when there comes a time you can't see your feet.

If you were already walking barefoot before pregnancy, congratulations—you've got a leg up here. Keep doing what you're doing if your doctor agrees, and it'll serve you well. But if you're already pregnant and would like to experience the benefits of being pregnant and going barefoot, always trust your doctor here, and when it doubt, be safe and ask.

NO EXCUSES!

Ultimately, there's almost no reason you can't or shouldn't go barefoot. Sure, if you have metal parts in your feet, are missing parts, or have had bones removed, then you may not get very far, but then again you may, if you start slowly enough. Barring this and diabetes (see Diabetes Control, page 292), trying barefoot is a great thing. It can help strengthen your feet, legs, back, and entire body. It can give you greater bone density, circulation, and balance. It can boost your immune system, decrease your blood pressure, and give you your health and freedom back. There are far too many benefits not to give it a try. So let's get going!

PART II

Free Your Feet and Experience the Earth

As I went walking that ribbon of highway
I saw above me that endless skyway
I saw below me that golden valley
This land was made for you and me.

—Woody Guthrie

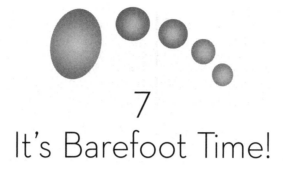

7
It's Barefoot Time!

Good walking leaves no track behind it.

—Lao Tsu

Are you ready to wake up muscles that have been sleeping for years? It's time to retrain your body to move in ways it likely hasn't since you were a child. In the process, you'll gain better circulation, strengthen all of your connective tissue, and grow strong skin and protective padding on the bottom of your feet.

But take the process slower than you ever imagined. Why? Because unlike muscles, which will feel relatively minimal strain in the upcoming coaching program, your ligaments and tendons have much more catching up to do and won't send as many warning signals.

This chapter is divided into two sections. In the first half, you train yourself to become more aware of your mind and your body. By emptying your mind of thoughts, you free up space to listen to the many cues your body is constantly giving you. And by listening more carefully to your body, you enable yourself to provide a self-diagnosis and dictate the best custom-designed walking program for yourself.

In the second half of this chapter, you will learn proper barefoot walking form, keeping in mind that there are two important areas to concentrate on. One, you will be encouraged to develop a natural alignment that minimizes injuries. Two, you will be coached toward the lightest, most efficient gait in order to minimize impact on your body.

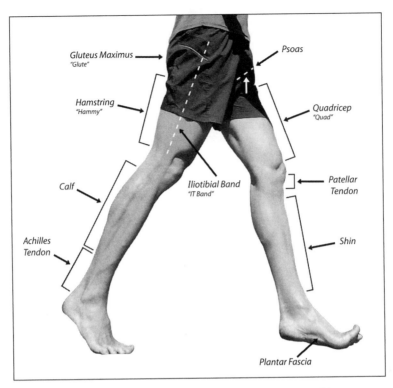

Get to know your body. These are approximate locations of key muscles, tendons, and connective tissue. It helps to know these parts for proper strengthening, stretching, and injury prevention.

From time to time throughout this book we'll refer to certain body parts. In case you're unsure of the location of some of these parts, above is a useful diagram of the lower body. Refer to this page if you're ever in doubt.

Read this chapter once through, and practice the exercises that don't require walking as much as you can before you head outside.

Let's start with a preliminary self-assessment of your body.

CHECKING IN: HOW DO YOU FEEL?

As we've said before and will say again, walking barefoot is walking awarefoot. It's not a matter of just stepping outside your door. Do you know how your body feels right now? How are your feet, legs, lower back, and shoulders? Are you holding tension anywhere? Is anything sore or not quite right? Barefoot walking and some simple exercises will help you reawaken self-awareness and your mind-body connection.

When you first get out of bed, do you ever ask yourself, "How do I feel?" or "How am I doing?" Your body knows a lot more than you realize, and it doesn't take rocket science to discover what it knows. The clues are always there, or as Michael likes to say, the answers are always on the inside.

If we only listened to our bodies, we'd have a much better idea of how we're doing and what we should plan for the day. It's very simple. If you feel a tweak or the slightest twinge of pain, don't think about it or intellectualize. Just stop what you're doing. If you feel a bit worn down, this means you should take it easy.

In general, people who are recovering from injuries have to listen to their bodies more than anyone else. That's because they're in a state of great growth or repair, but also at a tipping point. Consider a bone that's trying to heal—it needs a certain amount of stimulation or weight bearing in order to lay down new calcium. Too little and it won't lay down bone, too much and it'll rebreak the bone. So when it comes to healing of any kind, it's important to go slowly and listen to your body.

EXERCISE

Taking Inventory

We often forget how to breathe deeply. Tomorrow when you wake up, lie in bed for a few extra minutes. Practice taking long, slow, deep diaphragmatic breaths. To do this effectively, it's important not only to fully expand your lungs but to also allow your belly to expand as you inhale. Allowing your belly to rise lets much more air in. When you feel you can't inhale any more, exhale slowly. Deep diaphragmatic breathing returns you to the present moment, helping you take better stock of your body and relieve stress. If you think you may fall back asleep in bed, then get up for a few minutes, lie on a yoga mat, and do this on the floor. Better still, do this outside on the ground or on top of a sheet or blanket lying on the earth.

While you're breathing, try to empty your mind. Let go of all thoughts. If you hear a thought, notice it, or label it as "thought," as they do in many Buddhist meditation practices; then let it go. If this doesn't work, simply count between your breaths. For instance, inhale one, two, three. Exhale one, two, three.

After a few minutes, when the mind is clear, take inventory of yourself. Begin with your feet and work up through the body, examining each area in your mind between breaths.

As you begin to walk barefoot, you have great advantages as well as challenges compared to the average walker in shoes. Advantage: you can feel the ground and your body more, and adapt on the fly. Disadvantage: there is no protection if you're out when you should be home resting.

EXERCISE

Preflight Inspection

Either first thing in the morning or just prior to your workouts, do this short inspection to see how your body's doing. This exercise facilitates your mind-body-earth connection and helps alert you to areas in your body that require attention. Lying down so your body is relaxed, begin with your feet.

Take a deep breath and sense your feet; curl your toes if it helps. Hold your breath; then exhale and relax. Repeat this several times and get in touch with your feet. How do they feel? Are the toes doing all right? How about all twenty-eight bones in each foot and the countless ligaments and tendons? How does the skin feel? Rotate your ankles too. Does everything move freely, or do you feel resistance or tension anywhere?

Next move upward through your legs. Take a deep breath and inspect your calves. Breathe in, contract your calves, and then exhale. How do they feel? Next do your shins, then knees, quads, hamstrings, and glutes. Then move up and out of the legs: lower back, chest, shoulders, arms, neck, and everywhere else, even your face, sinuses, and head.

Are you getting a good sense or feel of everything?

Next, ask yourself how energetic you feel. Refreshed and relaxed? Did you get a good night's rest? Do you feel well fueled? Well hydrated?

Take mental notes. With practice, you'll start to know your body very well. You're like a pilot inspecting a plane before each and every flight. Soon with a quick check in the morning you'll know if your body is ready for a long flight or just a quick dash, or needs a day of maintenance.

Listen to your body in each and every moment. Don't be afraid to skip a walk, change a workout, or even turn for home. You're not being lazy, but being smart.

Michael notes, "I've headed out anticipating tremendous workouts, only to turn around within the first ten minutes or less. Of course, if I'm feeling good, I let myself go long as well. I just need to listen to the still voice on the inside."

WARMING UP FOR BAREFOOTERS

The human body can do some amazing things, but it doesn't like to do them cold. That's because cold muscles and tendons are tight. We want them loose to allow your joints to move freely and so you don't tear anything (even a finely tuned athlete can get hurt trying to go full speed when cold). Like the engine of a car, your body likes to get the oil pumping and be properly lubricated first. This means warming up.

The tighter you are, the more you want to warm up. After you feel things good and loose, you're ready to head out.

Walking is a very gentle exercise, which is why you don't need a big warm-up. However, since it's your feet that are going to be carrying your body weight, rather than your shoes, you want to be extra kind to them. This prevents injuries or soreness later on.

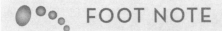
Never stretch cold muscles, as cold muscles don't stretch—they tear. Instead, walk slowly until you've heated up a bit; then stop and gently stretch things out if you need to. More on when and how to stretch in chapter 12.

EXERCISE

Waking Up the Feet

Warming up for barefoot walking is simple, and you don't need to break a mighty sweat.

What's the simplest way to warm up the feet? By rolling them out. Simply roll out one foot at a time back and forth and side to side on a tennis ball or foam roll, first slowly and then quite vigorously, for a minute or two each. Blood flow will begin increasing from your feet up to your calves, throughout your legs, and up to your hips.

EXERCISE

Golf Ball Grab

Want a fun way to warm up your feet *and* strengthen them at the same time? Here's a favorite at our clinics.

Get a golf ball and start working on picking it up with your toes. Practice this every other day before each of your walks, to warm up your feet and strengthen your arches. Work on grabbing the ball with your toes. If you can, grab for a count of five seconds, relax the foot, then grab again. Do this for a minute or two, maximum, to begin. Notice how your arch naturally raises and tightens? Just as you lift weights to tone arms, legs, or even abs, you can build those arches by grabbing with your toes.

If you're recovering from injury or plantar fasciitis, just be wise. Never go to the point of pain, and if there's a dull ache, *stop*. You're probably not ready.

When you begin, start with every other day, increasing by a minute with each scrunching session. You'll begin to feel power, dexterity, and flexibility return to your feet and toes. And before you know it, you'll be throwing golf balls with your feet and their happy, healthy arches.

GRASS FOR STARTERS

Consider this chapter a one-on-one coaching session with Michael.

"Although I like beginners to feel a hard surface," he says, "a swath of fifty to a hundred yards of gently sloped park or a well-groomed grassy area is great for your first time out. You can even begin on Astroturf or a well-groomed baseball field. There are sometimes hidden sharp things in the grass at parks. Be sure there's nothing hiding in the green stuff by walking it first in shoes. Then shed the shoes and have a little fun."

Why not head straight for a hard path or sidewalk? You can, but there's something universal about how great grass feels barefoot. It's like a long-lost childhood experience.

After your first session, allow yourself to rest the following day (go back to your supportive shoes and/or insoles); then get yourself out on a bike path or smooth sidewalk every other day for just a few weeks. The grass may be softer, but it's not actually easier on the muscles, and in the beginning we're not ready for that. However, after we're ready (give it a good month or so), walking on grass becomes a great uneven surface for working on muscle strength, core strength, and form. Hard surfaces are ideal for building technique quickly. They force you to feel the ground and find the lightest, softest step possible.

Once you've found the patch of grass you'll use just for your first time out (walk it first in shoes to be sure it's safe), check in with your body and apply these five essential steps to proper barefoot form.

STEP-BY-STEP GUIDE TO PROPER BAREFOOT WALKING FORM

We've broken proper form down into five easy steps.

Step 1: Addressing your pelvic tilt
Step 2: Tightening your core
Step 3: Opening your chest
Step 4: Getting your arms in position
Step 5: Standing tall

To begin walking barefoot, you must first unlearn a habit you've learned in a shoe. You see, the modern shoe isn't just a shoe but a high heel. The average walking or running shoe has a one-to-two-inch heel. And all high heels create a dangerous tilt in our pelvis that strains our backs, hamstrings, iliotibial (IT) bands, feet, and knees, and causes us to walk painfully and unnaturally, often leading to overuse injuries. There's no way to avoid it in a high heel, because as we've seen, you have to tilt at the waist if you don't want to fall forward on your face.

The higher your heel, the more you bend forward at the waist, stressing and straining joints, ligaments in the back, feet, and knees, not to mention completely throwing off your natural gait.

The challenge with a pelvic tilt is that it can become a permanent habit, even if you're not wearing a high heel. So the first thing you need to learn how to do is get your waist level, or what yoga and Pilates instructors call "pelvis neutral."

○°°° FOOT NOTE

Look at your children. Even children as young as two or three years old start to stand with this pelvic tilt caused by their sneakers. With continued use of these shoes, by the ages of five or six their butts stick out way behind them, and they have an unnatural and dangerous sway to their backs. That's because a tiny heel under a toddler's feet is equivalent to a two-to-three-inch heel under an adult's feet. So keep kids out of anything but the flattest of shoes. There's more on selecting proper footwear for children in chapter 14.

Step 1: Addressing Your Pelvic Tilt

You've seen them walking everywhere—people with their butts sticking out. To some it may seem sexy; however, it wreaks havoc on the kinetic chain of your body, putting stress on your knees, hips, back, neck, and more. You can't walk well if you're bending forward and sticking out your butt.

From now on, whether you're in or out of a shoe, make sure your waist is level and your pelvis is not dipping forward. Unfortunately, high heels and especially today's taller running shoes have habitualized a forward-dipping pelvic tilt.

If you walk with this tilt, you can't use your core as an anchor and your body as a human spring. Instead, by bending at the waist, you alter your center of gravity and increase the jarring your body undergoes. You have turned yourself into an inefficient and heavy walker, no matter how light you are.

By leaning forward at the waist, you place undue force on your quadriceps, knees, shins, and ankles, changing the force dynamics through the

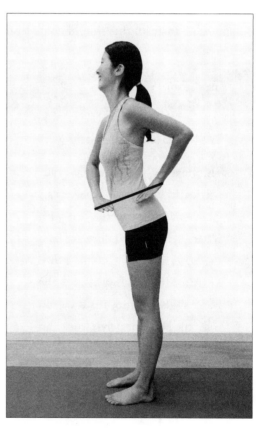

Avoid an awkward forward bend—a common habit developed by wearing shoes. To break this habit, work to get your pelvis level by placing one hand in front and one behind you at waist height. With both hands in position, work to bring them level or even in height.

foot and dangerously overstretching and straining your hamstrings. If you've ever experienced tight hamstrings from walking or running, this would be why. And unfortunately, tight hamstrings pull directly on your knees.

To correct this problem you must become conscious of your pelvic tilt. Take one hand and extend your thumb, making it into the shape of an *L*. Place it centered beneath your belly button, just above your waistband. Take your other hand, make it into the shape of an *L*, and place it centered over your spine, just above your waistband as well. Check in a mirror to see if your hands are level with each other. Is the front lower than the back? Then use your abdominal muscles to tilt your pelvis back. Is the back hand lower than the front? Then tilt your pelvis forward. Note: never tighten your glutes (butt muscles) to tilt your pelvis. Walking with tight glutes fights against your body and strains your muscles. Instead, this should come from your core or abdominals.

EXERCISE

Water Bowl Imagery

This imagery helps eliminate your pelvic tilt. Picture your pelvis as a giant bowl filled to the rim with water. Lean too far forward and the water spills out of the bowl. Lean too far backward and the water spills out too. Instead, you want the bowl (or pelvis) nice and neutral, with the front of your waist the same height as the back of your waist.

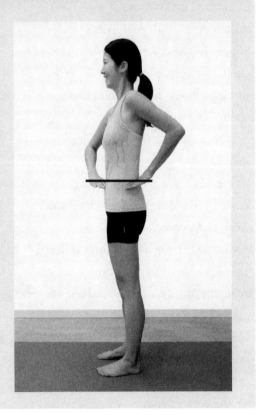

If you're still struggling with this one, you're not alone. It often helps to practice this exercise with a partner or while standing in front of a mirror with your shirt off to see your waistband. Pilates classes can also help you learn how to get in a pelvic-neutral position.

Step 2: Tightening Your Core

Barefoot walking gives you natural abs of steel. How? When you're wearing shoes, you rely on those shoes to hold you upright and balanced in position, albeit quite precariously. Without shoes, your own musculature and skeletal systems are responsible for keeping you upright, stable, and in proper alignment. Your core muscles (abs and lower back) now take on the bulk of this responsibility, as they should, and this is why you need to spend more time strengthening

EXERCISE

Snap Your Belly Button

Picture an imaginary giant metal clothing snap, about six inches in diameter. The front of the snap is on your belly button. The back of the snap is centered on the small of your back at your spine. Now, snap the two pieces together, snapping your belly button in toward your spine. You'll pull in your gut, pull in your back, and snap them together.

This exercise will help you produce a nice, very gentle slope in your back. If you were to lie down with your belly button

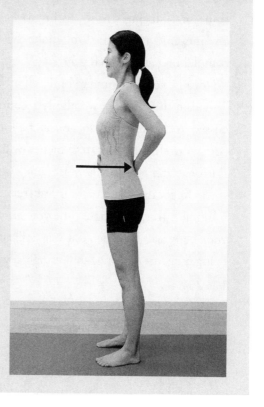

snapped to your spine, you'd actually find a small pocket beneath your lower back through which you could slide your hand.

As you tighten your core, it's important to remember to stay relaxed and continue breathing. Be careful not to hold your breath. Instead, keep your chest rising and falling naturally, while focusing on pulling in the muscles *beneath* the chest and lungs.

This action holds everything tight to keep the body from moving from side to side when you walk. This position also helps naturally strengthen and protect your back during any movement taken during the day, especially reaching for things off to the side, or precariously perching with outstretched arms (say, to get that big bowl from the top shelf or lift that heavy box). Grasp the idea of snapping your belly button to your spine, and you've just saved yourself from a plethora of potential injuries and future doctor bills.

your core. Having strong abs improves your balance and helps protect you in any movement you do throughout the day. And we've never heard of anyone complaining about having a six-pack either.

Ideally, you're aiming to build all movement and activity upon a strong core. To aid in this process, we highly recommend practicing balance exercises, discussed in chapter 11. Also, consider a Pilates class, which helps you engage your core more effectively than crunches or sit-ups. For now, use the Snap Your Belly Button exercise to engage your core.

So forget those late-night infomercials and videos selling abs of steel. Barefoot walking is free. The more time you spend barefoot, the more naturally sculpted your body will become. You may still need to lose a few pounds (or more), but being fit, getting strong, and losing a few pounds all go hand in hand.

Step 3: Opening Your Chest

Humans are the only true bipeds. Standing or moving upright on two legs gives us the ability to breathe without restriction as our arms and legs move.

Our ability to adjust our breathing patterns according to speed, terrain, heat, and stress is unique in the animal kingdom. This is one reason you hear about humans outrunning horses over great distances, or why indigenous peoples are able to run down animals in persistence hunting. Let's make the best of our biological advantage and open up our chests and lungs.

Here's one thing to watch for. When you open up your chest by bringing it up and wide, you may feel inclined to raise or shrug your shoulders. Don't do this, but also don't hunch in an effort to counter it. Either action tenses and strains the shoulders, back, and neck, while throwing you off balance. Instead, keep your shoulders down, yet wide and relaxed. Shrugged or hunched shoulders constrict your breathing and throw off your arm movement, resulting in a choppy, unnatural, imbalanced stride.

EXERCISE

Inflate the Balloon

Keep your belly in while bringing your chest up and wide. Picture your chest filled with a giant balloon, expanding and contracting with each breath. The bigger you practice inflating the balloon, the more air you'll take in for each stride.

Your chest adapts over time, growing stronger and wider. As you learn to coordinate a tightened core with expanded lungs (belly in, lungs expanded), you become an incredible breathing machine, drawing fantastic power from the air, while remaining firmly anchored and perfectly erect.

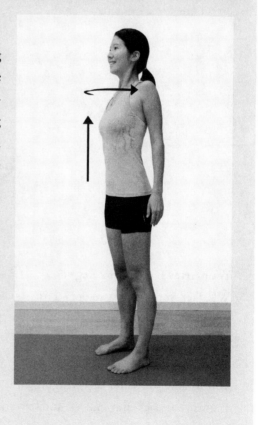

Step 4: Getting Your Arms in Position

To set the stage for a proper stride and to keep the shoulders relaxed, you want your arms to fall into a symmetrical, natural position by your sides.

EXERCISE

Stick 'Em Up

Bring your arms up above your head and out to the side in the shape of a *W* to form the natural bend. Then drop your arms to your sides. This is a good starting position.

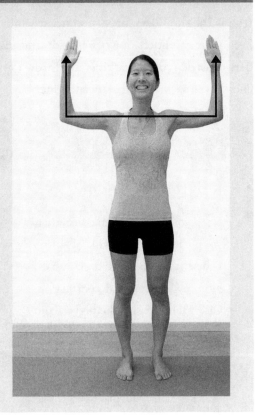

Your Arms Drive Your Legs

Whether you walk barefoot or in shoes, your arms and legs should move in near-perfect opposition as well-balanced counterweights. Whatever your right arm does, your left leg does, and vice versa. Realize, too, that subtle changes in your arm movement make big changes in your stride. For instance, swing your right arm in and you wind up swinging your left leg in. This unbalanced movement strains your back, hips, knees, and feet and can lead to a whole slew of injuries.

When you're barefoot, your arms work harder to balance your stride. This means barefoot walking is a more complete body workout, helping tone your arms as well as your legs.

However, this doesn't mean you have to exaggerate your arm movement. Instead, imagine a weight on a pendulum dangling off the ends of your middle fingers. With your hands facing inward (almost brushing your hips), let your arms naturally swing forward and back with the weight. You'll feel as if you have two pendulums for arms, one swinging forward, while the other swings back.

At its best, walking is a nearly effortless glide, even at speed. The lighter your arms, the lighter you'll be on your legs, feet, and all of your joints. So it's best to relax your arms, shoulders, and back and let them carry you along.

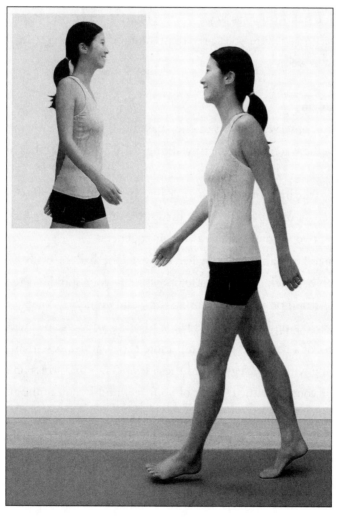

A gentle and relaxed arm swing keeps you light on your feet.

Here are a few key points to keep in mind as you let your arms swing naturally.

1. Keep your arms dangling by your sides. The more relaxed they are, the more you'll walk like a feather.
2. Let your arms swing back and forth like pendulums.
3. Don't lock your elbows. Allow the arm to naturally fall and bend where it may.
4. Make sure your arms aren't crisscrossing in front of you, but instead only moving forward and backward in the direction of travel.
5. Shoot for symmetry and balance in your arms. If you carry something in one hand (such as keys, a cell phone, a water bottle, or an MP3 player), make sure you carry something of equal weight in the other hand as well.

Pocket Problems

Michael often observes walkers as they pass by. On one brisk winter morning in Colorado, he watched a woman walking by his office with her hands in her pockets.

She was strutting with each step, a forced movement, hands in her pockets, using her shoulders to carry her forward. While this likely kept her hands warm, it had two serious, unintended consequences.

First, since her hands were in her pockets, she had to push her shoulders forward with her back to drive her legs. Swinging your shoulders to walk puts a great deal of strain on your neck, back, hips, and even your knees.

Second, swinging the shoulders tends to bring your legs out wide and bow-legged (think of a cowboy who spends more time on his horse than on his own feet). Walking with your legs out to the sides puts undue stress on everything: the inside of your legs, the outside of your feet and knees, and especially your hips.

In this walker's case, an overuse injury is likely if she makes this a regular habit. It's only a matter of the weakest link: which ligament, joint, or tendon will catch her first?

Step 5: Standing Tall

Now that your body is in proper alignment, you will want to pull yourself up nice and tall so that you're incredibly light on your feet and walking like a human spring.

EXERCISE

Silver String to the Sky

Picture an imaginary silver string. The string starts at your feet, passes through your tailbone, spine, chest, and neck, and comes out through the center of your head. This string will keep you light on your toes and help you maintain proper position and balance.

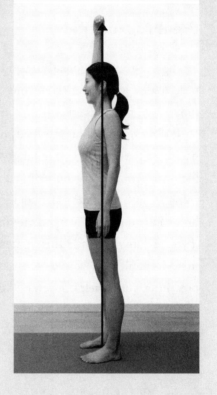

With an imaginary fishing reel, wind that string tight and pull yourself tall, as if you're being yanked up so high you're almost pulled onto your tiptoes.

Keep your head facing forward and your chin and jaw relaxed. Remember, the string pulls up through the center of your head, not the front.

You'll always want to walk with this silver string pulling you to the sky.

Our bodies also have memories—meaning what we do when we're not walking carries through to our other activities. From now on you'll always want to stand, and even sit, as tall as possible, with your core engaged. Try to stand this tall in all activities throughout your day.

One way to really emphasize this posture is to give away your office chair and sit on a balance ball; if not, try adding an inflatable disk to your chair. I can't think of a better way to engage your core during your workday even when you're doing a relatively sedentary task. You're forced to sit tall.

Before you begin walking, always pull yourself up as tall as you can. You can even pull yourself up onto the very tips of your toes before lowering your feet back down and preparing to begin.

Breathing for Life

Strange as it sounds, breathing will take some work in the beginning. First, you need to develop awareness of your breath. There are many different breath techniques and rhythms; over time you'll develop your own style.

For now, we're going to focus on a breath that helps increase your lung capacity and strengthen your lungs while tightening your core. When walking, focus on bringing in your belly button to your spine as you inhale. Draw everything in. When you exhale, hold in your belly button, but relax your chest and lungs (if you place one hand on your chest, and one on your belly, you'll know if you're doing it right). This tightening of the core may seem counterintuitive at first, particularly if you've been taught to expand your belly for diaphragmatic breathing. But it helps in several key ways.

1. By consciously expanding your lungs with each breath, over time you expand your lungs. It's like stretching and restretching a sock or your favorite pair of jeans.
2. You begin to strengthen the muscles around your lungs.
3. You teach your diaphragm to relax. When it relaxes, it drops down, giving you more room to breathe. A great way to help your diaphragm relax is to smile or laugh while you walk. The more we expand and strengthen our lungs while relaxing the diaphragm, the more air we can move.
4. Last, you tighten your core. This gives you more power when walking and helps protect you throughout the day. Learning to tighten your

core when breathing and walking doesn't stop when the workout's over, but carries through to all of your activities.

As an advanced technique, you can work on breathing in through the nose, and out through the mouth.

Focusing on your breath is one of the greatest gifts you can give yourself, and it's not just great for exercise—it means you breathe easier and deeper throughout the day. And deeper breathing has been directly linked to stress reduction. Focusing on your breath gives you confidence, quiets your mind, brings in great health, and helps you through all activities in life.

THE $40,000 EXERCISE

We learned this one from Dr. Maureen Traub and Darshan Zenith while out on Maui. Both teach the healing power of laughter, which is amplified by getting in touch with the earth.

Stand on the earth with your feet at least shoulder's width apart. Switch your weight from one foot to the other as you begin to breathe deeply. Take huge breaths as you feel the ground beneath your feet while shifting or stomping back and forth. Make yourself smile, and begin to laugh on the exhales. Smile big, breathe big, and watch the laughter grow. As you continue to breathe deep, you'll soon find yourself spontaneously laughing louder than you ever have, a contagious, raucous roar. You'll be giddy and feel light, wondering if perhaps you should be committed. Don't worry, though—you're just waking up the child inside you and releasing $40,000 worth of "happy drugs" with each laugh.

THE THREE METHODS OF BAREFOOT WALKING

There are three basic techniques to walking barefoot: the feather walk, the tiger walk, and the walk and roll. All three strides have the same basic premise: pelvis aligned, core tight, open chest, standing tall, and imagining a string pulling us to the sky. Where they differ is where the foot meets the ground.

In order to develop the best overall walking form possible, we'll begin by focusing on the feather walk, which encourages a light step, and the tiger walk, which helps strengthen the feet. On your very first day, limit yourself to a maximum of a hundred yards of barefoot walking on the grass. (Yes, just a hundred yards or less on your first day. We'll outline a progression plan for your first ninety days barefoot in the next chapter.)

A great way to do your initial walks is by breaking them up into sections of ten to twenty yards. For example, feather-walk for ten yards; then turn around and tiger-walk back ten yards. If you feel your feet beginning to fatigue, by all means feel free to resort to the walk-and-roll method.

For the first few weeks we're going to concentrate on these two techniques exclusively. Once your foot strength improves, you can begin doing some walk-and-roll exercises as your distances increase and/or you start to encounter more challenging terrain. However, the walk and roll should be your backup walk (for when things are difficult or when you are tired), rather than your default.

Feather walking is the lightest stride and the one you should concentrate on first. It will take the most time to develop but is helpful for the entire body.

Method #1: The Feather Walk

The feather walk is most like the walk used by Native Americans of old, whose stealth was legendary as they made their way through the woods with nary a sound.

This is the ideal method of walking under most conditions, and is still practiced by indigenous people deep in the heart of the Amazon rain forest, on the African savannah, and in other places where the influence of shoes hasn't changed this timeless practice.

But you needn't travel far to see the feather walk in action. Just turn your attention to a nearby barefoot toddler and you'll see the child up on his or her toes, almost from day one, doing a feather walk.

All of these feather walkers have one thing in common: they stay light and

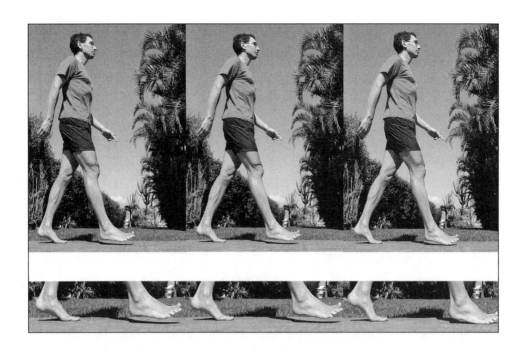

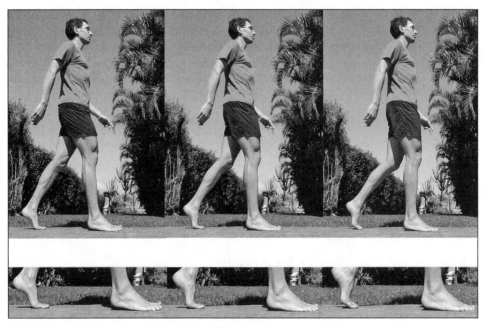

The feather walk. Note the gentle landing of the forefoot with the heel just barely off the ground.

tall, with barely any pressure on their feet. They do this by walking gently on their forefoot, using their entire leg as a shock absorber or spring.

Their walk looks incredibly graceful and light, with perfect posture almost like that of a ballet dancer. This is what we'll aspire to.

With the feather walk, you land just slightly up on your forefoot, with your heel between half an inch and an inch and half above the ground. I call this front part of your foot the landing zone. Conveniently, it has the most cushion. Don't fret if you don't have much cushion beneath your landing zone just yet. As you spend time walking barefoot, you'll stimulate growth

○°°。 FOOT NOTE

The foot is a true marvel of nature. The metatarsals, or bow-shaped bones behind our toes, are designed to compress just slightly and then spring back. The arch acts as a spring as well. It is one of the only shapes in nature designed to get stronger under pressure. The more you push on the arch, the more it pushes back.

Everything on the foot is attached to everything else and acts as a giant spring, compressing and springing back. It's then all attached to the Achilles tendon at the back of the heel, which is the only tendon capable of holding a ton of force. When you land on the forefoot, you load the Achilles tendon, which too acts as a spring.

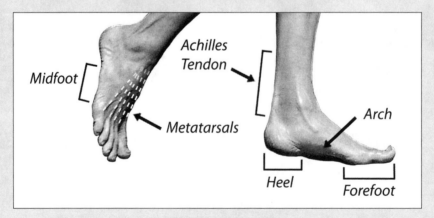

Parts of the foot.

of this fat pad. Additionally, don't worry if your heel brushes the ground initially; this helps keep you from overworking new muscles that aren't used to the feather walk.

This, along with your Achilles tendon, calf muscles, quadriceps, hamstrings, and glutes, gives you an amazing shock absorber, allowing you to gracefully walk on the harshest of terrain without a jarring impact being transmitted up through the body.

Think of it this way. When you land on your heel while wearing running shoes, it's like you're hitting your heels with a hammer with each step. The force of the hammer sends a shock wave directly up through your feet, ankles, shins, knees, hips, lower back, shoulders, and neck. And since your bones are long hollow tubes, it focuses the force at the head of each bone it passes through.

By contrast, when you land on your forefoot, it's as if you're stepping on a trampoline. Not only is the shock wave eliminated, but there's no impact or dangerous force being driven up your body. You may even bound back with each step. Remember when you were jumping rope as a child? You'd always land and spring off of the forefoot.

Walking lightly on the forefoot, having the heel slightly off the ground, helps engage the entire leg as an amazing shock-absorbing mechanism. And this technique does something very kind for you: once your feet have grown strong, they can return over 90 percent of the energy put into them. When you land on your forefoot, your entire foot compresses like a spring. As your foot rebounds, it propels you forward. With good form this means you don't have to work as hard. The gentle springs help you walk with less effort.

By landing on your forefoot, there's also no crashing impact with the ground—something Dr. Dan Lieberman of Harvard called an *impact transient* when he was comparing shod and unshod runners. He found that the group wearing shoes was hitting on the heel, transmitting a shock wave of force up through the body, while the barefoot running group was landing on the forefoot, with no initial impact transient or shock wave at all. This same effect takes place when walking.

When do you use this form? All the time, though build up gradually. You can use this both in and out of a shoe. However, I recommend you do it first fully barefoot, letting your skin be your guide, so you adapt slowly, without undue stress and strain to the foot, Achilles tendon, and calves. Try the many exercises in this book to help you strengthen your feet.

Feather walking promotes the lightest, most effortless stride or gait possible, but it also takes a lot of work in the beginning to support your body weight on your forefoot. Start with a few minutes at a time, practicing every other day, until your feet grow strong. In the beginning it's hard to use this form for all your walking because the muscles, ligaments, tendons, and even bones of the feet need to strengthen first.

When your feet fatigue, it's okay to lower the springs in your feet, but just realize that the rest of your body will now be taking on the impact. If you have weak knees or a sore back, you'll feel the impact there. So instead of reverting to your original shoes and way of walking, I'd recommend the gentle walk and roll (discussed later).

EXERCISE

Ninja Walking

Here's an exercise to practice walking lightly in your feather walk.

Head out for a walk without headphones. Simply focus on the sound of your footsteps during the walk, trying to adjust how you land to make the least noise possible. Barefoot walking is an exercise in awareness, in listening to yourself and in seeing how quiet you can become.

Try rolling off the heel, rather than smacking the ground. Hear a difference? Now try landing just on the forefoot, rather than on the heel. Notice another difference? Now try standing as tall as you can and practice both strides.

You'll find that the taller you stand, the more relaxed you are, and that the more you shift toward landing on your forefoot, the quieter you become.

You might also practice this exercise on an old wooden floor. You can often hear the floorboards creak beneath your feet. Figure out how to sneak down the hall without making a sound, and you're walking like a ninja!

Method #2: The Tiger Walk

Practice the tiger walk to keep your feet strong on even the toughest surfaces and to help you stay balanced on the most challenging of terrain. For this you'll land with your heel just barely off the ground, focusing on grabbing with your toes.

For all barefoot walking techniques, you want to grab with your toes to support your arch and protect your foot. In this case, however, you're exaggerating the toes to gain more support, strength, or traction underfoot.

This walk doesn't have quite the suppleness or springy feeling of the feather walk, but it supports you when you're carrying a heavy weight, walking on a challenging or slippery surface, or just want to work on strengthening your feet.

"I use all three walking methods interchangeably," says Michael, "primarily switching back and forth between the feather walk and the tiger walk. These are the two most preferred methods, and are much better than the walk and roll if you have a leg length discrepancy too. In wintry conditions or anywhere it might be slippery, I'm tiger walking. And if I'm carrying things in from the car, shopping, or anywhere I'm carrying anything, I'm tiger walking. But if I'm out in nature, doing a walking meditation, or effortlessly walking away the miles, then I'm feather walking instead. Or when I'm walking up steep hills and want to rest my calves and Achilles tendon, I'm using the walk-and-roll method. It all depends on what you want to do."

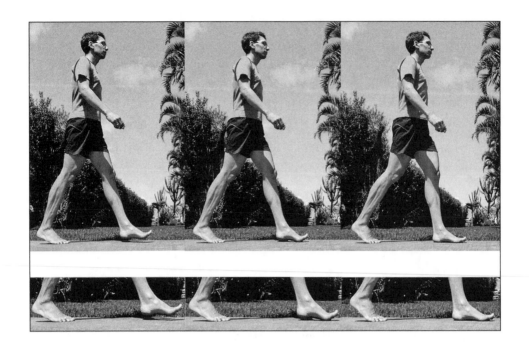

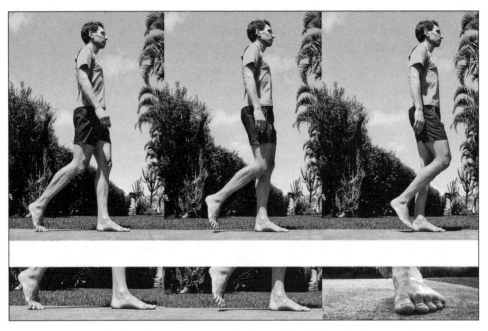

As you grab with your toes, your heel should barely brush the ground.

To do the tiger walk, pretend you have claws. Extend those claws, spread your toes apart, and, with each step, land on your forefoot with your heel slightly lifted off the ground, pulling forward with your claws.

EXERCISE

Advanced Tiger Walk

Walk ten steps as you normally do. Now walk ten steps while you're grabbing with your toes and pulling through behind you. Feel the difference? Visualize pulling through at the end of your steps with your toes. Picture an animal kicking up dirt behind itself, or perhaps the tail end of a paddle-wheel, drawing water up and out. The more you kick up the dirt behind you, the more you're using your toes, foot, and entire leg to gently and efficiently propel yourself forward.

Method #3: The Walk and Roll

Sometimes you'll find yourself in situations where the feather walk isn't appropriate, such as when your feet are tired, when you're traversing uneven surfaces, or when you're carrying a heavy load. Since you can't always feather-walk, particularly in the beginning, there has to be another way to walk light.

There is, and that's the walk and roll.

For this walk, you meet the ground with your heel as if you're seated in a rocking chair, gently lulling a baby to sleep. You're not slamming your heel into the ground, driving it into the ground, or even letting it slap onto the ground. Instead, you're gently rocking over the

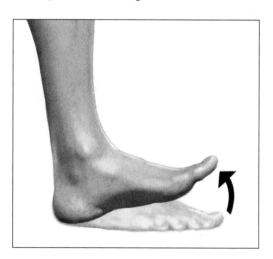

When using the walk-and-roll technique, dorsiflex—lift your forefoot up before you land, which aids with a gentle rocking motion.

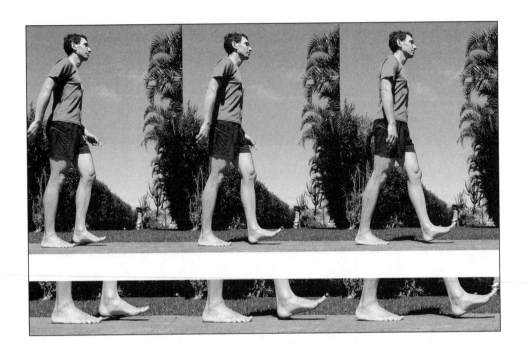

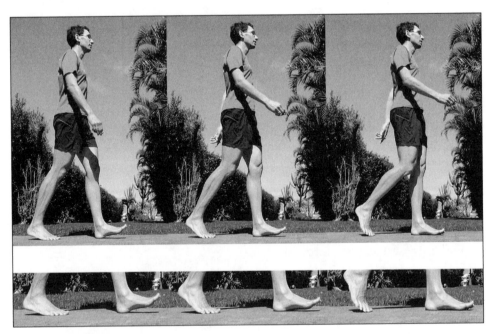

The walk-and-roll technique. Gently roll your heel over the ground as if your foot's a rocking chair.

ground. I call this walk a gentle handshake, because while there's no springing action when you meet the ground, it's like greeting an old friend. In essence, as you roll your foot on the ground with each step, you're shaking hands with Mother Earth.

Bring up your toes and forefoot before you land, with your heel gently touching down almost directly beneath you. Work on rolling or rocking your foot just before you roll over your heel. This gives you a gentle gliding motion, helps you stay graceful and tall, and allows you to use your heel as a rocker, rather than as a hammer.

Another way to think of this is as if your foot's a rocking chair—you gently rock forward with each step.

To keep your feet strong, make sure you grab the ground with your toes at the end of each step. Ideally, it's roll, grab, and release; roll, grab, and release.

The walk and roll doesn't give you nearly the shock absorbency of the feather walk, nor is it compensatory if you have a leg length discrepancy, but it takes less effort, at least in the short term. While you can't use your forefoot, Achilles, and calf as a great shock-absorbing mechanism, the more directly you keep your legs under your body as you roll off the heel, the less impact you'll transmit through your body.

Duck Walking: A Nationwide Epidemic

If you or someone you know walks like a duck, you're not alone. Today, millions of Americans are suffering from duck walking, and the vast majority have no idea. Don't know if you're a duck walker? Try walking a few steps and then stop. Now look down. Are your feet aiming forward or slightly off to the sides? If they're off to the sides, you're a victim of duck walking. The good news is you don't have to be just another statistic. Michael, too, once waddled like a duck, but he no longer does.

When Michael was a speed skater, he worked very hard to train his legs to push off side to side, not forward and back. The more he trained, the more his legs turned outward—ideal for speed skating, but terrible for walking. This created big problems for his feet, stressing them unnaturally when he walked and ran. Orthotics only exacerbated his condition. Had he not worked to correct his waddle, over time he would have hurt his knees too.

What else causes duck walking besides unnatural motions? Footwear's the number one culprit, along with weak feet and tight hips, psoas, or glutes.

Habits created over a lifetime take time to change, so be patient. If you see your feet pointed outward, it's something you'll want to correct very gradually. Changing too quickly could cause an injury because your body is not used to the new movement. Some poor habits take up to a year or more to fully rectify, so don't get discouraged, and don't rush things.

The best way to correct this is by giving your feet time out of your shoes. When your feet are out of shoes, you'll be able to better feel and sense if they're

EXERCISE

The Pigeon Strut

Due to a combination of tight hips, a titanium hip, and years spent in over-supportive shoes with arch supports, Michael once suffered from walking like a duck. Duck walking creates stress and strain on your hips, knees, IT bands, and elsewhere as you walk, run, or even just stand.

However, it can be corrected—over time. In addition to deep tissue massage, doing the Rolling over a Ball exercise, and stretches, you can also do this simple drill, either walking or standing, to help gently correct things. Remember, if you've spent the better part of a lifetime this way, you want to change things slowly. This isn't about forcing it today or tomorrow, but gradually over months if not longer. Our Tibetan Buddhist teacher Lhop-pon Rechung uses the analogy of straightening bent bamboo to illustrate changing things "slowly, slowly." If you force the bamboo to straighten too fast, it breaks, but if you soak the bamboo and gently straighten it over time, you will succeed.

The simplest and easiest way to work on this is to work on pointing your toes inward (or more like a pigeon) when you stand. You can do this while washing the dishes, sorting laundry, brushing your teeth, or for guys, standing in front of the toilet. Becoming conscious of how you stand at these times will affect all movement of the body.

You can also walk with your toes pointed in for very short sessions, a maximum of one to two minutes on your first day; then increase a minute every few days afterward. Introduce this gradually, or you'll start to feel twisting strains in your legs anywhere from your shins to your hips. If you feel these strains, it's a hint to back off.

For an easier version of the Pigeon Strut, try keeping your feet pointed straight as you walk along a painted line, or imagine walking along a balance beam.

Again, this is a long-term process to get your feet tracking straight again.

pointed anywhere but forward. This instant feedback from the bottom of the feet helps you naturally correct your stride. Barefoot walking is all about awareness: once you feel and see what's going on, you're more aware and can naturally correct any problems over time.

Working on hip flexibility can often greatly relax your legs and help you more naturally bring them in. Deep tissue massage and some of the stretching exercises later in this book (see Rolling over a Ball, chapter 10) can help. Additionally, examine your footwear. Do you have motion control shoes or arch supports? Either of these may be causing you to rotate your feet outward. (All of the negative effects of modern footwear are discussed in chapter 19.) Finally, give the Pigeon Strut a try.

Start slowly and watch yourself get true as an arrow. Every joint in your body will thank you.

How About Walking Sticks?

Unless used on steep or slippery terrain, I'm not a big fan of walking sticks, also known as trekking poles or Nordic poles. Although in certain situations walking sticks provide much-needed additional balance and control, many people use them as crutches unnecessarily. If you're recovering from sickness, injury, or surgery, by all means use them. But if you're strong and healthy and have a habit of relying on walking sticks when you don't need them, you can actually weaken your body. You also throw yourself off balance and rewire the mind so it can only balance itself by leaning on poles. Eventually you reduce your ability to balance yourself.

EXERCISE

Walk Softly and Carry a Balance Stick

Don't toss out those trekking poles just yet. You can use your trekking pole or, better yet, a stick you find on the ground for this exercise.

Find a fairly straight stick, between two and four feet long, and approximately the diameter of a broomstick. Now hold it in your hands with a

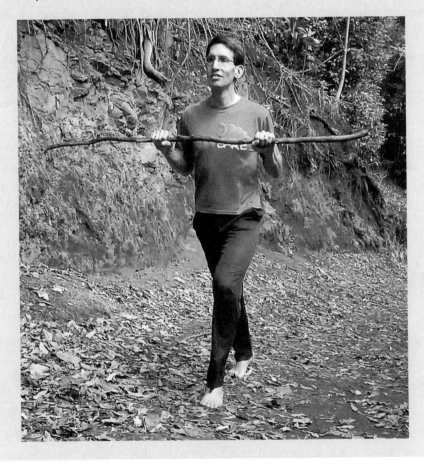

90-degree bend in your arms, at about mid-chest height, pulled in close against your body. Holding the stick here slightly shifts your weight forward.

If you don't engage your core, gravity will pull you forward, and that's the point. You'll need to keep your core engaged to keep that silver string pulling you to the sky. Just by holding the stick, you automatically work both core strength and balance.

Carry your stick for a few minutes each walk, and you'll be making great progress. You can even work up to longer durations or a heavier stick to progress even further. Just remember to rest your body in between.

This stick play helps develop strength, balance, and body awareness. It also helps keep you in the moment, as you focus on your core and the stick.

Checklist for Proper Barefoot Walking Form

Before you head out the door, review these key points.

- ☐ **Warm things up**—begin with Waking Up the Feet and the Golf Ball Grab.
- ☐ **Get neutral**—bring your waist to level by imagining your pelvis as a water bowl.
- ☐ **Snap it in**—snap your belly button in toward your spine.
- ☐ **Think up and wide**—open your lungs by bringing your chest up and shoulders wide.
- ☐ **Stick 'em up**—position your arms in a *W* above your head, then drop them by your sides.
- ☐ **Stand tall**—imagine a silver string pulling you tall.
- ☐ **Stay symmetrical**—keep your arms symmetrical and tracking straight and your legs will follow along.
- ☐ **Relax and have fun**—if you tense up, you're fighting against your body and the terrain. Keep your head, jaw, neck, shoulders, and every part of you relaxed. Flow with the ground and with your form.

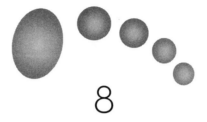

8
Ninety Days to Barefoot Freedom

An early-morning walk is a blessing for the whole day.
—Henry David Thoreau

To help you transition safely and easily, we've built an entire three-month program. From where to walk, when, and even how long, it'll get you going day by day. Since everyone is unique, this program is meant as a guideline, meaning above all else, listen to your body. If every inch of your body truly feels great, keep on going. Conversely, if you're tired and sore, go shorter and slower or perhaps take the day off.

MICHAEL'S TWO-QUESTION RULE

Here's a very important safety rule we always teach our students, about when to go home. If you're tired and thinking of heading for home, if you feel sore, achy, or tender, or if you have even an inkling of doubt, ask yourself, "Should I stop?" If the answer is yes, then head straight home, but chances are you'll say no and want to continue a little bit farther.

At this point, double-check your form, go through the checklist for proper walking form, and make sure you've re-snapped your belly button in toward your spine, relaxed your arms, and are staying tall. Did the soreness or fatigue go away? If so, great. If not, the next time you ask "Should I stop?" don't even finish the question—just turn around and head for home.

While the first question may be a fluke, the second time you ask if you should stop, it's your intuition, that small still voice that never lies and never steers us wrong (if only we would listen to it) telling us we've had enough. So *please* don't ignore it!

"HAND WEIGHTS," AKA SHOES

When Michael begins a barefoot clinic, he always picks up a pair of shoes and gives a pop quiz. "What are these?" he asks.

The creative responses range from "foot coffins" to "door stops" to "cruelty chambers." The answer Michael's looking for, though? Hand weights.

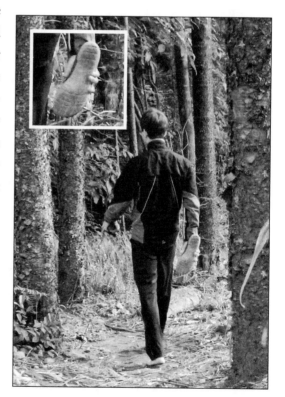

Yes, we have a new purpose for your shoes: they're now hand weights. You can strengthen your arms by carrying a pair (one shoe in each hand) as you walk barefoot. This helps keep your body balanced and symmetrical, helps strengthen the muscles of your back, and tones your arms. And it means your shoes are available to protect your feet in case you need them. When the going gets tough or your feet get tired (particularly the skin, early on), shoes will be there if you need them.

Now, we're not talking about carrying a heavy boot. We're talking about your regular walking shoe, and over time a more moccasin-like shoe. Since the arms have to swing forward and back with each step,

Even as an experienced barefooter, carry your "hand weights" with you just in case you need them. Here Michael is carrying a pair of flexible, lightweight shoes called Lems.

even a small weight makes a big difference. Here less is more—carrying too heavy a weight or a clunky heavy shoe throws everything out of balance. So the lighter the shoe you carry, the better it is for your walk.

Five Simple Rules for Safety

1. Stop barefoot walking once you stop having fun.
2. Stop barefoot walking once you feel the slightest tweak or twinge of pain.
3. Never let your pride get in the way of stopping, whether it's to brush off the foot, pluck out a pebble pressed into your skin, or put on footwear.
4. Don't walk on an open wound.
5. Always bring footwear (aka "hand weights") just in case.

START WITH ONLY 100 YARDS

First, do a three- to five-minute warm-up with a golf ball (see chapter 7) or with an inflatable ball (see chapter 10). Next, as you walk, begin with thirty seconds of slow tiger walking, followed by thirty seconds of slow feather walking. For the first few weeks, alternating between both strides is your best plan as you strengthen your feet and develop a strong, light feather walk. Over time you can build up to switching every minute to two minutes between strides.

Start with only a hundred yards; then progress by adding about a hundred yards, or approximately three minutes, to your walks every other day. This means you'll be walking for about ten minutes barefoot after your first week, twenty minutes after your second, thirty after your third. You'll be comfortably up to about an hour of barefoot walking, every other day, by the end of your first month.

In our clinics we have participants repeat a mantra. We'd like you to do the same here. Repeat after us: "I will start with only one hundred yards." Now repeat: "I will start with only one hundred yards."

Thank you.

THE FIRST THIRTY DAYS: GO SLOW TO GO FAST

The first thirty days are the most important of the program. We need to wake the feet up slowly, without doing too much. This means very short periods of barefoot activity one day, followed by a non-barefoot day the next. Always wear your shoes and/or insoles or orthotics when you're not working out barefoot; this allows your feet to rest and recover. While you can go barefoot on grass for your first workout, we recommend that most of every session after that for the first two weeks is on a hard bike path or sidewalk. This will help you find your lightest stride. During this time try to spend about 10 percent of your time on a more uneven surface, such as a dirt path paralleling the bike path.

Progression:

Grass → Smooth flat paths → Hard-packed trails → Hills → All terrain

Week 1

Day 1: Start on a flat bed of nice green grass for the fun of it. Walk for ten to twenty yards, rest for thirty seconds, then repeat, for a total of three to five times. Total distance should be no more than a hundred yards, or the length of an average parking lot. Actual walking time should be only one to three minutes. After your barefoot time, go back to your regular shoes, with insoles or orthotics if you usually use them.

Day 2: No barefoot walking. For every day you are asked not to walk barefoot, you may continue your daily walks (if you're already a daily walker) in your shoes. This is also a great time to stretch and consider cross-training activities; just let your bare feet rest.

Day 3: Find a smooth flat bike path, jogging path, or sidewalk (we'll be spending the next couple of weeks here), or better still, a path around a local park or lake. Walk barefoot for about two hundred yards, or a total of three to five minutes, before you slip back into your shoes. You can walk twenty yards of this on an uneven surface such as grass or a dirt trail. Remember to carry your shoes with you as "hand weights."

Day 4: Same as day 2.

Day 5: Increase your barefoot time to approximately three hundred yards (with thirty yards on uneven terrain), or approximately five to seven minutes.

Day 6: Same as day 2.

Day 7: Increase your barefoot time to seven to nine minutes.

Week 2

Day 1: No barefoot walking.

Day 2: Barefoot walking for nine to eleven minutes on a hard path.

Day 3: No barefoot walking.

Day 4: Barefoot walking for eleven to thirteen minutes on a hard path.

Day 5: No barefoot walking.

Day 6: Barefoot walking thirteen to fifteen minutes on a hard path.

Day 7: No barefoot walking.

Week 3

You can stay on man-made surfaces if you'd like; it's also the perfect time to find a hard-packed path or hiking trail (perhaps one that parallels a smooth bike path you've been walking on, or a quiet nature trail not too far from home). In an ideal world, you'd alternate between a few minutes on the tougher stuff and a few minutes on the smooth stuff.

If that's not possible, then use the following timeline as a guideline— meaning don't be afraid to put your shoes back on and head for home if the trail's too tough. Uneven surfaces are the best for getting blood flow back to your feet but can be tough on the skin until it adapts. Always let your skin be your guide.

Day 1: Take your time and go slowly with your new, all-terrain feet: fifteen to seventeen minutes max, but don't be afraid to back down the time if it's a big challenge.

Day 2: No barefoot walking.

Day 3: Barefoot walking for seventeen to nineteen minutes, preferably on a hard-packed path.

Day 4: No barefoot walking.

Day 5: Barefoot walking for nineteen to twenty-one minutes, preferably on a hard-packed path.

Day 6: No barefoot walking.

Day 7: Head out for a gentle hike. Go explore a new hiking trail. Do twenty-one to twenty-three minutes, or a bit more if you stop and start a lot (this helps the feet recover). Try out your new all-terrain feet.

Week 4

During week 4 of your initial training period, you will build on progress made in week 3.

Day 1: Rest and recover from your week 3 gentle hike.

Day 2: Barefoot walking for twenty-three to twenty-five minutes, on a hard-packed path.

Day 3: No barefoot walking.

Day 4: Barefoot walking for twenty-five to twenty-seven minutes, preferably on a hiking trail.

Day 5: No barefoot walking.

Day 6: Barefoot walking for twenty-seven to twenty-nine minutes, preferably on a hiking trail. Take a hike!

Day 7: Rest.

Congratulations—you've reached the thirty-minute mark! From here on out it's up to you. You can mix and match trails and paths. You could even do two walks of twenty minutes a day, such as one on the trails and one on the roads. Once you've hit the thirty-minute mark, your body is well on its way to adaptation.

Your greatest changes will occur over the first three to six months, but at thirty minutes of barefoot walking, you've hit a milestone. You'll be working on walking taller, walking stronger, increasing the pace, and venturing into even more challenging terrain.

○°°₀ FOOT NOTE

When Do Drills and Exercises Fit In?

There are many valuable drills and exercises recommended in this book. However, we suggest holding off on these for the first month. Beginning in your second month, you can start doing the supplementary drills and exercises *after* your barefoot walks and *never* on your non-barefoot days.

Here are some suggestions for the next few months.

MONTH TWO: WALK AWAY FROM THAT SHOE

You've now been walking barefoot for a month. Your feet are likely starting to feel stronger, the skin is growing tougher, a bit of padding is beginning to return, and you're standing taller than ever. The sky's the limit, and over the next few months you'll gradually be increasing the time or distance you go and work toward barefoot walking four to six days a week. How far and how fast you progress is up to you. There really is no ultimate goal other than your own health, so take days off as you need them. Keep up the gentle progression, listen to your body, and have fun.

This is hill-climbing month. Have you wanted to explore the area, try out new paths, new trails, new hills? Then now's the time to do it. Continue increasing your barefoot walking time up to three minutes every other day and start bringing in the vertical routes.

One of the greatest workouts in the world is walking up steep hills. However, hills are *significantly* more challenging on the body than flat terrain, so baby-step your way into hills. When you first start walking hills, begin with only a few minutes, walking uphill barefoot, and then putting your shoes on for the downhill. Very gradually introduce downhills to the bare feet, as they're the hardest of the bunch. Remember not to use your heels as brakes, and don't worry about getting to the top of a big hill in the beginning. It's far more important to finish fresh, rather than cooking yourself.

For this month, consider doing hills once to a maximum of twice a week, and never two sessions in a row. By the end of the month, you should be tromping the hills without trouble, or at least gradually making it to the top.

MONTH THREE: TIME TO SAY WHEE!

By now you're moving up and down hills with ease, or at least getting up and over them. You've worked your way onto some easy trails. (If you're not cresting the hills or on the trails yet, don't sweat it—everyone progresses at their own pace. You'll get there soon enough.) Now you can work on challenging yourself even more. It's time to expand your horizon.

Start looking for trails outside of town, or ones you were avoiding for their difficulty. Really dive in and start to head out into nature. You may be up to an hour's walk right now and are ready for some real hiking. So grab that pack (start carrying a light pack on your back—you'll need to build up to this as well) and head out.

During month 3 you can also work on walking up to six days a week. Remember, though, that the body always needs a chance to rest and recover. So if you do a long or challenging walk or hike one day, make sure it's a shorter, easier one the next.

As for the progression, let your body be your guide. By the end of month 3 you could be doing perhaps an hour of walking on your long days, and thirty minutes on your easier days. Just make sure you keep the easier ones easy. For instance, if you're tromping up your local hills on Monday, make sure Tuesday's walk is on flatter, easier terrain. Never forget to alternate, both in intensity and in duration.

And remember that intensity and duration are inversely proportional. What in the world does this mean? It means that if you start doing walks that are much harder, faster, or fatiguing, you need to back off on the distance. Never change or greatly increase the difficulty *and* distance of a walk or hike at the same time, as the body needs time to adapt.

Congratulations! You're well on your way to exploring this fantastic new and eternally old way of walking. You'll never view your form, or anyone else's, in quite the same way. In fact, you'll likely find yourself watching others while you walk, helping you to reinforce your own newfound natural form and freedom. And you'll never walk the same way again. Welcome to your new world, a world with a new form, a new stride, and new possibilities.

FOOT NOTE

Focusing on Time

While almost all of us can get caught up in the gadgetry of the day, don't get caught up in how far you walk. You don't need to map your walk or pack your favorite GPS or pedometer, at least for now. These devices only encourage you to go too far and too fast in the beginning. Instead, after you've graduated beyond a few hundred yards, focus not on how far you've walked but simply on how long. Focusing on time helps you avoid walking too far and allows you to let go of the outcome.

When you focus on a distance, your mind has a funny way of slipping into the "more" game. You start wanting more speed and miles to add to your log, more distance to tell others about—more, more, and more. Remember, though, when it comes to barefoot walking, less is more, at least in the beginning. The more you let your body adapt naturally, the farther (and faster) you'll go in the long run, and with much less chance of injury.

We have deliberately sculpted our step-by-step program to focus on time, rather than distance, to help you ease in without pushing yourself too much. But if you really love tracking numbers, just remember that this is a game of awareness. So observe yourself and ask the tough questions: "Is the watch or pedometer encouraging me to walk farther or faster than I normally would?" Put another way: "Is it causing me to ignore my body's signals?"

The 10 Percent Rule

One of the things to keep in mind while building up your feet is the 10 percent rule. It states you should never exceed more than a 10 percent gain in activity (a total of duration, distance, and intensity) in a given week.

For example, if you walk for twenty minutes one week, then you can walk twenty-two minutes the next (duration). Or if you walk ten miles one week, you can walk eleven miles the next (distance). Or if you walk 3 miles per hour one week, you can walk 3.3 miles per hour the next (intensity).

Of course, 10 percent is just a rule of thumb. For example, if you haven't exercised at all for a while, change it to a 5 percent rule.

The point is to set an appropriate limit and not go beyond it. Otherwise, you risk a cumulative overuse injury. You might not feel pain right away, but mounting damage can sneak up on you and result in a severe tear or break down the line. That's what happens when many people—bare or shod—go for an easy walk and, seemingly out of nowhere, experience their feet or legs giving out. Nothing special happened during that particular activity; it was just the last straw in a series of abuses over the course of weeks that finally pushed tendons, muscles, or bones too far too fast.

BAREFOOT BEADS

Want a simple way to walk light *and* stay mindful?

If you don't mind stashing your "hand weights" in your backpack to free your hands, try carrying a bracelet in each hand.

Barefoot beads are simple bracelets made of alternating patterns of large and small beads (all about pea-sized) that help you repeat a mantra to a rhythm as you walk. We like those made of all-natural materials (such as wood, stone, or seeds) threaded onto an elastic string that makes it easy to pass individual beads through our fingers one by one.

Simply carry one of these bracelets in each hand, allowing the bracelet to

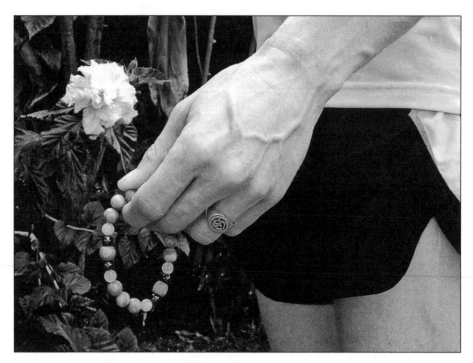

Holding barefoot beads in each hand helps you stay mindful and light as you walk.

loosely dangle between your thumb, index, and middle fingers. If you can keep the bracelets swinging forward and backward and not side to side, it's a sign that your arms are tracking straight. These bracelets also help you stay in a place of gratitude or mindfulness. When we walk, we often repeat a mantra as we scroll through the beads with our fingers. For instance, Michael is often repeating, "Thank you for my happy, healthy feet," while Jessica repeats, "Thank you for this beautiful walk." This reminds us to stay in a place of gratitude rather than ego, walking gently and with proper form.

BUILDING A BASE

You may wonder why I recommend a three-month program for getting into barefoot walking. It's because for any exercise routine you need to both (a) build a base and (b) make it a healthy habit or routine.

A base is like the foundation of a building or the roots of a tree. A solid base of several months helps you grow stronger and keeps you injury resistant.

After you build your base, you can work on going faster or farther, or on doing back-to-back walks or hikes. Building a solid base means working out, then resting and recovering.

And it means a term Michael came to love in training back in the early 1980s: LSD. No, this isn't a mind-altering drug. It stands for "long steady distance." It means that to build a healthy base, you don't need to go fast, but just to put in time on your legs.

This is the time when you'll get to know your body, your breath, and your mind. So build that base strong—get yourself good and healthy and injury resistant. And play! We're sure there's a trail that's calling your name!

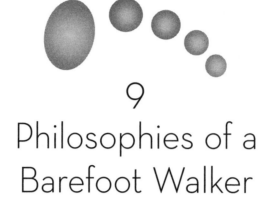

9
Philosophies of a Barefoot Walker

If you are seeking creative ideas, go out walking. Angels whisper to a man when he goes for a walk.

—Raymond Inmon

Jessica shares: "On my journey to barefoot freedom, I've learned many life lessons along the way. The hardest lesson came from my struggle to heal my left foot.

"In the fall of 2010, just two weeks after our wedding, I was tromping around in a pair of old two-dollar flip-flops that I picked up at a gas station somewhere in Kansas while on our book tour. I thought they were great—bright green with yellow flowers and a translucent rubber pink strap. I'd use them for those inconvenient times when I'd need footwear, such as public restrooms, grocery stores, and restaurants. They'd seen their day in the sun and were begging to be retired, especially the left flip-flop. The little knob at the end of the strap was threatening to pull through the bottom of the sole.

"On this particular day I was sporting them for the task of moving furniture. If ever there's a time for wearing more substantial footwear, this is one of them. Maneuvering heavy furniture through our overstuffed storage unit, I tweaked my left foot. The next morning I looked down and saw what looked like an inflated marshmallow.

"With constant touring and obligations for nine months, I struggled to heal.

I'd get a bit better, only to be knocked down again. Eventually I began hobbling around in a postsurgical boot, then in an air cast, and finally on crutches. One day my foot would look fine; the next it'd be swollen again. I couldn't figure out what was helping and what was hurting it. I saw podiatrists, but they all said the same thing, time after time: rest. More and more I was becoming a recluse. I was too embarrassed to be seen out and about on crutches. Boulder has a tightly knit running community. Everyone knows everyone. On my own, they might not recognize me, but with Michael's bare feet by my side, it was a dead giveaway. I didn't want to give people the opportunity to say, 'See, that's what happens when you run barefoot. You get injured.'

"By spring I was done being cooped up. After a liberating road trip down to Taos, New Mexico, with my best friend, Diane, I fell in love with New Mexico. I was enamored with the artistic and free spirit vibe, the Native American culture, and the open skies and desert lands. The following month, I introduced Michael to Taos and told him my heart said we needed to move there.

"The locals will be the first to tell you that if the sacred Taos Mountain doesn't like you, it'll spit you out. Conversely, sometimes the mountain doesn't let you go, so if you try to leave, your car might break down each time. As I felt the mountain drawing me in to help me heal, I wasn't frightened of being spat out. Instead, I felt embraced. As for the potential for getting stuck, I figured if that happened, it meant I hadn't quite learned all my lessons yet.

"So less than a month later, we were moving our lives into the Earthship we described in the introduction. (Actually, I just watched as I leaned on my crutches.) Two days after unloading the moving truck, Michael went off to Arizona and California. With running season in full swing, we sent him out on the road solo, while I stayed back hobbling, cleaning, unpacking, organizing, and coordinating the book tour from our new home base—on crutches.

"Each week, I was on my own five out of seven days in a new home in a new town (technically, twenty miles from town, out in the desert next to the famous Rio Grande Gorge and Bridge), where my only friends were our dog Sawa, a wild desert rabbit we named Junior, and at least a dozen hearty mice who had declared our home theirs. Despite my ever-growing list of things to do, I slowed down. It was my last hope for healing.

"One morning, exhausted from the move and the relentless howling wind that brought dust and smoke from New Mexico's largest recorded fire, just thirty-four miles away on the outskirts of Los Alamos, I finally took a break. I left behind the wind-worn desert, driving up a winding road to Taos Ski Valley, up in the mountains. In the summertime, the resort area with its brisk clean air is a welcome cool reprieve from the heat below. There's an extensive network of trails running all over the mountain, but like the previous nine months, I could only admire them from afar—wistfully.

"Instead I parked at the base of the resort and crutched my way to a gravel trail along a mountain stream carrying water from the peaks down to the arroyos below. I sat down on a bench, lay down my crutches, and released my left foot from its air cast. I rested my two feet on the ground beneath me and closed my eyes. I thanked the mountain for bringing me there and thanked it for my healing. And then a steady flow of tears began to stream down my cheeks. I didn't know what to do. I had another appointment with a new podiatrist the following Monday, but I highly doubted he could give me any new answers.

"I wanted to give up. 'I surrender,' I cried. I knew I needed to learn a lesson from my ailing foot, but I had learned so many already: compassion for other injured people, gratitude for my healthy foot, acceptance of help from others, and humility. What more could I possibly learn from this struggle? I knew the answer wasn't going to come from me, so I pleaded for help.

"Eventually the tears subsided and I felt an urge to walk the gravel trail barefoot, without the cast and crutch-free. I had never walked so slowly and tenderly before, as if I were learning to walk all over again but even *slower*. I moved slowly to be conscious enough not to flex my foot and thereby protect it from injury. The time allowed me to feel every stone, pebble, seed, and twig and see every leaf, stem, and flower.

"Most important, I felt absolutely no pain, only the pleasant feeling of reflexology at work on the soles of my feet. Suddenly, it dawned on me. This was exactly how slow the universe had wanted me to move this entire time. *This* was the true meditation walk.

"The medical devices of the boot, cast, and crutches were tools intended to protect me from myself and my inability to slow down. Instead I had used them as tools to propel me faster despite my injury. They couldn't heal my foot. Even *I* couldn't heal my foot. The healing was always taking place. I simply needed to get out of the way and allow it to happen.

"Sometimes we think we're being present and listening to our bodies, when in reality we can be even more present and aware.

"You just have to listen to your body and allow."

BE PRESENT

In the movie *Way of the Peaceful Warrior*, the main character, a know-it-all gymnast, is thrown off a bridge by his teacher into a river. When he gets out of the water, he screams at his teacher, "What the heck is wrong with you?"

The teacher retorts, "I emptied your mind."

"You threw me into the river!"

"And while you were falling, tell me . . . what were you thinking of? Were you thinking of school . . . grocery shopping . . that thing you had to hurry off to? No . . . [you were] present. Devoted 100 percent to the experience you were having. You even had a word for it . . . 'Ahhhhhhhh!' "

The student replies, "You're out of your mind. You know that?"

Says the teacher, "It's taken a lifetime of practice."

When you get out of your mind and into the present moment, you're truly living. You're not worrying about tomorrow or thinking regretfully about yesterday, but instead focused firmly on the present moment. And it's here, in the present moment, that the magic really happens. It's where all of our creativity comes from, all of our joy, and where we gain a richness of experience we can't find from our memories or future dreams.

It's in this moment, not a later one or an earlier one, that everything we do takes place. It's why meditative practices have you focus on your breath or a mantra to help you clear your mind.

Being present enriches the experience, any experience, and helps us shed all the junk that's going on in our minds. Truly, the only moment we have, or that the entire universe has, is the moment we're presently in. It's where all the action is happening!

And barefoot walking can help. When you walk barefoot you can focus on exactly what's going on beneath your feet. By doing so, you begin to leave the junk behind, as Jessica did on that New Mexico mountain trail. And when you are focused on what's beneath your feet, you're also focusing on the sound your feet are making, where your feet are going, and what's going on all around. That's the present moment.

BAREFOOT MEDITATION WALKS

Barefoot walking, almost by definition, is a walking meditation. When you focus on your breath and the ground beneath your feet, you can't help but be present. The next time you head out walking, take five or ten minutes to place one hand over the other, either in front of you or behind, and focus solely on your breath as you walk. Go about one-half or even one-quarter of the speed you normally travel. Make sure you're doing this someplace quiet where it's easy to walk; here grass (where no objects may be hiding) is ideal. This exercise helps reduce stress, quiet the mind, and bring everything into focus.

As an advanced version of this, we like to focus on a distant object, such as a tree, as we walk along. We repeat a mantra, typically of thanks, as we walk toward the tree, and then continue past. Each time we pass, we focus on the next tree, followed by the next. In this way we don't let any other thoughts come into the mind. We're focused solely on the path before us and the next tree coming our way.

With each of these meditations, be kind to yourself. All of our minds wander. If you catch your mind drifting away, just repeat a word, such as "thought" or "present" or even "tree," and bring your mind back into focus. There's no scorekeeping in meditation, just a beautiful "ahhhhhhh."

Problem Solving

If you want to be creative, brainstorm, or have your best ideas possible, or if you simply need to problem-solve and find a solution, don't think about the issue or problem that's on your mind. In fact, don't think about anything. Instead, go for a barefoot walk, feel the ground, clear your mind, and watch the answers come to you.

Be the Buddha

Walk as if you are kissing the Earth with your feet.
—Thich Nhat Hanh

There's a Buddhist legend that talks about how when the Buddha walked, he didn't leave footprints, but instead lotus flowers where he stepped. The lotus has represented fertility, rebirth, or life throughout history across many cultures.

It's natural that when you walk barefoot, you walk more softly and are more aware, and therefore you are kinder and gentler to our environment. You're less likely to kick loose stones and branches, trample over flowers or bushes, or generally wreak havoc to a trail than you are when you're wearing overbuilt shoes and boots.

To walk lighter still, walk like the Buddha and envision a flower beginning to grow wherever you place your feet. This symbolizes the connection or the dance between ourselves and the earth. For as the saying goes, when your feet meet the ground, the ground meets your feet. Walking barefoot is an exchange between you and Mother Earth.

Practice walking like the Buddha from time to time, and you'll find yourself walking lighter, smiling brighter, and growing an even stronger connection with the earth.

BE PATIENT AND LISTEN TO YOUR BODY

When it comes to transitioning into barefoot walking, the tortoise will *always* beat the hare. So what's the easiest, safest, most effective way to transition? Take off the shoes cold turkey. No transition shoes, no easing in. Dive off the deep end and into the water.

"But wait!" you may say. "Won't I get an overuse injury right away?"

Yes, if you don't listen to your body and go too far or too fast.

You have the most amazing biofeedback mechanism already built into you. It's your skin. Walk too far on bare skin, and blisters, bruised skin, or tenderized pads will alert the thousands of nerve endings embedded in your feet and stop you in your tracks. If you walk too far barefoot one day, you'll certainly be unable to do it the next. But if you watch your feet, particularly your skin, you'll stop well in advance of pain.

As soon as your skin feels too sore, or you get even a whiff of a hint that a blister is coming on, you should stop, put on your shoes, and turn for home.

Let your skin be your guide. This skin advice goes beyond your first few excursions too. Let it be your guide for training in general. If your skin feels strong, head out on a walk. If not, stay home.

Letting Go of Outcome

When it comes to barefoot walking, you need to let go of the outcome, which means letting go of goals, whether they involve time, fitness level, or distance. Transitioning into barefoot walking is highly individual, though it usually takes three to six months, after which you'll be stronger than ever before. During this process, you're changing more than your body—you're almost becoming a new person, sounder of mind, stronger of body, and more connected to the earth. That's because barefoot walking is more than a physical activity. It's a journey to discover the capabilities of your mind and your body. It's developing the discipline of being aware, letting go, and turning things over to a higher power.

When you are barefoot walking in solitude, it's a lot easier to stay in the zone, in that quiet place where the material world fades away. Ego takes you out of the zone. It unplugs you from that silent inner voice and vetoes your awareness. You're no longer thinking about your breath, the road, hazards, form, or stride. Instead, you're intent on going longer, faster, and farther. And that's precisely when you might walk into trouble.

Letting Go of Expectation

Barefoot walking is not about forcing things, but about flowing like water and letting nature guide you where she may. Some days you'll want to walk longer or faster. Other days you'll want to keep your walks short and sweet. When it comes to barefoot walking, listen to the earth, to the stillness, to your body, and to the silence. Let these forces guide you along. If you go out without a plan, without any expectation, deadline, or specific goal in mind, it's amazing how far you'll travel and how fresh you'll be.

This is also the premise behind a beautiful book by Dr. Majid Ali called *The Ghoraa and Limbic Exercise.* He talks about how the African messenger lets go and can run effortlessly almost without breaking a sweat, mile after mile, while the American businessman labors, toils, and struggles to run his doctor-prescribed twenty minutes at 70 percent of his maximal heart rate. The messenger lets go and can fly, while the businessman, stuck focused on his goal, struggles and may even hurt himself.

Having no expectation or plans is a plan unto itself—one of letting go. Without expectation you will never push yourself too far or too fast. You become one with the earth and simply flow.

So walk without ego. If you head out for thirty minutes but realize five minutes is all your feet can handle, take a break. If you're walking with a group and the pace is too fast, don't be afraid to drop back. Conversely, if you're walking along, feeling light as a feather, don't be afraid to go a bit farther. Chances are that over time you'll far surpass the distance you once thought possible for yourself.

BE THE HUMBLE BAREFOOT WALKER

Know where you're going—and bring your shoes. Even if you're an experienced barefooter, there are times you may want your shoes. So if you're headed out with friends for what appears to be an easy walk, if you haven't been there before and don't know the terrain, bring your "hand weights" to be safe. You never know what you're in for, and if your skin or feet get tired, you'll be thankful you brought them with you.

This is also a way of saying leave the ego behind. It's fun and "different" to be a barefoot walker. Some people even define themselves by their activity; however, tempting as it may be, don't fall into the trap of saying, "I always go barefoot," or worry that your friends will say something to you (as they do to us) if you show up with your shoes. It doesn't make you weak, and it doesn't mean you don't love to go barefoot; it just means you're being smart!

The Magic of the Maze: Labyrinths

Labyrinths, as first described in the introduction, are a special and sacred place to us. They help us clear our minds, reflect on the past, and gain direction for our future.

Our favorite experience with a labyrinth was while teaching a multiday retreat at Kripalu in the Berkshires. On the final day, participants navigated a labyrinth blindfolded.

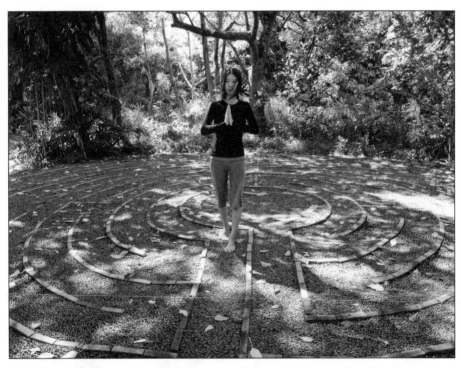

Jessica experiences greater inner awareness while walking barefoot along a labyrinth at the Sacred Garden on Maui.

It took courage and trust. The giant maze was lined with shrubbery and flowers, and it took over 15 minutes to walk to the center, even in shoes. For people who were blindfolded, it would take at least twice that time. There was no assistance aside from the natural boundaries of the labyrinth itself. And yet all the participants made it. They all relied on their senses and their inner voices to guide them through.

It was a silent experience, with the exception of a few childlike giggles. And when people finished, they were tears of joy and laughter as if they were children all over again.

Walking a labyrinth is a metaphorical experience: the farther we walk toward the center, the deeper we venture inwardly. It teaches us lessons as we go. Going toward the center, we learn about the obstacles in our path and the journey through life we're on. In the center we typically take some time for quiet contemplation, and the way back out serves as a time to integrate what we've learned.

If you ever get a chance, try a labyrinth barefoot; if you're daring and it looks safe, try it with your eyes closed. It's a life-changing experience. You'll learn about yourself and how to listen on the inside, let go, and trust the earth.

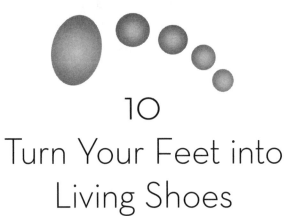

10

Turn Your Feet into Living Shoes

The foolish man seeks happiness in the distance,
the wise grows it under his feet.
—James Oppenheim

I f you want to walk better, have fewer aches and pains, and be healthier and happier in general, then you need strong, healthy, happy feet—not just for walking, but for every activity in your life.

Did you know the average 150-pound person puts 2,000 tons of cumulative weight on his or her feet every single day? That's just getting around. Even if you aren't active, you're likely to get back, hip, neck, and other injuries if you never strengthen your feet.

In cultures where people don't wear shoes, approximately 2 percent of the population has foot-related injuries, compared to 70 percent among shoe-wearing societies. And people wearing shoes have feet at least 40 to 50 percent weaker than shoeless populations. In other words, the average American's foot is only half as strong as it should be, if that.

As we've so often heard, perception dictates reality. If we think of the feet as weak and fragile, then we end up with weak and fragile feet. If we think of them as inflexible, unbendable stubs, we act as if they're inflexible and unbendable. But our feet aren't fragile, and they're far from unbendable. They're dynamic, changing, multisensory devices—that is, *until* we stuff them into shoes.

It's in a shoe that perception becomes reality. In a shoe, our feet lose the ability to sense, adjust, adapt, flex, and stay strong; instead, they become weakened, inflexible stubs we need to protect.

According to evolutionary biologists, it's our magnificent two feet that helped us evolve into the amazing species we are today. The foot made us who we are, made us strong, light, smart, and agile, and helped us to be mobile, thrive, and survive.

In this chapter we'll look at this magnificent marvel, help you understand how it works and why, and then explain how to build your strongest feet ever. We will dig deep inside, looking at the structure of the foot and the physics behind its design.

MICHAEL'S STORY

Custom insoles and orthotics are inserts that go inside shoes, and they are designed to help give greater support and stability. Custom insoles are the non-prescription "supportive" baby brothers of orthotics, which are available by prescription and are considered "corrective" in nature. In essence, once your feet have weakened sufficiently from the insoles, you graduate to full-on orthotics.

I got my first pair of custom insoles at the Olympic Training Center in 1988. I'd been participating in a training camp for speed skaters, and after a twelve-mile run on a chewed-up granite trail (aka scree) around Rampart Range Reservoir, high above Colorado Springs, my calves were killing me. I don't remember my feet being in any pain, but the trainers on staff there cooked me up my first pair of insoles from a toaster oven.

I used those over the next ten years, and even made similar things, custom-molded footbeds and insoles, for my customers and clients at the ski and rollerblade shops where I worked.

I believed in them.

I made them.

And I used them.

And when I began to date a podiatrist, trained at one of the top programs in the country, who taught me even more about orthotics and insoles, I became almost religious about their value. I wrote about them, studied them, and even based both my master's degree thesis and a senior project on the manufacture of orthotics.

Yet, through it all, no orthotic ever felt right to me. I met my former girlfriend just after my first Half-Ironman, after her colleague at a running store had looked at my old, tattered insoles and told me I needed proper orthotics. My feet weren't bothering me much, but it made sense to me.

So after the race I visited their clinic and my former girlfriend made me a $600 pair of hard-plastic orthotics. Looking at my feet, she was dismayed I was running. "You have the world's flattest feet," she told me, later calling me "Mr. Plantar Fasciitis."

"You should never, ever go anywhere barefoot. You shouldn't even get out of bed barefoot. And you should throw away your sandals; those are killing you." Who was I to argue with a medically trained expert? So, I flung myself fully into the world of foot support. I got hard plastic orthotics for my running shoes, taller orthotics for my walking shoes, cork orthotics for my gym shoes (and occasionally for running when my feet were too sensitive for the plastic), and even über-lightweight carbon fiber orthotics for my cycling shoes.

And you know what? My feet got worse. Much worse.

I didn't know it at the time, but the very thing I believed in so much, that I thought was helping me, and helping others, was actually killing my feet.

It wasn't the cause of our breakup, but became a very sore topic of conversation, because I couldn't accept the fact I couldn't heal or strengthen my feet, and why none of my orthotics ever felt right.

During this time I did the California Ironman, a contest that involved a 1.2-mile swim, a 112-mile bike ride, and a 26.2-mile marathon run to finish things off.

My feet had been hurting so much in training that I'd substituted snowshoeing at a high altitude for the running. It felt great, but you can guess the result. I finished the competition, but I had to walk the second half of the course *backward* because my feet were in such pain. It was a combination of weak feet, plus new, squirmy, heavily cushioned shoes that did me in, though at the time I didn't know it. Instead, I thought we just hadn't gotten the orthotics right.

During our entire time together, we couldn't get the orthotics figured out. Afterward she sent me to a new podiatrist and I asked him for foot exercises. Instead, he scoffed at me, saying nobody can strengthen their feet. His advice: stop running, never go barefoot, and don't skate. My feet were too weak and would never improve. I didn't follow this advice, of course, but a year later, while still struggling with my feet, I was injured in my near-death accident. Out of that, things changed, and through barefoot walking and running, I began to grow stronger. I ditched my orthotics, and eventually all support under my feet. Yet my feet never fell apart. Instead they grew stronger, wider, and healthier.

To build your strongest feet ever, it helps to understand what the foot really is, its integral parts, and how these parts work together.

Our feet are incredible massive springs that are meant to coil and recoil with every single step. They're also dynamic—able to handle different contours, surfaces, speeds, and angles, all in an instant. They house thousands of nerve endings that enable us to sense or feel for the ground, giving us fantastic balance and the ability to handle challenging three-dimensional surfaces. There's nothing in the mechanical world—not even robots—that matches the sophistication, complexity, and multitasking ability of the foot.

AND NOW ... THE FOOT

The human foot is a masterpiece of engineering and a work of art.
—Leonardo da Vinci

Let's look at the inner workings of this marvel. Since this isn't a high school biology class, we'll just briefly cover the basics, starting from the inside out, and head to specific parts of the foot.

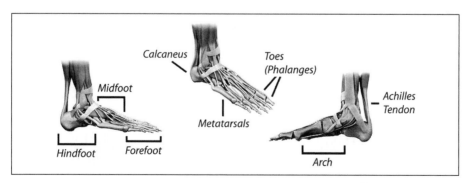

A sophisticated and remarkable design of nature, the foot provides strength, stability, and amazing shock absorption when allowed to work and move freely.

◐°°°₀ FOOT NOTE

Helpful Terms to Know

BONES. Your feet have more than one-quarter of all of the bones in the human body—fifty-six in all. Each foot has twenty-eight bones, each with its own unique purpose and design. There are fourteen toe bones that grab, five midfoot metatarsals that act as springs, and seven bones of the hindfoot or heel, which help support weight and hold everything together. Plus there are two little ones in each foot, called sesamoid bones, under the big toe's joint, which protect its large tendon. Consider the bones the foundation of the foot. They're what hold it together and help turn it into a spring.

JOINTS. All bones connect or hinge at joints. There are thirty-seven different joints in the foot.

LIGAMENTS. There are 107 ligaments that crisscross the joints in the foot. They're semielastic fibers that help the joints move at hinges. Since they stretch a bit, they allow the joints to expand or open up a bit when you move, helping with shock absorption and handling weight.

CARTILAGE. This resilient connective tissue covers and connects bones, providing cushioning and protecting against shock.

MUSCLES. There are nineteen different muscles of the foot. Each pulls on an individual tendon that attaches to a bone to provide support and move joints.

TENDONS. Each foot has nineteen tendons—highly elastic fibers that connect muscles to joints. Each muscle has a connecting tendon. This is where the majority of the energy is stored in the foot, as tendons can store and return up to 93 percent of the energy they receive.

SWEAT GLANDS. Your foot has more than 250,000 sweat glands, capable of producing over a half pint of sweat from each foot daily (an important reason to wear breathable footwear if you must wear shoes at all).

PLANTAR FASCIA. A broad span of ligament-like tissue which fans out across the sole, covering the foot from the forefoot to the heel. This tissue, the plantar fascia, helps hold the foot together and provides cushioning.

These three main sections of the foot work together:

1. **Midfoot**—made up of slightly bow-shaped bones, called metatarsals, which help absorb energy
2. **Forefoot**—comprised of toes and joints that grab
3. **Hindfoot**—made up of the largest bones of the foot, which help with weight bearing and providing stability

The Midfoot Bridges

One way to view the foot is as a living, breathing bridge. It absorbs energy, returns it, and despite a heavy load always returns back to center. You can think of the foot as a two-level bridge: above is a high-tension suspension bridge, and below are giant stone arches.

The five metatarsals of the foot and their ligaments, tendons, and connective tissue act as giant energy storage devices and shock absorbers. They're held together under tension, and when you add weight, they get even tighter. Step down, and your midfoot stores energy. Step up, and it snaps or springs right back into place again.

The metatarsals are also special because each one can move independently of the others, allowing the foot to change shape and mold to the terrain. This helps you keep your balance and stability even on the harshest of terrain. (That is, unless you keep your foot in a shoe, in which case you lose all of this midfoot flexibility and strength. In essence, you lock out your adaptable spring, which hinders your ability to absorb impact and handle uneven terrain.)

Beneath the metatarsals are two giant arches. There's one stretching the length of the foot, and one stretching the width of the foot. An arch is defined as a weight-bearing structure that gets *stronger* under load. This is particularly important because your arches don't collapse under weight, as you've likely been told, but instead get stronger. Trouble is, if you don't use and strengthen the muscles that hold the arches up, they become atrophied and inflexible. Once this occurs, the connective tissue, commonly plantar fascia, is forced to hold the arches up. Since plantar fascia were never intended to do the work of muscles, they become stressed, strained, inflamed, or torn. And voilà—you have a recipe for plantar fasciitis.

If you keep your muscles strong, however, and allow them unrestricted movement, the suspension bridge above and the arches below will take almost all of the force you apply on landing and return it right back. In essence, your foot can turn gravity into forward momentum. What an incredibly efficient device!

A note about arches and bridge design: Stone arches work fantastic under compression, but don't do well with twisting, pulling, or shearing. Human bones work just the same way. They're one-fifth the weight of steel, but can handle twice the compression force of granite and four times the force of concrete. However, just like granite and concrete, human bones can't handle shearing, pulling, or torsion forces, the *exact* forces amplified by most shoes.

Look at your foot. Lift your toes, then curl them. As you flex things, can you see the cables of your foot (your muscles, tendons, and to a lesser extent your ligaments) tighten and release? This is your suspension bridge. Your foot is a series of cables or wires working in harmony under tension. In combination with your arch, these cables work to absorb energy when you land or step down and rebound this energy when you lift off the ground.

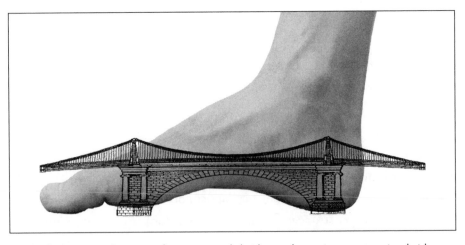

The foot is a combination of a strong arch bridge and a springy suspension bridge, providing incredible support, flexibility, and propulsion.

The Forefoot Anchor

For a bridge to be strong, it needs support at both ends. This helps anchor the arches and tie in the cables of your suspension bridges, known as your feet. The two ends of your bridges are your toes and your heels. The small bones of the toes (three in each small toe, two in the big toe) connect to eighteen of the nineteen muscles in your feet. This is important, as strong toes strengthen and hold together your entire foot.

Few people realize that when you walk, your toes should be active. Barefoot, you pull up your toes (dorsiflexion) before meeting the ground (which ensures they clear obstacles), and upon landing your toes push down (plantar flexion), grabbing the ground and bracing the arch.

Additionally, when you walk you naturally roll your foot gently from the outside (landing around the fifth metatarsal, or behind the fifth toe (your pinky toe), inward to the first, or big toe. It should be a subtle movement, like lightly tapping the keys of a piano, that further helps absorb and dissipate shock while loading the springs of the foot. By rolling your foot and tapping the keys, you're landing lighter than you ever could in a shoe, even a minimalist one. That's because a shoe has a stiff, rigid bottom that doesn't allow you to gently land from the outside to the inside (with the exception perhaps of moccasins or moccasin-like shoes).

When you work your toes, you strengthen your arch and your entire foot. Conversely, when your toes are weak, your entire foot is weak. This is exceptionally important, because in almost all modern athletic shoes your toes are eliminated from your stride. There's just no place for the toes to move up or down. Additionally, toe spring, the upward curvature found at the front of shoes, keeps your toes off the ground and out of the action, while stiff shoes further prohibit your toes from experiencing even a limited range of motion.

A last thought on the toes: Your toes naturally spread. If you look at the toes of someone who's been barefoot an entire lifetime, you'll see a natural large gap between the big toe and the second toe. The more your toes spread, the wider your forefoot, the greater your stability when you stand, walk, or run, and the more you spread out the impact.

Picture the difference between a narrow foot and a wide foot as the difference between sinking through snow in a regular shoe and staying on top of the snow in a snowshoe. When your toes can spread, you have a bigger paddle for propulsion, balance, and weight distribution, keeping you from harm.

Unfortunately, when you're in a shoe, your toes are bound in a very narrow passageway, keeping them from spreading. Over time, this can even change your feet to where your first and fifth toes tend to point inward. By keeping your feet from spreading, you're not only losing surface area for balance and stability but reducing the landing zone of the foot, forcing tremendous pressure onto a very small part of the foot.

The Hindfoot Anchor

At the other end of your bridge are the seven big bones of the foot, all intricately wedged together like fine masonry. While these bones have some ability to rotate the entire foot slightly inward like a screw, overall they have limited mobility, because their purpose is to anchor the foot and bear heavy weight.

These seven bones give your feet great strength and stability for carrying heavy loads or walking on very uneven or challenging surfaces. What they do *not* do is store energy. That's the combined job of your forefoot and midfoot. And that's important because when you strike with your heel, you're not taking advantage of your foot's natural spring.

Your foot and leg work together as a natural shock absorption system. The midfoot and arch constitute your first shock-absorbing spring, while your Achilles tendon—the strongest, most resilient, and most elastic tendon in your body—acts as your second. Your Achilles tendon connects your calf to your heel and can handle nearly a ton of weight. This tendon is essential for efficient movement and forward propulsion. Unfortunately, when you strike with your heels, you lock out almost all of its abilities.

Our feet are efficient because each part is allowed to move independently, and everything works together to move and adapt to the terrain. Each part of the foot is integral to the whole, and each has its own independent job. Yet when you put that foot in a shoe, you turn a multisegmented, dynamic, spring-loaded device into a solid block of wood. The foot can only work its magic if you promote its strength and flexibility, allow it to move freely, and, in particular, allow natural motion of the toes.

CONDITIONING EXERCISES

This unique sequence of exercises was adapted from Pat Guyton and Jan Dunn, who teach the Eric Franklin conditioning method (www.franklinmethodtrain ing.com) along with Pilates for rehabilitation and dancing. It's a great way to warm up the feet, get the muscles firing, and help train the connection between your mind and feet.

In short, the following exercises, all of which can be done on their own or as part of this warm-up series, do four key things:

1. Warm up foot muscles
2. Stretch out the foot
3. Strengthen foot muscles
4. Establish a kinesthetic loop between your brain and your foot

In essence, these exercises help wake up the neurological connection between foot and brain, which is essential for strength, movement, coordination, and balance.

P.S. You can do many of these exercises while seated at your desk while working on other things. Don't tell the boss.

Step 1: Loosen up. Obtain a small inflatable ball, just bigger than a tennis ball (we use the Eric Franklin 10 cm textured balls and 10 cm smooth balls and equivalent RunBare balls). Begin by moving the arch of your foot back and forth across the ball for a minute. You don't need to bend or move your knee to do this. Just roll your foot from front to back slowly.

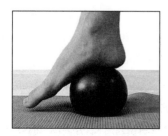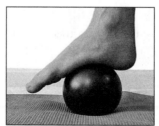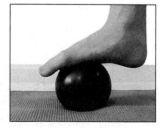

Rolling your foot back and forth on a ball helps wake up the nerves and muscles of your feet.

Step 2: Stretch out your metatarsals. After a minute, begin moving your forefoot from side to side over the ball. Move it down to one side, and then back down to the other, repeating five times. This is also a great exercise for building flexibility in the forefoot, as it relaxes and stretches the ligaments and tendons between your metatarsals, important for keeping your feet supple and healthy, particularly when walking on uneven terrain.

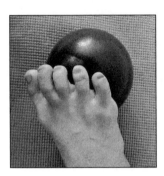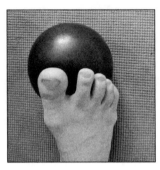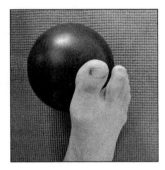

Wake up your metatarsals by rolling your forefoot sideways and down while hugging the sides of the ball. Roll down one side, then back up and down the other.

Step 3: Wake up your dorsiflexors. After you've awakened and stretched out your metatarsals, continue rolling your forefoot slowly sideways across the top of the ball, but this time raise your foot as you raise your toes. This is the reverse of the previous exercise. Repeat this for a set of five to each side as well. This helps reawaken the flexibility and strength of the extensors in your toes, which is particularly important for keeping your toes above the ground (before impact). In other words, you'll prevent toe stubbing.

Step 4: Get jiggy with the heels. Next roll your foot forward on the ball until your forefoot's on the ground and your heel is on the ball. Then roll your heel side to side over the ball, repeating five times. Again, you don't have to flex or move your knee. All movement should come from the foot. This helps awaken rotational control of the foot, something that's dormant in a shoe.

Step 5: Say hello to your toes. Next, roll your heel back and put your toes on top of the ball. Grab and dig into the ball with your toes for one minute, grabbing and releasing.

Before we get into the strengthening exercises, Michael has another personal favorite warm-up exercise you may already be familiar with: Foot Circles. With your leg extended on a bench, rotate your foot counterclockwise for ten circles without moving your leg. Then reverse direction for another count of ten.

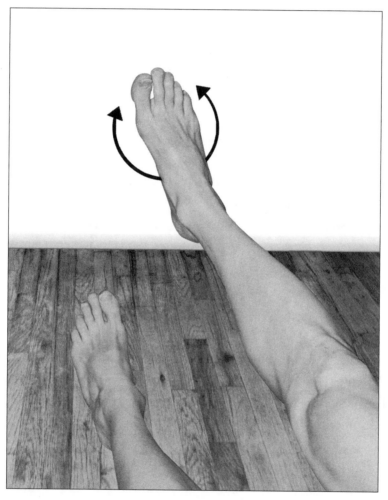

Draw circles with your feet, moving only from the ankles (try to keep your leg still in the air).

STRENGTHENING EXERCISES

This section describes exercises for building foot strength, coordination, balance, and flexibility. *Grabbing exercises* can be practiced daily over time. However, more intense exercises, such as *raising exercises, resistance band exercises,* and *toe movement exercises,* should be practiced at most every other day, just like lifting weights.

Remember, you build muscle by stressing the fibers, which then rebuild and become stronger. Because of this process, you never want to work muscles that are still sore; you won't make them stronger, but simply delay recovery at best, or tear muscles at worst.

In a nutshell, the process is as follows:

Step 1: Overwork your feet very slightly. A small percentage of muscle fibers in your feet are torn down.

Step 2: Stop and rest, providing your feet time to recover. Your miraculously adaptable body responds by growing the muscle fibers back stronger than before.

Step 3: Repeat steps 1 and 2. Very slowly but surely, your feet grow stronger and stronger.

As you continue this process—gradually and patiently, over the course of several months—you're likely to develop marvelously strong feet that let you walk bare for long periods, and even under extreme conditions, without significant harm.

◐°°₀ FOOT NOTE

Delayed-onset muscle soreness (DOMS) is muscle soreness experienced on the second and third days following the start of a new exercise, movement, or exercise program. Anytime you tax your muscles, whether you're walking or running, doing bicep curls or bench presses, you are essentially creating microscopic tears to the muscles, which take time to heal. Beginner barefoot walkers commonly experience DOMS in the feet and calves, though it's not unusual to experience DOMS elsewhere. It's not something to worry about; however, never repeat the offending exercise that made you sore until you're 100 percent recovered.

While it may seem counterintuitive, this process of going slowly is actually the fastest—as well as the safest—way to develop your feet.

Grabbing Exercises

By strengthening the toes, you strengthen the entire foot and help build healthy arches. These exercises help you warm up before barefoot activity and help sustain healthy circulation levels in your lower legs and feet while sitting at a desk or on a plane.

- **Golf Ball Grab.** Described in detail in chapter 7, this is one of the best exercises for your feet. Simply grab a golf ball with your toes. Hold for five or ten seconds; then repeat. Do a set of ten to twenty grabs your first time; then build up from there. As we've seen, almost every muscle of your foot attaches to your toes. By grabbing a

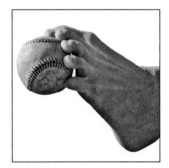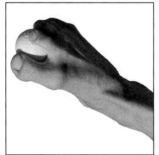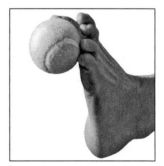

Strengthen your feet by working to grab a golf ball. Jessica has worked her way up to tennis balls and baseballs.

ball, you're working nearly every muscle of the foot, and in particular, you're waking up and strengthening your long-dormant arch.

Variations: If you get really good, you can try picking up the ball, passing it from foot to foot, and even work up to larger balls, such as tennis balls and baseballs. Try walking around your house holding golf balls with your feet, or do a Pilates or balance routine without letting go of a ball. Want to work on toe coordination? Consider lifting marbles as well. Try to lift them with each toe, rather than just with your big toe.

- **Towel Scrunch.** This is a simpler version of the golf ball grab. Simply roll up a towel, place it beneath your feet, and grab it with your toes. Hold for five to ten seconds; then repeat for a set of ten.

- **Desk Grab.** When you find yourself stuck at a desk for hours at a time, try grabbing the desktop or legs of the desk with your feet. Hold for a count of five to ten seconds. Then release. Or keep a golf ball under your desk, kick off your shoes, and strengthen those toes while no one is looking.

- **Inch Worm.** This is a more dynamic version of a scrunch or grab. It's easier to do this sitting rather than standing when you first begin. Grab the ground (any surface will work) and pull your foot forward and repeat, inch-worming along, until your leg is extended out in front of you. Then reverse direction and push your foot back with your toes. You may not be used to moving your toes this way; however, this aids with dorsiflexion (lifting up) with your toes, critical for a good stride.

Raising Exercises

- **Lifting Your Arch.** While standing with your foot planted firmly on the ground, imagine a string pulling through your arch and through the top of your feet. Lift your arch to the sky *without* moving your toes. Imagine your arch as a bridge that grows taller with each upward pull. Hold for a count of five and repeat for a total of ten times to begin.

• **Straight Toe Stands.** Standing in front of a mirror with both feet pointed in front of you (shoulder width apart), slowly raise yourself onto your toes, then lower your feet back down. Do this on a five count to begin, two seconds to raise your feet, and three to lower them. Concentrate on control over speed, going slowly and stopping just shy of your heels hitting the ground. Repeat for a set of ten to begin.

This exercise is also commonly referred to as a calf raise. While it does have the benefit of strengthening your calves and Achilles tendon, it requires the firing of nearly every muscle of the foot and ankle to do so, building foot strength, coordination, and balance.

Over time you can progress to three sets, then begin doing this exercise with one leg at a time. However, make sure you have your balance first—engage your core and make sure you do the exercise *without* holding on to anything. Too difficult in the beginning?

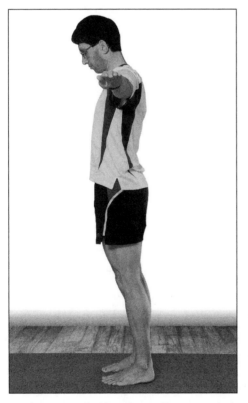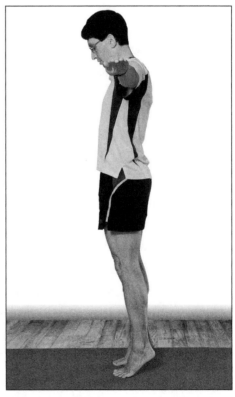

Slow, controlled barefoot calf raises with your arms extended give you greater muscle and balance coordination while strengthening your core.

Then hold on lightly (with your arms close to you so you're not leaning), and keep yourself tall and straight. If you're gripping too hard, you'll negate the benefits for your feet.

- **Ankle Rolls.** To begin, it's best to lightly hold on to a chair or counter for support. Stand in position as if you are about to do calf raises. Your feet should be set no farther than shoulder width apart, pointed forward. Begin by slowly lifting your feet off the ground, until you are standing only on your forefeet and toes. Then simultaneously rotate both feet in a circle (around the ankle) inward for ten repetitions, and then outward for ten repetitions. Do this to a count of two seconds per roll.

Resistance Band Exercises

These exercises can be done with physical therapy bands such as Therabands (different colors for different resistance levels), or even cut up old inner tubes. Start with very little resistance. Build up your number of sets, and then begin increasing resistance.

- **Rotating In.** Sit on the floor with your legs stretched out in front of you. Affix one end of a band to an object directly to your side and place the other end around your foot near the ball of the foot—up high, but where it won't slip off your foot. For the left foot, keep the band to your left side; reverse for your right. Gently and slowly rotate your foot inward while pivoting on your heel. Keep your leg on the ground and make sure there is no leg movement. This may feel awkward or jerky at first. Do the rotation on a count of three: one second to rotate in, two seconds to rotate back out. Repeat for a set of ten.
- **Rotating Out.** Repeat the same exercise but with the band and direction reversed. For your left side, place the band directly to the right of you, and vice versa. Here, slowly rotate your foot outward while pivoting on your heel, again with your leg on the ground and without leg movement. Repeat for a set of ten.

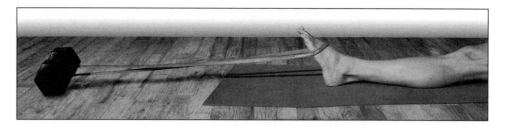

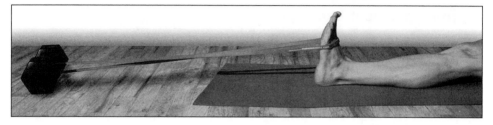

Make sure the band won't slip off your foot; then gently pull your foot up and toward you while keeping your heel on the ground.

- **Pulling In.** With the band directly in front of you, dorsiflex your foot (bring your forefoot toward you). This should also be done on a count of three and repeated for a set of ten.
- **Alphabet.** This should be done without resistance to begin, and then over time can be done with a resistance band of your choice. Keep

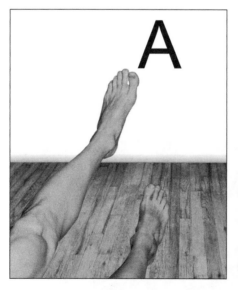
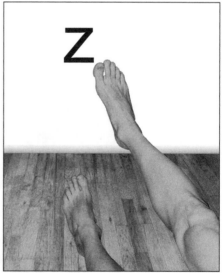

Draw the letters of the alphabet with your foot. Make sure you do not move your leg, only your foot and ankle.

your foot in front of you with your heel two to three inches above the ground. Using your forefoot, draw out the individual letters of the alphabet. Make sure you do not draw the alphabet with your leg. Try not to move your leg; this is a foot and ankle exercise only.

Toe Movement Exercises

People who are born without arms or have impaired arm ability often turn to their feet to do almost every daily skill others do with their hands. Our feet are capable of holding, writing, painting, cooking, turning doorknobs, and more, if we work on it diligently.

Babies use their feet as hands, grabbing and moving things with their toes, and even putting their feet in their mouths, until they're taught not to or have their feet put in shoes. Until that point they essentially have four hands, not two.

For these exercises, you must reawaken the coordination and movement of each individual toe. This can be challenging and take quite a bit of time and dedication. Start slowly and be patient.

- **Raising Toes.** This is the simplest one of the bunch. You want to be seated during this exercise with your foot firmly planted on the

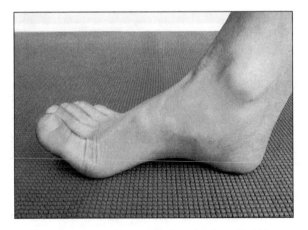

Raise your toes with your feet on the floor. Hold for a count of five, then repeat.

ground. From here raise your toes away from the floor and hold for a count of five. Repeat for a set of ten. As an advanced exercise, work on raising each toe individually, fanning out from your biggest toe to your smallest.

• **Toe Pump.** We learned this exercise from a Jamaican barefoot walker at a clinic in Baltimore. Simply scrunch or clench your toes together and hold for a count of ten. Then, instead of relaxing, spread your toes apart as wide as you can for another count of ten. Repeat three

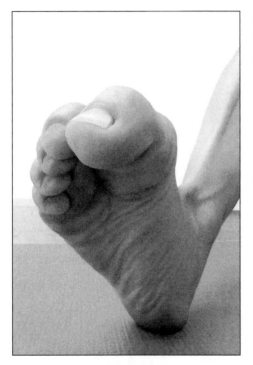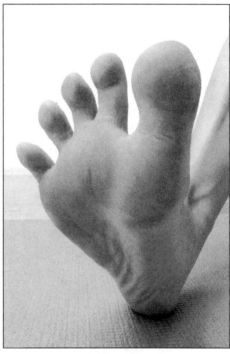

Scrunch your toes like a fist for a count of ten. Then spread your toes for another count of ten. Repeat three times.

times. If it's hard to get your foot to cooperate, do this with your hands at the same time: clench and hold, then spread and hold. By working opposing muscle groups, this exercise helps your toes relax, let go, and begin to spread again. In essence, you're helping your foot regain its natural shape and natural strength all at once! Repeat this every other day for best results.

• **Tapping Keys.** Pretend your toes are your fingers, and you're playing the piano. With your heel firmly on the ground, raise and lower each toe individually from your biggest to your smallest. You may have to visualize this in your head for many practice sessions before you can do it, but keep working at it, and you may amaze yourself!

◉°°· FOOT NOTE

Designed by foot surgeon Dr. Ray McClanahan, Correct Toes are a soft silicone toe-spreading device you slide gently between your toes. They're great for reversing the damage that's been done in a shoe, particularly for conditions such as bunions. Think of Correct Toes as braces not for your teeth, but instead for your feet. They work well if you gradually tighten them. However, you don't want to crank them down too aggressively or too quickly.

When using Correct Toes, Yoga Toes, or any similar device, add three to five minutes of usage every other day. Adding small increments of time is the safest way to progress and gradually help your feet return to their natural ways. If they get uncomfortable, you're probably going too long.

Use your Correct Toes right after you've taken off your shoes to help your feet relax after being cramped in shoes all day. You may also use them at the end of the day before heading to bed so your toes can get proper circulation and recovery while you sleep.

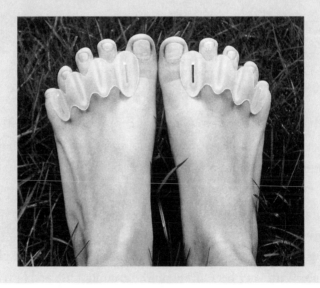

- **Toe Wiggles.** Whenever you get the opportunity—such as when you're sitting at a desk, attending a meeting, or riding in a car—simply spread out your toes and flex them up and down as much as possible. This helps with flexibility, dexterity, toe spread, and blood flow. The more you're moving your feet, the greater their circulation, and the more they heal and grow strong.

DYNAMIC STRETCHING

So far this chapter has discussed foot conditioning and strengthening, but foot conditioning extends well beyond the feet. Your body is like a marionette with interconnected strings (muscles and tendons) pulling to hold and move you.

If you've been stretching like crazy but your feet are still getting tight, or if you feel as though you can't overcome internal resistance in your feet, it may not be your feet at all. Another part of your body may be pulling on your feet. Your feet are your weak link, as they have the smallest muscles, ligaments, and tendons and are likely where you might feel a "problem" even though you may not have a foot problem at all. For instance, once Michael identified a weakness in his hip that manifested as foot soreness, he was able to stretch out his hips more, and the soreness went away. The key is to work on balancing and symmetrically strengthening and stretching the rest of your body. Grab a foam roll and tennis ball or RunBare ball and make sure you're stretching out all parts of your legs, plus your hip flexors, psoas, and glutes.

Here are some exercises to help you smooth out some weaknesses:

- **Rolling over a Ball.** Earlier we suggested using a golf ball for strengthening exercises, but golf balls and other similar balls (such as the RunBare foot ball) can also be used for stretching too. Rolling your feet over a golf ball or other hard ball is a great foot massage that helps loosen up your muscles and tendons. With the golf ball under your foot, slowly roll the ball around the bottom of the foot while seated or standing lightly, for a total of a minute or two. If you find any tight spots, keep the ball there for a few extra seconds; then move along slowly. Make sure you start this slowly (meaning don't use your full body weight or force on the ball) and work up very gradually, or you may bruise or strain the bottom of your foot. Over time this exercise will help keep your plantar fascia loose, as well as give additional flexibility between your toes.

- **Rolling Arches.** Standing with your foot firmly on the ground, roll your arch inward toward the ground as you gently squish your foot down to the inside, and then roll your foot back up to the outside. Repeat ten times. After a week or two, progress to two sets of ten, then eventually three sets of ten.

- **Log Roll.** Sitting in a chair with your foot out in front of you, hold your foot with your opposing hand, with your fingers on top of the forefoot, and your thumb under the ball of your foot. Picturing your foot or metatarsals as a series of logs, gently roll the logs (and your foot) as you roll the logs back and forth. Hold in each direction for a count of three; then repeat in the opposing direction. Move slowly and repeat for a set of ten. After a week or two, progress to two sets of ten, then eventually three sets of ten.

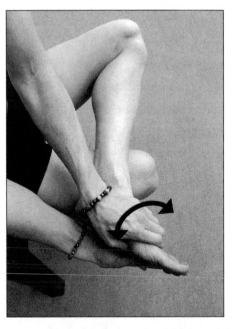 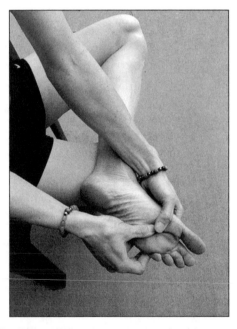

Gently roll your foot to the outside and then back in, imagining your metatarsals as logs rolling back and forth.

Work on moving slowly with proper form, rather than rushing through these exercises. It's best to teach your muscles to move individually and correctly, rather than using brute force and muscling through all at once. In all foot movement, you're shooting for gaining mobility, flexibility, strength, and control. You don't need to do all of these in one shot. Mix it up as often as you can to give your body as much variety as possible. Whatever you do, take your time, and have fun with these!

THE FOOT EXTERNALS

Feet have eyes—in other words, the sole has the ability to sense the terrain and maintain balance. It's said our soles have a "dynamometric map" for balance and control. By feeling the ground, they greatly assist in keeping us upright. In short, the feet act as an incredible biofeedback mechanism, sending valuable information to our nervous system to help control the incredibly sophisticated task of staying balanced.

In essence, "the feet at the ball and the heel act as two antennae that repeatedly scan the ground," according to *The Human Foot*, a textbook written for podiatric school students.

Feet were meant to feel the ground. They're not just equipped with more nerve endings than almost anywhere else on the body, but with more *types* of nerve endings. There are four different kinds of mechanical receptors or mechanosensors in the sole of the foot, including sensors for vertical pressure, local pressure, skin stretch, and rapid tissue movements. If you've ever stepped on a very sharp object or come down hard on a rock, you also triggered nerve endings or pain sensors that respond to high levels of force and pressure. Other types of nerve endings respond to lesser, dull pain in already damaged or inflamed tissue, such as when you've formed a blister from repeated stress to the foot. Both of these sensors work together to keep you out of harm's way from acute injury or overuse.

Unfortunately, when you place your feet in shoes, you deaden the effectiveness of your entire sensory feedback system.

Stages of Pad Development

1. Soft and tender skin gets compacted (moisture is squished or packed out) and begins to thicken for natural puncture protection.
2. Fat begins to get deposited under skin to act as a natural shock absorber.
3. Skin begins to harden to protect against blisters.
4. Skin begins to get shiny and "plasticized," particularly if walking on man-made surfaces.
5. As layer after layer of skin is deposited, the foot becomes thicker, even on the sides. Over time, you can expect up to half an inch of growth beneath your feet. (Yes, you literally do grow taller!)
6. Extra cushioning continues to be deposited to your thickened skin.
7. Gains become permanent—meaning the padding you've grown will last even through the winter.
8. You'll notice additional creases in your foot padding, especially beneath the transversal arch, the second arch that stretches across your forefoot. As your foot increases in flexibility, it will start to "fold" inward along the midline of your foot, allowing your foot to mold around objects such as rocks for stability. This folding action creates creases or lines (like palm lines) where the skin most often folds. (Check out a baby's foot sometime—babies haven't lost their foot flexibility yet, and therefore still have their handlike creases!)

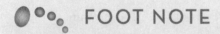 **FOOT NOTE**

Super Skin

How do you build stronger skin? Your plantar skin (skin on the bottom of your feet) is naturally 600 percent stronger than skin elsewhere on your body and can grow even thicker—up to half an inch—but only if you use it. (Think of being a half inch taller just by strengthening your skin! And that's before you begin to work on your posture too!)

As you start to go barefoot, you wake up this potential for "safety skin" on your feet. Being barefoot both stimulates additional skin growth on your feet (layering) and pushes the moisture out of the skin (strengthening). Together, by adding layers of skin and by strengthening the skin, you thicken the soles of your feet.

Grow Your Own Safety Skin

During the adjustment period, you can expect to experience scuffs or potentially even small cuts (we've found this quite rare, but it's worth a mention). As long as you're not rushing things, though, these will be minor nuisances rather than serious injuries. And whenever your skin heals from such nicks and tears, it will grow back stronger. Note: Never continue walking barefoot if you have an open cut. Always bring your "hand weights" with you in case of the rare boo-boo.

It will take months until you have "living shoes" that are both highly in tune with the environment and able to shrug off collisions with unexpected objects. Once you toughen up, though, you'll be surprised at what your feet can tolerate.

One important caveat is to beware of substances that reduce the hardiness of your feet. For example, walking on water- or snow-covered surfaces will soften your pads. That's okay if you remain on such mild surfaces for the remainder of your walk. But if you switch to a rougher surface while your feet are tender, they're likely to become raw and injured. This also goes for walking barefoot along the water's edge at a beach and then heading for higher, drier ground.

The same goes for walking in shoes—even minimalist shoes—that make your feet sweat and thus tender. If you take your shoes off in the middle of the walk, your feet may be extra sensitive to the ground. Always consider the state of your skin when selecting what ground to walk on, and always walk barefoot first, then put on the shoes—never the reverse.

As long as you maintain continual awareness of both your walking surface and your body, your "living shoes" will reduce your chances of a serious injury.

When you're in shoes, you can see these receptors at work because you develop calluses, or thickened, hardened skin, wherever you have an irritation with the shoe. What happens is the sensory receptor sends a message to the brain saying there's an irritation, and the brain sends a signal back to the foot to grow the skin thicker at the area of irritation. Calluses and corns then grow, which is nature's way of protecting your feet from that pressure spot.

We use this same feedback mechanism to grow thicker pads on our feet for barefoot activities. When you first go barefoot (no more than a hundred yards), you gently stress the bottom of your feet. This sends signals to your brain to lay down more skin to protect the feet. As new layers of skin are laid down and as you continue to be out of shoes, you push the moisture out of this skin. The thicker your skin, the more protection you have; the less moisture in your skin, the stronger it is and less susceptible to wearing down or being punctured.

To grow this thicker skin, you must work the skin (walk barefoot) and then rest the skin. If you don't give at least a day or two between barefoot workouts, you'll just keep wearing down the new skin you're trying to build. Expect your skin to feel hot and tender after your early workouts. This is your body's way to both stimulate growth and throw additional blood flow to your feet to grow additional skin. Respect this heat and the growth by resting between these workouts. It'll be a few months before you're ready to walk daily on your bare feet, but if you give the skin the time it needs, you'll be there before you know it.

Surefire Ways to Stimulate Pad Growth

Want to grow pads fast? While you can't rush Mother Nature, here are some elements to consider exposing your feet to. Just remember, your skin grows slowly for a reason. It's to keep you from doing too much. But with that said, the following list may help with your pads.

- **Pressure.** The more pressure you put on your skin, the better. Now this doesn't necessarily mean going out with a backpack full of bricks. This does mean that walking uphill or on coarser surfaces will stimulate pad growth faster than walking on flat, smooth ground, as you are forced to put down more pressure per square inch. Just remember that the more pressure you're putting on your skin, the more you're putting on the rest of your feet as well. Let it happen naturally, until your ligaments, tendons, and bones can handle the pressure. Resist the urge to build too quickly.

- **Pressure and pain.** If you step on something that makes you wince, as long as you're not bleeding on the spot, rest assured you're doing your feet some good. Those small pressure points will heal to grow stronger, thicker, and faster. Unfortunately, it's often the outsides of your big toes that take the biggest hits from pebbles. Ouch! This does help the feet, but can hurt like a bugger!
- **Duration of contact.** Over time, the more distance you put on your feet, the better. Time on the feet is essential. Just be sure not to walk too far and scuff your feet raw. Build up slowly and rest in between.
- **Intensity.** Walking uphill on the balls of your feet is a way to grow your own shoes quickly. Why? Because you're really pushing into the ground to lift yourself up the hill.
- **Dirt and trails.** We recommend spending time in the dirt. When you walk on the roads, only your contact points with the roads get stronger and tougher. The skin under your arches stays far too soft. This can be dangerous for stepping on sharp objects or rocks on the path. Not only do dirt surfaces provide natural pressure spots (small rocks and other things) to stimulate quick growth, but the dirt seems to aid thickening of the skin. Dirt and trails have the added benefit of positively affecting and protecting more of the foot.
- **Heat.** Our bodies are amazingly adaptable, if we start slowly enough. For Michael, nothing beats heat for quick skin and pad development. The hot pavement also feels good underfoot, once you're used to it. But you must start slowly, or dance with the heat in extreme moderation. Moderate or even excessive heat can stimulate fast skin growth as long as you don't go too far. In springtime or on your first walks in heat, pay careful attention to pain, and let it be your guide. Avoid blisters or burns by stopping early and putting on your shoes. By the time your feet feel toasty, you're already doing damage.
- **Cold.** In moderation, cold is another great stimulator of foot changes and growth. As long as you don't expose your feet to frostbite conditions, cold temperatures can greatly increase pad development and vasculature to the foot. (More on adapting to heat and cold in chapter 16.)

Top Seven Ways to Maintain Pads During Inclement Weather

1. **Walk whenever possible.** Walk on dry pavement or dirt any chance you get as long as your feet aren't too cold. Dirt's preferred over pavement, but take whatever you can get. Go at a good pace, but not too fast, and warm up your feet first. If there's a chance of salt on the ground, make sure to wash your feet afterward and use an oil or balm to protect the skin and prevent cracking. Note: Avoid products designed to soften the skin and any foot products that appear to be laden with chemicals. We also avoid applying anything on our skin we wouldn't ingest—these do not promote long-term healthy skin and can be absorbed into your bloodstream.

2. **Head for the mall.** Do you have a mall with stone or tiled floors? People are often found walking in malls during early morning hours. Consider walking barefoot at your mall once or twice a week. While it's always best to wash feet after workouts, make sure to wash your feet after the mall. These floors are not as clean as nature and are washed with chemicals and solutions you don't want to leave on your skin.

3. **Make friends with a treadmill.** While treadmills can change your stride (more on this in chapter 11) and overall aren't the best, they're far better than nothing when it comes to maintaining your pads. Start slowly, vary the incline, and work those pads. Just don't go too far or too fast, particularly in the beginning, or your feet can become raw or blistered. (If you smell smoke on the treadmill, that really *is* your feet burning!)

4. **Protect your pads.** If you walk in snow and water, make sure you don't hit coarse dry pavement immediately afterward. Instead of protecting your pads, you'll end up scuffing skin off. These conditions may feel cool, but they don't promote pad growth.

5. **Feel the ground.** When you can't go barefoot, use shoes with an ultrathin sole, no thicker than a thin sock, to feel the ground. This helps maintain and stimulate fat padding growth just beneath the skin. With very thin shoes, such as those by Feelmax (with only a 1 mm sole), you can be building fat padding even during months and conditions where you dare not go bare.

6. **Keep your feet dry.** If you're stuck in shoes or in boots, make sure you

keep your feet dry. This helps you hold on to the skin you've worked so hard to get. Consider chalking your feet (with real chalk, not a synthetic version) before and after each time you put them in a shoe (never baby powder, which softens the skin). And make sure your shoes keep your feet dry. Better yet, consider shoes that allow your feet to breathe! Breathable shoes are a key to foot health if you must be in a shoe, but if at all possible, get out of the shoe.

7. **Beware of rock salt.** Rock salt is incredibly sharp and dangerous for bare feet. Salt breaks down tissue, and rock salt can quickly turn toughened skin to mush. It's insidious too because it can hide in melted snow, run off, or even coat dried sidewalks and roadways long after visible crystals disappear. If your feet have touched rock salt, make sure to wash them off!

PAMPERING YOUR FEET FOR RECOVERY

With all of these exercises, and with barefoot walking in general, your feet may get sore and tired. This is to be expected. As long as you start slowly and vow not to work out again until your feet feel fresh and recovered, you'll do fine. Take these additional steps to aid your recovery.

- **Ice down.** In the beginning your feet may get noticeably sore after a walk or strengthening exercise. We recommend cooling your feet off after workouts with five to ten minutes of icing, and repeating two or three times if necessary. Personally, we like the Mueller cold/hot wraps. They're inexpensive, are usually found at your local grocery or sporting goods store, are infinitely reusable, and allow you to Velcro the ice pack to your foot. It's clean, easy, and fast. We always keep a few packs ready in the freezer.

  For a relaxing alternative, if it's not too cold out, head to a local stream or creek, and soak your feet and legs in the water. This is not only soothing and healing for the body, but for the mind and spirit as well!

- **Mud up.** Even better than ice, we love healing mud for cooling things down and reducing inflammation. The healing benefits of mud can't be overstated. You can paint or dip your feet (or anywhere that's sore) in mud after a workout. We like a bentonite clay called Aztec Secret Indian Healing Clay, though there are many other brands available. You could even collect your own local mud too—the closer to home the better! This gives you instant vitamin G benefits, reducing inflammation and greatly accelerating the healing and recovery process. After the mud dries, flake off or wash off, and repeat as necessary.

- **Elevate.** If you've had a really good workout and your feet or legs are wobbly, prop them up on a chair, against a wall, or better yet on something found in nature, to let your feet and legs drain lactic acid, lymphatic fluid (from inflammation), and toxins so they can be removed from the body through the liver and kidneys. Our preferred support is a tree out on a trail or in our front yard. Using something outdoors allows us to take advantage of vitamin G, killing two birds with one stone, and expediting our recovery process even more. We simply lie down on our backs, and prop our legs straight up (at a 90-degree angle) against a tree for about twenty minutes or until our feet get tingly. This leaves your feet feeling lighter after your workout and gives you a chance to rest, relax, quiet the mind, and breathe.

- **Foot massage.** You never need an excuse for a good foot massage, but if you've been working your feet hard, we especially recommend you get one. A foot massage helps loosen the muscles, aids with flexibility, relaxes tense muscles, and aids with circulation—in other words, it doesn't just feel great, but helps your feet recover and grow back stronger. You can have one done professionally or by a partner, or you can even do a self-massage.

Nature's Foot Massage

Ready for some challenging terrain? Stone paths, pebbles, logs, and other uneven surfaces do an amazing job at massaging the bottom of your feet.

Think of uneven surfaces as the world's best massage, for the benefits are similar. First, they begin to wake up the nerve endings on the bottom of your feet, reestablishing the connection between your feet, your brain, and your body's sense of balance. Second, they help your feet gain new flexibility and return to their natural, pliable shape. Third, they may break down old scar tissue in the foot. And fourth, walking on uneven surfaces increases blood flow to the feet, particularly to parts that historically have had poor circulation. This additional blood flow is the cornerstone for overcoming injuries by bringing additional nutrients and oxygen to the feet.

Just make sure to introduce uneven surfaces slowly and never force the foot to flex in any way it doesn't want to.

How *Not* to Pamper Yourself

- **Pedicures.** Feel free to trim, buff, and paint your toenails as often as you like. However, avoid that pumice stone like the plague. For all the pedicure virgins out there, pumice stones are used to exfoliate or remove dead skin on your feet. In a matter of minutes they can sand months of your hard work away, reverting you back to the status of tenderfoot. We highly recommend avoiding this. (Note: We also recommend opting for nontoxic nail polish free of carcinogens such as formaldehyde—or, better yet, letting your true colors shine!)

- **Hot tubs.** Until gains become permanent, pads wear down quickly if your feet are wet. We've all seen our skin look like a prune after we're out of the water (this is actually an amazing design of nature, as your softened skin has greater traction on wet surfaces). Even a long shower or bath can temporarily soften our skin. Make sure you don't go barefoot on any dry or coarse surfaces until your feet are completely dry and your skin has unwrinkled and resumed its regular tautness.

- **Moisturizing socks.** Apparently there are two categories of moisturizing socks these days—those that come with lotion built in and those that are pulled over an already well-lotioned foot. If you get a pair of these for Christmas, we recommend repurposing the gift again the next Christmas. Soon moisturizing socks will become the next ten-year-old fruitcake that never gets eaten. A heavily moisturized foot becomes a highly sensitive and tender foot when it comes to barefoot walking.

GETTING TO KNOW YOUR FEET

Make your feet your friend.
—J. M. Barrie

Get into the practice of examining your feet daily and after your barefoot activities. If you take the time to look and touch, your feet can tell you a lot.

Inspect your feet. Is the skin still soft and tender? Are there any cracks that need attention? Any nicks or scratches you may not have noticed or areas of concern? Any tweaks of pain you hadn't noticed? And are they ready to actively walk barefoot again? By watching your feet, you'll learn about your body, figuring out what's right and what's not, what's working and what could be improved.

Self-knowledge and awareness are the keys to barefoot walking and perhaps to life as well. The better you know your feet, the happier and healthier you'll be. Take care of your feet, and you'll go far.

PART III

Tips for Strength, Nutrition, and Total Health

The best six doctors anywhere
And no one can deny it
Are sunshine, water, rest, and air
Exercise and diet.
These six will gladly you attend
If only you are willing
Your mind they'll ease
Your will they'll mend
And charge you not a shilling.

—Nursery rhyme quoted by Wayne Fields, *What the River Knows*, 1990

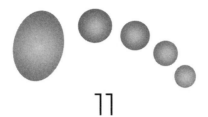

11

Conditioning the Barefoot Walker for Strength and Balance

If you built castles in the sky, your work need not be lost; that is where they should be. Now, put the foundations under them.
—Henry David Thoreau

When we first founded RunBare, a wellness center devoted to helping people experience the spiritual and antiaging benefits of reconnecting with the earth, we were told we could make a fortune selling our own line of clothing, fitness products, and health aids (such as skin care products). Ironic as it seems, nearly everyone suggested we design our own "barefoot-like" shoes and start selling those too. Well, unfortunately for us, we're not big on manufacturing more stuff that ultimately finds itself in a landfill. You could say we try minimizing our footprint on the planet when we can.

We are, however, big on using what nature provides. Sticks and stones really are the perfect tools for getting ourselves in shape. They're like nature's massage sticks, chin-up bars, balance beams, inflatable disks, and more. They don't require assembly, storage, maintenance, or cleaning. Best of all, they're completely free! And when you grow tired of them, there's no guilt in just leaving them where you found them. After all, that root and branch belong attached to the tree, that log will decompose into dirt in the woods, and that smooth round stone belongs alongside the river.

Says Jessica, "Spending quality time in the outdoors while I was nursing my foot back to full strength helped me discover this 'earth gym.' While I never looked forward to heading to the neighborhood fitness center, I always looked forward to discovering what natural tools I could find outdoors. My inability to run (or even walk quickly) was a true blessing in disguise, because slowing down encouraged me to be resourceful and be even more aware of my environment and connect with it in a new way.

"I started with simple exercises like rolling my feet over tree roots and round stones on the ground. This helped me warm up my feet and work out any knots in my arches, especially in my left foot, which hadn't been used in months. My entire left leg had weakened too during that time of healing, as I shifted the majority of my body weight to my right side. I needed to rebalance myself. So as my feet grew stronger, I started building strength in my ankle and leg by balancing on these same natural massage tools. Eventually, I progressed to balancing on logs. After six months, I found myself walking across low-hanging tree limbs.

"Six months may seem like a long journey, but the fun started from day one. That's the wonderful thing about the 'earth gym'—it's never boring."

We're always finding new toys to play with. Many of the tools mentioned in this chapter can be replaced with objects found in nature. See what you can find outdoors and enjoy the added benefits of vitamin G and dirt. Discover and create your own "earth gym."

The human body can handle almost any challenge or stress if it gets accustomed to it gradually enough. That's why karate experts can chop through cinder blocks with their bare hands and why great barefoot walkers can trek for many miles over extreme surfaces. But they didn't develop such skills overnight—and you shouldn't try to either.

This applies even if you're just getting started in a walking program or already an accomplished athlete. That's because your body adapts to very specific activities. So no matter your skill level, you'll need to slowly get used to landing on the balls of your feet.

You also know there's a lot more you can do to improve your health and stride than mere walking alone. To become the healthiest you can be requires work on alignment, flexibility, strength, rest, and proper nutrition.

In this chapter we'll look at fun ways to help you achieve your health goals. We'll get you fitter and stronger. We'll do drills, balance work, strength training, games, and more, helping you get started on the right bare foot (and then the left).

THE DANGEROUSLY WRONG WAY
TO CONDITIONING

Unfortunately, we often hear such slogans as "No pain, no gain" and "What doesn't kill you makes you stronger" misinterpreted to mean that it's a good idea to push yourself relentlessly without carefully listening to what your body is telling you. We even read popular books that immortalize athletes (most often runners) who have "broken through the barriers" and "pushed past the pain." The philosophy behind these slogans and stories causes people to do too much too quickly.

As a result, people overwork their feet, and then overwork them some more, without providing adequate periods for rest and recovery. Since the damage is cumulative, even if they don't feel pain right away, they're injuring themselves further and further as the days and weeks go by. So their attempts to rush through a transition to walking barefoot actually have the opposite effect by preventing them from being active at all.

Pain is your body's signal that something is wrong. Stop the cycle of pain by resting—days, weeks, whatever it takes. Give your body a chance to rest and recover. Our friend Zach Bergen was forced to take time off from barefoot activities because of an unrelated health issue that required surgery. Instead of weakening him, it gave his feet time to grow stronger.

Best advice: Don't do everything at once. Rather, pick and choose what seems like the most fun and go for it. Try new things out and feel free to mix up the routine. Your body is incredible at adapting to new challenges. So don't get stuck in a rut. Instead, change up your routine and mix and match drills and exercises as much as you can. This helps work muscle groups you never knew you had and loosens you up in ways you once thought impossible, so you can build a well-balanced body.

BAREFOOT DRILLS

Drills actively help you gain strength, coordination, flexibility, and balance. In the beginning, do drills on the same day as your walks, but only if you're not too fatigued. Don't do drills on your recovery days, as you need non-barefoot time to rest.

You can choose from an infinite number of variations. Just focus on proper body position or form, as described in the earlier chapter on getting started. These drills can be done with any of the three strides mentioned early in this book, though a feather walk (up lightly on your forefoot) is preferred. Whichever you choose is up to you and your strength. Remember, you don't need to push it to get into the best shape of your life, so err on the easy side. Keep your pelvis neutral in all exercises and keep your belly snapped in toward your spine, your chest wide, and that silver string pulling you toward the sky.

Remember, you're training your mind as much as your body—building that mind-body-earth connection, in essence rewiring your mind with each step. When you make a movement, you connect two neurons in your brain and each movement becomes a new physical connection. Over time, the neural connections become more permanent, and the movements more fluid. The trick is, if you perform the exercises in a sloppy fashion (such as bending forward or landing flat-footed), you'll wire sloppy connections. Focus on proper form over quantity. Less is more. Hardwire good moves and stop if you start getting sloppy.

Where to Begin

Consider practicing these drills out on the path every few walks. Once you get the hang of things, work on quick, fluid, yet snappy motions. Before you're done, you should feel as if you've been doing a dance.

You may incorporate the following drills into or before your walks two to three times a week. Part of the goal is to keep you flexible, strong, and balanced by doing different movements. So if you feel like hopping, skipping, or walking sideways during your walk, then go for it. The more you work your feet and legs in different ways, the healthier, more economical, injury-resistant, and stronger you'll be as a barefoot walker.

The following drills are particularly important for injury prevention. They help strengthen your hips and other stabilizing muscles, helping you prevent falls and giving you the anchor and stability you need to move without excess motion or wobbling.

EAGLE WINGS

Purpose:	Builds core, arms, and shoulder strength, balance, coordination, and efficiency. The more you engage your core, the easier all other movement becomes, whether walking, running, or any other activity.
Do this:	Lightly walk and extend your arms straight out to your sides at shoulder height. Concentrate on a tight core and keeping your upper body from moving, bending, or wiggling. Make sure you're not letting your head wag from side to side. Walk for approximately fifty feet. Over time do a little more, and then a little more, until you're incorporating at least a few minutes of Eagle Wings into your regular walks.
Imagine this:	Visualize your arms out to the sides like the wings of an eagle or a plane.

SIDE-TO-SIDE CRISSCROSS

Purpose:	Gain lateral coordination and learn to keep your weight centered as you strengthen your external obliques (side abdominal muscles).
Do this:	Instead of walking forward, walk directly to your side for fifty feet while crisscrossing your legs with each step. Going first to your left, cross your right leg over your left leg. Then, bring your left leg out from behind

your right. Repeat for fifty feet, then return in reverse, now crossing your left leg over your right leg.

Imagine this:	Picture yourself dancing like Gene Kelly in *Singin' in the Rain*.

THE REWIND

Purpose:	Keeps opposing muscles strong and helps prevent injuries by working on stabilizing muscles. This exercise also helps strengthen your feet, Achilles tendon, and calves by encouraging you to stay on your toes.
Do this:	Walk backward for fifty feet. Land on your forefoot to go backward with grace. Concentrate on staying relaxed and fully upright. Do not bend forward at the waist. This is another drill you can practice at length during your walks, particularly if your legs need a break to recover. Simply turn around and walk backward. Just make sure you keep checking behind you for safety, alternating looks from one side to the other.
Imagine this:	Backing away from a mama bear and her cub.

THE BALANCE BEAM

Purpose:	Improve balance, gain control of small muscle groups, and tighten core muscles.
Do this:	Simply see how long you can walk barefoot on the curb, putting one foot in front of the other.
Imagine this:	Visualize yourself up on a balance beam. Keep one foot in front of the other and make sure you don't fall off the beam.

BAREFOOT GAMES

Hot Potato

Work on passing a golf ball from your foot to your partner's foot as fast as possible. Or turn this game into a team competition and see which team can pass the ball around first. You can also do this solo—just work on passing a ball from one foot to the other while seated at your desk. It's more challenging than it sounds, but it builds dexterity, strength, and balance through coordination.

Slacklining

Slacklining is like walking a beginner's version of a tightrope and can be done right in your backyard or at your local park. We had a chance to try slacklining

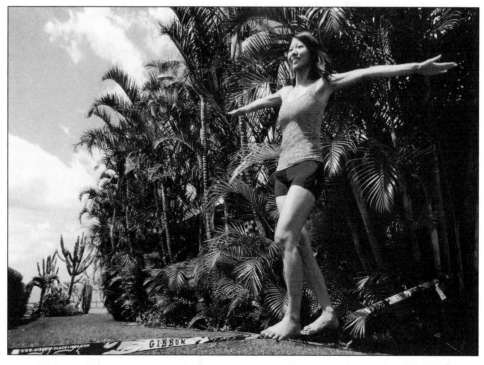

Slacklining is a great way to gain balance, strengthen your feet, and have fun. A Gibbon slackline kit is pictured here.

while spending some time in Boracay, Philippines, after holding a series of barefoot wellness clinics in that country. While there are more sophisticated (and stable) ways to go, the instructor simply took a piece of one-inch climbing harness webbing, attached it to two trees just a foot off the ground, and ratcheted it taut.

The goal was simple enough: try to walk barefoot from one end of the line (about twenty feet) to the other without falling off. Danger wasn't an issue, since it was so close to the ground and had soft sand underneath.

Walking a tightrope requires incredible balance and great sensory perception from your feet. However, slacklining is much simpler with two-inch-wide webbing beneath your feet. Companies such as Gibbon Slacklines sell slacklining kits with this wider webbing to make it much easier to get started (watch YouTube videos to see this in action). You can even buy a slacklining system that lets you set up a line in a large room or basement of your house. This is fun for the whole family, particularly in the wintertime, and boy, will the kids get creative given half a chance!

BUILDING CORE STRENGTH

To become an effective and efficient barefoot walker, you must work on core strength, stability, and balance, balance, and more balance.

Balance Exercises

Work on balance exercises either on a flat surface or using an inflatable disk or an inflatable half ball (also known as a Bosu ball). Try the following exercises standing on the floor or ground for one to three months (depending on how fast you progress) before graduating to an inflatable disk or half ball. Once you graduate to the inflatable device, start with both feet on the disk or on the platform of the half ball.

The more one-legged exercises you do, the better balanced, stronger, and injury resistant you'll be. Start with a set of eight to ten repetitions to begin, but if the going gets tough, trust your gut and cut the workout short. Over time, work up to three sets of eight to ten repetitions or more.

These exercises are some of the best (and therefore most difficult) exercises for strengthening your core and directly translating your balance to barefoot walking. In the beginning, allow two days between each workout. If your legs or feet get sore, apply mud or ice after your workout, and never do this workout two days in a row. Maximum benefits will begin after your first two to three weeks and occur if you're doing these exercises at least twice a week.

Start with your feet no wider than shoulder's width apart. The closer they are together, the more challenging the exercises will be.

For each of these exercises, snap your belly button in toward your spine and snap your core together (both belly and spine) as tightly as you can with each movement. With all exercises, except for Hundreds, inhale on the outward or upward movement (the beginning movement) and exhale on the return. As you inhale, bring your core in tighter. As you exhale, continue to hold your core in. (You should feel as if your core is getting tighter and tighter.) At first this seems counterintuitive, but with time becomes quite natural. This will help build stronger lungs and teach your diaphragm to relax while keeping your core engaged. Begin each exercise with one set of five to ten repetitions (never force, strain, or push yourself; if your body tells you to stop, listen). The goal is to work up to three sets of ten repetitions, which may take a month's time or more.

JUMPING JACKS—ENGAGES YOUR CORE AND UPPER BODY.

Start by standing on the ground or on an inflatable disk with your arms by your sides. Your weight should be centered over the balls of your feet with your heels just slightly off of the ground, while you work on grabbing with your toes. Slowly raise your arms up above you, as if you were doing a jumping jack, until your hands touch palm to palm above your head. However, do not jump. Do this to a count of three, then return your arms back to your sides for a count of three.

HUNDREDS—ENGAGES YOUR CORE AND UPPER BODY.

While standing, bring your arms out to your sides at shoulder level, palms facing down, as if you were flying. Keeping your weight on your forefoot, with your heel just slightly off of the ground, pulsate your arms

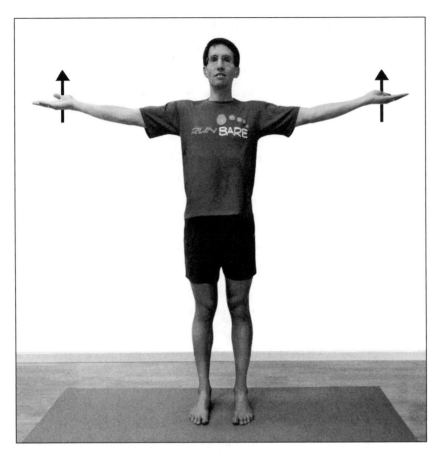

Hundreds.

downward five times with five short crisp exhalations. Next, flip your hands over so that your palms are now facing up, and pulsate your arms upward with five short crisp inhalations.

KNEE KICK—ENGAGES YOUR QUADS AND PSOAS.

With your arms out again to the sides, palms facing down, bring your left knee up in front of you slowly as high as you can to a count of three while inhaling and drawing your core in tight (as you'll do on all of these exercises). Return it to a count of three while exhaling, holding your core in. Then switch and bring your right knee up in front of you as high as you can to a count of three. Return it to a count of three as well.

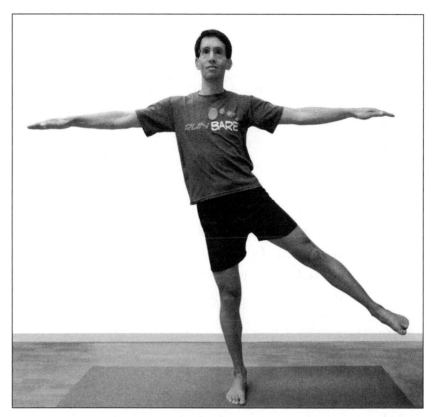

Side leg raise.

Maintain the same upper body and core positioning and breathing as in the Knee Kick, but now move your leg out to your side to a count of three, then return your leg in to your side in a slow and controlled manner to a count of three. Make sure you keep your arms level and do not lean. Lift as far as you comfortably can with your leg, then return.

Here you will use the same upper body, core positioning, and breathing as in the Knee Kick and Side Leg Raise. With your arms out by your sides, bring one foot up behind you until your knee is bent at a 90-degree angle. From here slowly kick your leg out behind you while maintaining the same bend at the knee. Bring your leg back slowly until you feel resistance, to a count of three. This is a very small movement exercise, typically no more than six to twelve inches to begin. Pay particular attention so that you don't bend forward at the waist to try to exaggerate your movement. Return in a very slow and controlled fashion.

PILATES

Another way to help hold your core in place and for a perfect warm-up is to do ten minutes of Pilates exercises before you walk. Pilates has a natural connection to barefoot walking because both require stability, balance, strength, and coordination that all come from the core. Pop in a DVD, follow along, and then head out the door.

Packs and Bags

If you really want to take your toning to the next level, consider getting a back-pack. Michael is a big fan of a small pack, particularly in the winter, as it helps him stay warm by making him work harder, and it carries a few extra pieces of gear (such as hand warmers, extra gloves, and dog treats) in case he needs them.

A backpack has several advantages when it comes to toning the body. First, it makes your whole body work harder to carry the additional weight and remain balanced. This means far greater fat burning and toning of the muscles of the entire body. Second, when you have weight strapped to your back, your heart and lungs have to work harder, thus you're getting a better cardiovascular work-out at the same time.

Michael's favorite packs are the ultralight models. No matter how much he wants to stuff the inside, he likes his packs light. He tends to get hydration packs (packs that are designed to carry water in addition to gear) and yank out the inner bladder unless it's needed. A few of his favorites are packs made by Inov-8 such as the Race Pac. They're superlight, sit on the back well, and, most important, don't bounce.

When it comes to choosing or using a pack, make sure it doesn't swing from side to side or up and down on your back. Look for one that has both a chest strap and a substantial waist strap (Some waist straps are too thin and flimsy to have any real benefit.) Once strapped in place, it should become one with your back. If not, it becomes a counterweight throwing off your gait and works against you, rather than with you.

If the pack causes you to bend forward at the waist, raise or lower the pack or stop using it in favor of another.

WEIGHT TRAINING

Weight lifting can help you gain muscle strength and balance in ways that are initially difficult for beginner barefoot exercisers. Over time, as you work on balance ball exercises and spend time on the trails, you most likely won't need weight lifting anymore. Sure, you don't really need it to begin with, but chances are you have some muscle imbalances. In other words, you may need to balance out muscles that are stronger, weaker, looser, or tighter than others.

Weight lifting can help particularly as you get into a barefoot walking program, or during the off-season (late fall through early spring in cold climates, when walking outdoors becomes more challenging). Weight lifting helps with injury prevention, proper form, greater efficiency, and endurance. Most important, weight lifting builds bone density and joint stability, and helps prevent falls at any age.

To get the most out of the gym, perform strength training two to three times a week. You don't need hard workouts here, just consistency. Work your muscles frequently, and they'll remember what you want and give you what you need.

The Overload Principle

As with all physical training, weight training works on the overload principle. Overload or strain the body slightly yet repetitively, and as long as you give your muscles time to rest and recover, they'll grow back stronger (this goes for our bones as well). This is the same principle that kept our ancestors alive for millions of years. Chase after prey today and struggle? You'll get stronger for your next hunt.

The overload principle works well as long as you don't overdo it and as long as you give yourself plenty of time for recovery. Rest for at least one day in between before heading back to the weights.

In order for the overload principle to work, you must teach or train the body on a regular basis. In other words, one weight-lifting session that gets you sore will do little to train and strengthen your muscles. You need to work muscles every few days in order for them to gain memory and strength. The first time you overwork something, it's unlikely the body becomes stronger. Instead, it just repairs the damage. But if done with frequency or repetition, such as two to three days a week, you'll become stronger, fitter, faster, and more resilient. However, if you don't give your muscles a chance to recover and grow back stronger, you'll just tear things apart instead of strengthening muscles.

Michael's Rules for Strength Training

- **Train in moderation.** Any extra weight you gain has to be carried by your feet and legs. Especially train your upper body in moderation.
- **Focus on form, not speed.** Anyone can throw a weight, but that's not the goal. The goal is to lift the weight slowly with control. Lift with a three count, lower with a three count. Your maximum gains come on the down part of the lift, or the eccentric muscle contraction, so return the weight slowly with full control.
- **Engage your core.** All of your power and strength comes from your core. It also helps protect your back and keeps you safe. So consider every weight-lifting exercise as an opportunity to strengthen your core. This means snapping your belly button in toward your spine with every weight-lifting move.
- **Build up gradually.** Even if your legs are strong from barefoot walking, the ligaments and tendons aren't ready for the new motions. They'll be foreign and create some strain for your joints in the beginning.
- **Listen to your body.** There's no set formula for how much weight to increase how quickly. Instead, just as in barefoot activity, you must become more aware of your body and its needs.
- **Think balance.** In every exercise you do, in each movement, seek balance between the right and the left, and each opposing muscle group. In other

words, work out each leg separately. We all have a weak side and a strong side. But barefoot walking is about a delicate, soft, balanced stride. This means you need to correct imbalances in strength and stride equally with both sides.

- **Concentrate on higher repetitions and lower resistance.** For example, if you're doing leg extensions using light weights, do a set of ten to twelve repetitions with your right leg, then the same number with your left. Remember to go extra slowly and controlled.
- **Recover, recover, recover.** Always rest at least one day between weight-training sessions.
- **The 90-degree bend rule.** Stay safe in the gym by never exceeding 90-degree bends with your joints. If you're doing a hip sled, standing squat, or lunge, don't bring the weights so far down you bend your knees more than 90 degrees. The same goes for leg extensions or any other exercise. Always stop at 90 degrees.
- **Never lock your knees.** When doing a hip sled or hamstring curl, never lock your knees or bring them fully vertical. Instead leave a slight bend in the knees so they're not forced backward or hyperextended . . . ouch!
- **Stop early.** Are your legs wobbly? Or have you done the suggested number of reps but think you can do more? Stop. Save it for next time. Your goal here is slow, steady building to help your barefoot walking, not to risk injury while becoming the strongest guy or gal in the gym. It's too easy to rip, tear, or overuse muscles, especially when you're just working for a bit of tone, strength, and balance. Remember your priorities, and live to lift another day!

Weight-Training Plan for Beginners

Walk on fresh legs *before* you lift weights if possible. Barefoot walking on tired legs not only promotes poor form but can lead to overuse injuries because your stride changes to accommodate your wobbly muscles, and your feet and legs aren't as elastic or flexible as you'd like them to be. Remember, walking is the priority, not lifting. You can lift weights on your days off from barefoot walking, as long as you're not also barefoot in the gym. Remember, for the first three months the feet need time to recover in between barefoot walking workouts.

For the first session in the gym, do one set of each exercise, with zero resistance. For instance, if you're doing lunges (an exercise where you squat down with one leg at a time in front of you), do a set of ten to twelve repetitions without holding any hand weights. A set of hamstring curls? Keep the pin out of the machine weight stack and again do one set of ten to twelve repetitions with zero resistance.

Yes, for some it may seem ridiculously easy at first. But remember, you're not building muscle strength in the beginning; you're building ligament and tendon strength. The neural pathways help the muscles learn the new movements and fire effectively.

At your second session (at least two days later), do two sets with zero resistance. If it isn't a struggle, move to three sets with zero resistance at your third session. On your fourth day of lifting (this should be after a week), add light resistance to your third set. On your fifth day, add light resistance to your second and third sets, and on your sixth day, you can add light resistance to all three sets. From there on out, the simplest rule is that if on your third set you can comfortably do ten to twelve repetitions at a given resistance level, very gently increase the resistance for the next lifting session (for example, if you could lift twenty pounds for three sets on Wednesday, go to twenty-five pounds for three sets on Friday).

Another option is to lift following a pyramid progression. Michael's favorite method: lift one set at fifteen pounds, one set at twenty pounds, then one set at twenty-five pounds.

For the first three months, wear shoes in the gym. After that, you can go barefoot if it's safe and acceptable. This helps you feel the exercise better and works your toes, feet, and legs for greater balance. However, if it's not comfortable for you or permitted by the establishment, then no worries. An alternative is wearing indoor toe socks, or a moccasin-like shoe. They still let you use your toes to grab the floor and allow free movement of your feet. However, they won't get you kicked out of the gym.

Being barefoot in the gym helps you feel imbalances and asymmetries in terms of strength, flexibility, and form. Think of it like a martial arts expert: they wear either nothing on their feet or the most minimal kung-fu slipper (another option if they're wide) so that they can sense what's going on. Lifting weights, even upper body movements, such as bicep curls, are felt through the feet. Lift one side better than the other, and you'll feel it. Jerk the weight around instead of moving slowly with controlled movements, and you'll feel that too.

An argument can be made that you want more protection for your feet in case you drop a dumbbell or weight on your foot. However, if you have the misfortune of dropping a weight on your foot, unless you're in a steel-toed boot, any protection is likely too little. Best to be extra careful in the first place, never to rush, and be mindful of what you're doing. And when you're barefoot, you are *extra* careful.

Toning the Arms

First the bad news: fat can't be toned. Unfortunately, there's no way to firm up flabby upper arms or magically turn fat into muscle. This means that to see the tone in arms, you need to lose some body fat.

Burning fat is a total body workout, and the good news is, so is barefoot walking. Just the very act of carrying yourself on the trails without the support of your shoes works to strengthen and tone your entire body—and burn extra calories.

You've heard the benefits recently claimed by the walking shoe companies. Well, those are real when it comes to barefoot walking. You're going to work extra muscle groups, tone your thighs, tighten those buttocks, and work on your abs, arms, and back.

This is especially great news for the arms. Walking barefoot means you need to use your arms as counterweights to keep yourself upright and moving forward. Even more than in a shoe, this means you strengthen your arms as you walk.

And the more you walk or hike on uneven surfaces, the more you need to balance, and therefore the more you strengthen your arms. Think of your arms as being the balancing pole held in the grip of a tightrope walker: the more challenging the crossing, the longer the pole the tightrope walker uses. Our arms are like the poles of the tightrope walker. We use the arms for balance, particularly in challenging situations.

Don't Be a Dumbbell

Michael says, "As a kid, I used to run around with ankle weights attached to my lower legs. As an adult, I tried holding dumbbells in my arms as I ran. They always threw off my stride, causing me to lumber along. My calves got sore, for sure, as did my biceps, triceps, and shoulders, and it never felt quite right."

That's because whether running or walking, weights inherently change your gait, and not for the better. In fact, carrying dumbbells and throwing the arms back and forth (or in a curling motion) throws your arms into opposition with your legs. It's as if you're in competition between your arms and your legs, creating twisting and torque throughout your body, and in particular your hips and back.

When you're walking barefoot, everything needs to work together and in proper alignment. We develop a strong core and toned arms, because everything is recruited to work together to help you find the lightest, most natural stride.

So for now, leave the real weights behind.

TREADMILLS

Are treadmills good or bad, and how do you get into them barefoot?

Approach treadmills with caution. They're a good winter training tool but can bite you if you don't use care. They are, however, a useful real-world compromise for barefooting in the cold.

If you start slowly, the friction on the nylon belt does wonders for pad development. But proceed with extreme caution. A treadmill radically changes your step and the forces involved and can wear off your pads in an instant. Having a belt coming toward you, a control panel before you, and a cushioned platform all change your gait and make you land hard. Add a little ego to the mix, or a desire to see your pace or incline go up, and you can quickly get yourself in trouble.

To safely traverse the treadmill, follow four simple rules.

1. **Let the heat on your skin be your guide.** If your feet start getting hot, even if the skin looks good, call it a day. Never go to the point of blistering, and if you've scuffed your toes raw, give them plenty of time to rest. If you smell something burning on the treadmill, that's your feet. Friction between your feet and the nylon belt can really heat up the skin.

2. **Never walk the treadmill two days in a row.** In fact, if you're scuffing your skin up pretty good, don't use the treadmill more than every third day until the skin's grown stronger. Remember, if your skin's cooked, so is everything else on the inside.

3. **Never exceed your form.** Consider glancing into a mirror and seeing how smooth and symmetrical you are. If your form starts looking sloppy or you start landing hard, slow down or hop off. Watch for a head bounce too. If you feel force resonating up through your heels, either check your form or hit the stop button. Walking with poor form not only habitualizes poor form but can lead to injury fast.

4. **Don't watch the TV.** If you're watching a TV while walking on a treadmill, you can't watch your form. On a treadmill or on a trail, being present in the moment is essential for proper form and for staying safe. Take off the headphones and ask, "How little noise can I make?"

Getting Started on a Treadmill

Instead of starting into treadmill walking once every other day, begin with every third day, at least for the first two weeks. Best advice: start with five minutes max, then adding two minutes, every third day. Here is a good general progression to follow (in minutes): 5 ➝ 7 ➝ 9 ➝ 11 ➝ 13 ➝ 15 ➝ 17 ➝ 19 ➝ 21. A key note, if this is your first foray into barefoot walking, please read chapter 8, Ninety Days to Barefoot Freedom, and start with a maximum of one minute at one to two miles per hour on the treadmill, or the equivalent of approximately 100 yards to begin.

During the first four sessions, keep the treadmill flat. After that you can begin adding an incline, but no more than a 1 percent grade increase per session. Start flat to warm up, add an incline for the first half, then lower the incline for the second half. After the first month a preset hill program or interval routine can help you mix things up and keep you changing pace. Never increase your grade or speed more than 1 percent or a tenth of a mile per hour per workout. You can hold on to the treadmill as needed, but do not lean forward or put weight on your arms. This encourages a pelvic tilt, hunched back, poor form, and over time, overuse injuries. You want to stand nice and tall, with that silver string pulling you to the sky.

These rules may seem quite stringent, but we have heard from countless people who've done too much, too quickly on a treadmill and have gotten injured (Michael included).

Alongside overall fitness gains, your first priority on a treadmill is to increase distance, rather than speed or grade, to build a base, and to accomplish this without sacrificing form. This gives ligaments, tendons, and bones a chance to grow stronger, without the risk of injury.

Minimalist Footwear on Treadmills

Many people use the treadmill to work their way into minimalist shoes. We prefer barefoot first, or even a pair of socks, before you use minimalist footwear. This is especially important on a treadmill where the cushioning, belt, and speed all conspire against you. In minimalist footwear it's easy to overdo it since you can't feel what's going on beneath you, adjust your stride, and let your skin be your guide.

CROSS TRAINING FOR BAREFOOT WALKERS

Cross training or doing activities other than walking is a smart way to build form, strength, and fitness. By working muscles you might not target with barefoot walking, you build a stronger, more balanced body, prevent overuse injuries, and keep your mind fresh.

Choose from an almost infinite number of possible activities for cross training. If it gets your heart rate up and works different muscles without impact, then you're probably on the right track.

Cross-Training Guidelines

When it comes to cross training, follow these key rules:

- **Do all exercises 100 percent erect.** This means standing tall without leaning forward at all. Never stick your butt out or curve your back, but keep your core engaged, your back strong, and your posture tall. Remember that silver string pulling you to the sky. Remember too that if you're leaning on a machine, you're not standing erect.
- **Stay light on your forefoot.** At first you may find it incredibly difficult to maintain balance on your forefoot, so work on this slowly. The lighter you are on your forefoot, the more you mimic the best barefoot walking form. However, depending on the machine, this may be very difficult to do at first and may require significant strengthening of your stabilizing muscles.
- **Watch your reflection.** Do the activity in front of a mirror if possible, and do your best to mimic your barefoot form.

Gotta Bounce!

If you're looking for a cross-training workout that'll help strengthen your feet, strengthen your bones, loosen your joints, and likely reduce the chance of many diseases, all with nearly zero impact, then you've got to try a mini-trampoline. Approximately three feet wide by nine inches high, these trampolines, also known as "rebounders," allow you to experience brief periods of weightlessness, while giving you a total body workout.

Years ago, astronauts were returning from outer space missions with weakened bones and weakened cardiovascular systems. In a search to return astronauts to health, NASA scientists discovered that bouncing on trampolines was the perfect exercise for counteracting the effects of zero-gravity living without placing stress and strain on the joints.

In our own experimentation, we've discovered childlike glee playing on a trampoline, as well as a lighter step when we walk. It greatly works the lymphatic system, a circulatory system that is involved in your immune system, removing toxins, recovering between workouts, and even helping fight cancer. When you bounce up and down, gravity works its wonders, helping clean and detoxify your body. Best of all, as we've seen with our ninety-year-old friend Jack, it's an exercise you can do at any age!

Cycling/Spinning

With Michael's cycling background, he still loves at least one long bike ride once a week. If you're injured and out of the walking game for a while, get to know your bicycle, as long as it doesn't aggravate your injury. It's one of the best cross-training tools you have. Just make sure to ride it barefoot . . . no, just kidding, but make sure you're using shoes that are wide enough for your evolving feet. If you need to, take your cycling shoes to the cobbler to get them stretched out or wear Correct Toes in your cycling shoes.

Aqua Jogging and Water Aerobics

Aqua jogging is a great way to get the legs moving with fantastic aerobic benefits, yet without putting any weight on the feet. This is a great exercise to do on your non-barefoot days or if you're recovering from injury. Wearing a flotation belt, head to where your feet don't touch the ground in the pool. Then move your legs as if you are pedaling a bicycle to propel yourself forward. Try to stay symmetrical and fairly upright with your core engaged, but don't worry about perfect form. For a more complete workout, you can add arm movement, as if you're running in place.

A great way to start working the foot muscles, but without full body weight, is water aerobics. You don't even have to be a great swimmer to participate in this activity. In the safe confines of a shallow pool, an instructor guides you through a series of exercises. You can be either barefoot or in a water shoe (if you're in a water shoe, get the widest ones you can). Either way, you're in an unsupported shoe or barefoot, waking up the muscles of the feet and lower legs.

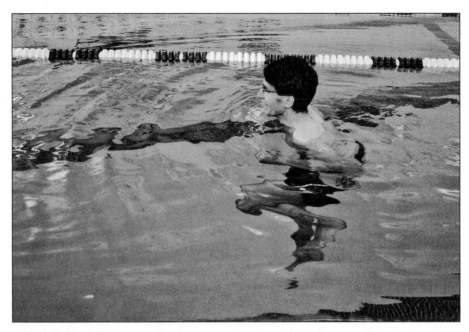

Aqua jogging is a great way to get in shape, tone neglected muscles, and hold on to fitness if you've been injured. All you need is a pool and a flotation belt.

Other Barefoot Activities

Did you know that Jazzercise started out as a barefoot activity? Founder Judi Sheppard Missett began teaching jazz-based exercise in 1969 and introduced the universally known name of Jazzercise in 1974. She originally took dance classes as a child to correct foot imbalances.

Today there are more excellent barefoot fitness options than ever. Martial arts have always been about bare feet or minimal footwear. Pilates and yoga too. Just about any activity you do in shoes you can do barefoot.

- **Yoga.** Yoga is a great way to gain flexibility, body control, and awareness. Done properly and with a good instructor, yoga is a perfect complementary exercise to barefoot walking. Just be careful to start slowly and not push it. Yoga should not be a game of the ego, seeing what you can do or how far you can push it. It takes time and awareness to build up to your poses (asanas). So seek a teacher who resonates with you and will take the extra time to understand you and your body and help you start in gently. If you're careful, not only will yoga strengthen your feet, but it will support your mind-body connection and help you quiet the mind.

- **Mall walking.** If you have the time, or if it fits in your schedule, early-morning mall walks, especially over uneven stone or tiles, can be a relatively more "natural" solution than the treadmill. You're moving toward a surface (rather than a treadmill belt moving toward you—see treadmills), you can walk up and down stairs, and you can walk in peace at any speed you want. You don't have to worry about the friction of a belt, or any of the other funny business a treadmill can present. Almost all malls allow walking before business hours. Most are barefoot-friendly, though some may not be. And, as Jessica says, the stores are closed, so you won't be tempted to shop.

- **Fitness classes, Zumba, step classes, slide-board classes, Tae Bo.** These and just about all other activity classes that do not have you throwing weights around are all cross-training opportunities. Just start slowly, listen to your body, and as much as possible do them barefoot.

- **Dance.** Choose whichever dance class interests you the most, but make sure you can do it barefoot or in a minimalist shoe. One dance method to try is modern dance, which is essentially done barefoot, as are many forms of African dance, which are a ton of fun! Note: if you try ballet, look for the widest slippers you can get your hands on and feet in. Check out the Eric Franklin Method classes, which were designed to help dancers improve their form. Aerobic dance conditioning classes, in particular, are another way to get in shape and improve lower-body (and foot) strength and flexibility. Dancing simultaneously works on balance and core strength. Even if the class isn't very aerobic, there are still great benefits.

- **Martial arts and tai chi.** There's a reason martial artists go barefoot or wear minimalist shoes that let their feet and toes feel the ground. Getting grounded, centered, and balanced by feeling the ground is essential for nearly every martial art. As you practice a martial art, you'll be developing foot strength and coordination, as well as core strength, and coordination between your feet and the rest of your body. Tai chi further develops the mind-body-earth connection. Although it's a total body workout, it does a particularly good job at improving body control, proprioception (your perception of movement and orientation in space), and balance, which can help you walk better, stay healthier, and stay safer (with less chance of falling). Studies are showing tai chi is ideal for seniors. By connecting you with the earth, tai chi helps remap, or rewire, your mind for balance and control.

- **Gardening** may not be aerobic, but it qualifies as a moderate physical activity under federal guidelines for exercise. Putting your hands in the dirt also helps you get grounded. And certainly gardening can be done without shoes. In fact, a nice squishy soil might be just the foot mask you need while tending the peas and carrots.

Our Barefoot Wedding

Almost anything you can think of can be done barefoot—particularly, or especially, getting married.

After we got engaged, we couldn't think of a better way to share our vows and our deep connection with the earth than by getting married barefoot.

And so, on October 10, 2010, at 10:10 a.m. (yes, that's 10/10/10 at 10:10), we got married barefoot on an organic farm. We asked all the guests to be barefoot too and enjoy this "perfect ten" experience with us.

The ground felt incredible, and it rained a bit too, a very fortuitous sign. And as we went under the tent for our meal, we sat, walked, and even danced on pea-sized gravel barefoot, which felt spectacular underfoot.

By getting married barefoot we weren't just sharing vows between us but showing our deep reverence or commitment to Mother Earth.

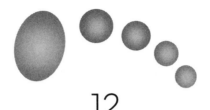

12
Stretching for Healing and Injury Prevention

Your hand opens and closes and opens and closes. If it were always a
fist or always stretched open, you would be paralyzed. Your deepest
presence is in every small contracting and expanding, the two as
beautifully balanced and coordinated as bird wings.

—Rumi

In 1992 I was racing bicycles in the French Alps trying to make it to the Tour de France. Climbing into the little mountain town of Hauteville, with a crowd cheering me on and blocking my view, I was waved through a blind turn by a safety official—and into an oncoming car. The crowd gasped as they watched the car flip me up and over the hood.

When I landed I thought I was okay. But then I saw my left leg. It was like a scene out of the movie *Misery*, with a right-angle bend where one didn't belong. In broken English, a French doctor later told me I "hurted the automobile," to which I replied, "Au contraire!"

At the time, it appeared to be a career-ending injury, though in hindsight it didn't have to be. But everything happens for a reason, and I learned more than I bargained for from that accident. In fact, it was learning to heal from this accident that helped me survive and soar after my inline skating accident in 2004.

However, it turned out not to be the leg that gave me the most grief. It was my lower back, an injury to the vertebrae and disks. They would burn and sear with pain, and cause the right side of my back (where there are ropelike muscles called the paraspinals) to tighten up anytime I tried to be active or work out.

For years I visited doctors, physical therapists, acupuncturists, pain centers, and anywhere I could think of in hopes of finding relief. They all told me the same thing—rest. I was resting, but I didn't want to become a couch potato.

And then I saw a true guru, someone who changed my life with a humble little tennis ball. Don Spence is an amazing former professional cyclist, a massage therapist, and a guru when it comes to helping people heal through Pilates. In my case, he found that a big part of my back pain was caused by tight muscles beneath my glutes. These tight muscles were pulling on my back, which was spasming in return. Once he started me rolling out over a tennis ball on my glutes, my back began to relax. After only a few weeks of daily work on the ball, my back pain was completely gone.

Barefoot walking is great for your back. It tones and helps hold everything in proper position, with great alignment and posture, and better balance. If I walk barefoot every few days, it helps keep my back nice and handy. But I always have a tennis ball at the ready and try to "sit on it" every chance that I get.

Stretching is an investment in yourself that pays huge dividends. And a tennis ball, a tiny investment, can be worth a hefty fortune.

When I was coming back from injury, it was a combination of stretching, foam rolling, rolling over a ball, and Pilates that really got me going again. I'd use a hot tub to warm and loosen my muscles and then stretch for hours. It was a big investment in time, but worth a fortune in health. If you're beginning a new fitness program (such as barefoot walking), or if you're just stiff after years of inactivity, these modalities will also serve you well. If you're recovering from injury, I recommend twice as much stretching. That's because stretching helps you get the body going again, lubricates the joints, reduces inflammation, can help prevent or heal many injuries, and just overall feels great. Consider stretching and core work (core exercises are discussed in chapter 11) to be as important to your fitness, health, and well-being as any aerobic activity.

As mentioned earlier, barefoot walking inevitably results in stronger muscles. The act of strengthening muscles, however, will also cause them to tighten, especially early on. That's why we recommend stretching one-for-one in the beginning. Commit to at least one minute of stretching for every minute of exercise you do, at least until you've reached thirty minutes of exercise or more. This stretching rule keeps your muscles limber and strong.

A LITTLE STRETCHING GOES A LONG WAY

It's a natural fact that walking strengthens your muscles. But what it doesn't do is loosen them up. Particularly in the beginning, keep your muscles loose and supple by allotting some quality time to stretching. This will not only help you walk smoothly and efficiently but also help relieve any aches and pains you've accumulated over the years.

If you're like me and have a titanium hip or other replacement part, congratulations—you've earned an obligatory membership to the professional stretchers club. In other words, expect to stretch much more than the average Joe. Or as I like to say, when you qualify for AARP (they've been sending me invites since I broke my hip at age thirty-six), it's time to become a full-time athlete. We tighten up more and faster, so we need to stay on top of it.

The more we stretch, the healthier, happier, and more pain-free we are. Ever wake up with creaky joints in the morning? If your muscles aren't loose, they pull on your joints, creating resistance. When you stretch, you allow your joints to move freely, rather than in stutter-steps that strain your entire body.

What you're aiming for is basic balance (like preventing one hip or calf from being tighter than the other) and knot-free muscles. Stretching helps bring blood flow to your muscles, which is especially helpful in achieving your goals.

If possible, stretch every day. Stretch after each walk or barefoot activity, after long travel in a car or on a plane, and especially on a day off from walking or working out. This helps the body recover and allows it to relax and hit the reset button for each new day and new week. And if you get the chance, stretch outside as well for the added benefits of vitamin G.

TYPES OF STRETCHES

As long as your muscles are warm, I find great benefits with both traditional and rolling stretches. Personally, there would have been no way to rehab my hip had I not spent a great deal of time working with traditional stretches to get my hip joint loose and mobile again. And it was only by stretching in a warm environment, such as a hot tub, that I was able to get the hip to relax enough for me to begin rehabilitation.

In essence, a traditional stretch is one in which you reach or extend as far as you can for a given period of time. These stretches are best at stretching out the ends of muscles but don't do very much to lengthen the belly or body of the muscle. To dig in or knead out the belly of the muscle, we need tools such as a foam roll, ball, or other device, which we'll discuss next.

Old-School Stretching

If done properly, traditional stretches can be quite helpful, but all too often, people push beyond the point of pain, stretch when their muscles are cold, or overstretch, digging so deep they tear their muscles or loosen their joints. These aren't real concerns if these stretches are done in moderation and done when muscles are warm.

For a traditional stretch, slowly and gently reach in the direction of your stretch, exhaling as you extend. Without going to the point of pain, stop when you feel resistance. Hold for at least thirty seconds to a minute. Then

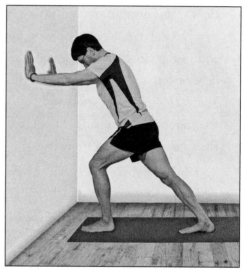

Traditional stretches, such as this calf stretch, should never be done with cold muscles. Warm up first and be gentle; never go to the point of pain.

rest and repeat, going a little further each time. Ideally do a set of at least three of each stretch for maximum benefit. Never go to the point of pain.

Also consider alternating between opposing muscle groups. For instance, work your quads and then your hamstrings. Going back and forth between opposing muscle groups helps loosen both. Here's a great technique with opposing muscle groups. If you've been stretching your hamstring (back of your thigh) and it won't relax, try tightening your quadriceps (muscles on the front top of your thigh) for ten to twenty seconds, and then restretch your hamstring. By tightening and then relaxing your opposing muscle group, you help the muscles let down their guard (for instance, often the hamstring protects the quadriceps, and vice versa), allowing you to get a better stretch.

Rolling Out Is In

I recommend that each of my clinic participants invest in a good foam roll and tennis ball (a stretching kit will be available soon on our website, RunBare .com). These tools are lifesavers.

Since traditional stretches often just work the beginning and end of the muscle, this means the attachments are loose, but the body of the muscle remains tight and at risk of injury. Additionally, we often have trauma or sore spots within the muscle itself that feel like knots. These points of inflammation can develop into scar tissue over time, creating muscle imbalances and chronic pain. You can get at these knots and scar tissue with deep tissue massage and other techniques, but you can't get at them with traditional stretching. This is where the foam roll and ball come in.

You can use this technique for any muscle group on your legs, or even your

EXERCISE

Foam Rolling

Your iliotibial (IT) band is a band of ropelike connective tissue that runs along the outside of your leg from your hip to your knee, and can pull all the way up your back and all the way down to your feet. It's commonly aggravated by poor form, poor shoes, or imbalances in strength or flexibility. Relaxing your IT band is a great way to ease tension throughout your hips, legs, and back. Lie on your side with the foam roll resting on your IT band, just a few inches above the outside of your knee. Then roll your leg very

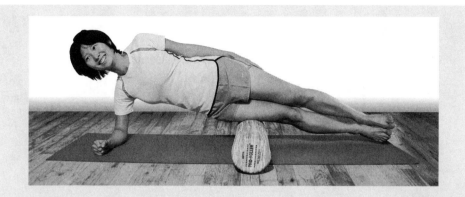

slowly down the foam roll, inch by inch. As you roll, become aware of any tight spots, and if you find one (it's usually accompanied by pain), stop on the tight spot and lean into it on the foam roll. Unlike traditional stretches, where you don't want pain, here a little pain is a good thing. It's letting you know you've found a knot and are working it out. After one to two minutes move on, seeking the next point of discomfort, tightness, or pain.

You can do this for your entire leg. As you start into barefoot walking, a few key spots to work on will also be your calves, Achilles tendon, and quadriceps. Work each of these areas out, doing the hamstrings as well, inner thighs, and even up to your psoas (the group of muscles just before your groin that help you bring your leg forward as you walk), which are often too tight, preventing a proper stride.

Note: Never roll over joints or directly next to a joint. Leave at least an inch and a half of room between a foam roll and a joint.

arms (and I've heard of some people using it for their back as well). Simply lie down on the foam roll on the muscle group you want to work on.

A Tennis Ball for Your Derrière

If you hold tension in your back or legs (as Michael did after his bicycle accident), or if you spend a large part of your day sitting, as most of us do, then you

◐°°₀ FOOT NOTE

When Michael started into barefoot activities, his left knee started tightening up on him. He thought, "Uh-oh, the doc was right. I'm not going to be able to do this anymore." But then he started rolling things out over his quad, and his knee began to feel better—100 percent better. It turns out it wasn't the knee at all but tight muscles caused by his leg length discrepancy. Once he loosened things up, all of the pain went away.

owe it to yourself to spend some time sitting on a tennis ball. Simply place the fuzzy yellow ball on the ground and sit on it with one of your butt cheeks. Roll around slowly on the ball until you find the spot that makes you grimace; then live there for a minute or two. Roll on the ball for the first day for five minutes on each side, and increase as necessary. You'll almost immediately feel muscle tension reduced in your legs and back.

GUIDELINES FOR STRETCHING

Many of the basic stretches done before an activity have been around for thousands of years. Stories of ancient runners, dating back to the time of the Romans and Greeks, tell the tale of runners pulling, pushing, and contorting their muscles with bouncing motions just before the start of a race. These stretches did little to help the runners and may have actually hurt them. Boy, do old habits die hard!

Unfortunately, these same stretches are around to this day and have as little effect now as they did then. They don't work for two key reasons. First, bouncing (or ballistic stretching, as it's called) is a surefire way to hurt yourself if you don't build up to it slowly and with proper form. Second, stretching cold muscles, particularly by pulling on them, tears fibers.

Bouncing when stretching is a big no-no. And cold muscle stretching is incredibly traumatic to the body. It should never be done, particularly by barefoot walkers, who rely so heavily on stability and balance from muscles and joints.

The Three Best Times to Stretch

- **After a warm-up.** Stretch after you've been walking for at least ten minutes. If you have a sore muscle, such as a tight calf or hip, walk for ten minutes, then stop and ever so gently stretch things out. This'll help you have a better walk and keep you from injuring yourself or changing your stride due to tightness. You can even walk around the block, head for home, and roll yourself out on a foam roll before your walk to increase blood flow and circulation to your muscles.

- **After a walk.** After walking, your muscles are nice and loose, as long as you haven't overdone things. Now is the time to work out the knots, keep things supple, and allow for the best possible recovery. Again, make sure you don't bounce, but with warm muscles you'll likely find you can easily stretch twice as far and with half the effort as stretching without a walk. Stretching after a workout is one of the best things in the world you can do for recovery and to keep muscles from tightening up. Of course, if you've gone too far or too fast, stretching after a workout will only help so much. And if you're in pain or sense swelling, skip the stretch and head straight for the ice.

- **Once a day.** Stretch as part of a daily routine. Consider this maintenance stretching, perhaps the most important kind. You can stretch any time of the day, although do it at the same time each day. This helps you get into a rhythm or routine and ensures you get it done. Perhaps you do it after some core work in the morning, or after a Pilates class, or even in the evening when it's time to wind down. Warm up the muscles for five to ten minutes (a mini-trampoline works wonders), and then go through a regular stretching routine, preferably emphasizing your foam roll and tennis ball. For instance, you could warm up on the tramp, do a brief balance workout, and then head for the stretching mat.

YOU DESERVE A MASSAGE

The value of a great deep tissue or myofascial release massage cannot be overstated. They help break down scar tissue, the result of unhealthy habits, a sedentary lifestyle, or injuries from the past that prevent us from moving pain-free. These sessions are often quite grisly (particularly if you find a good, strong, intuitive, experienced therapist) but work miracles. Things that seemed tight or "stuck" for years suddenly work again as they once did, and are pain-free. Of course, you may find yourself begging, pleading, or even crying (as I have) during a great massage, but in the long run, it's worth it.

If you don't have a great massage therapist near you, or if you can't find an affordable option (on that note, students at local massage schools often work on a donation basis), you can look to your spouse if you trust him or her to go digging into your muscles. Doing massage with a spouse helps build a special bond and intimacy between you, and helps him or her learn how best to help.

As another option, there's perhaps no better way at finding the spots than a deep-tissue self-massage, but you're going to have to be committed to actually digging into yourself.

Self-Massage

Michael occasionally struggles with a tight left IT band—it's forced to do more of the work of holding his left knee stable, since that knee doesn't have a functional ACL. He also has a tight right calf on occasion, from two years of driving nonstop on a book tour. When he takes the time to massage these things out, not only does he feel better, but he moves more fluidly, without any pulling on his joints.

Warm up the muscles slowly with gentle kneading motions, using a natural oil or healing salve to keep the skin or hair from being torn or chafing. Never massage into a joint. To focus on recovery and returning circulation to the heart, try to always work the muscles toward rather than away from the heart. Gradually go deeper, feeling for lumps, knots, or the tightest spots you can find (you'll know when you hit them). When you find them, hold pressure there for at least a minute or two, until they feel like they're loosening up or going away. This is the tough part, but if you can, slowly bend at the nearest joint over a period of three to five seconds while holding pressure on the knot; this helps break things up. After your massage, drink plenty of fluids to help your muscles stay loose.

The same techniques above can be used on your spouse. Added benefit: it brings you closer together.

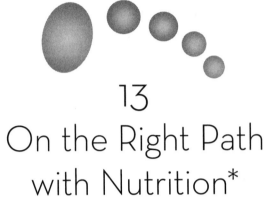

13
On the Right Path
with Nutrition*

*I eat the ground. I will tell you that [in] every wine-growing
region . . . the first thing I do is put my hand in the ground
and eat it. . . . I always feel a connection.*
—Gary Vaynerchuk, *Dirt! The Movie*

MICHAEL'S STORY

Throughout my life, I've had a love-hate relationship with food. I've struggled with food for as long as I can remember. As a child I was fed a diet of processed foods, sugary cereal, and TV dinners. Making my own dinner typically meant microwaving a can of Chef Boyardee. Before I could even walk, I was chugging prune juice to purge my digestive system. And throughout childhood, I struggled with a bloated belly and blood sugar lows. On top of that, I *hated* veggies. The only kind I would eat were those drowned in butter, sitting next to the dessert in the tray of my TV dinner.

* Michael Sandler and Jessica Lee are not registered dietitians. Advice given here is gleaned from the athletic world's experts on sports nutrition and Michael's professional athletic experience. As with all medical advice, consult your doctor before making any changes in your diet.

As a cyclist, I experimented with almost every legal supplement, protein powder, and recovery drink out there, which were no more than chemical soups designed to stuff your muscles with sugar.

In 1993, recouping from cycling injuries in Europe, I took a vacation to Morocco. There I got food poisoning. As the cab driver taking me out of the country said when he heard my story, "You ate fish in *Fez*? Fez is a desert! What, they bring in fish by camel?" Whoops. To add insult to injury, I got giardia after drinking the local tap water because I was too weak to walk to the store. I was sick for several months and put on antibiotic after antibiotic. Ever since, my stomach has never been quite right.

I've been hospitalized twice for a gastrointestinal system that stopped working, requiring . . . well, you can guess what, along with multiple colonoscopies. I've seen internists, specialists, allergists, holistic docs, Tibetan docs, Chinese medicine docs, and some specialists I can't even recall. Not one had a solution for me.

On top of that, I've struggled badly with hypoglycemia, or low blood sugar, for nearly my entire life. I'd be perfectly fine one minute, then crashing hard the next. I once literally crashed a car, totaling it after passing out behind the wheel, exactly thirty minutes after a glass of orange juice. Try as I might, until recent days, I had not succeeded in getting my blood sugar under control. It's been hard on me, and harder still on my family.

I'm doing much better now, better than I have in my entire life. My bloated belly, or "Buddha belly," as I call it, is almost nonexistent now. I digest foods better, have better energy, and get sick far less often. My stomach feels *worlds* better than it ever has, so I know I'm on the right path.

Here's the biggest lesson I've learned: food can work either for you or against you. It's that simple. Foods that work for you are those that give your body what it needs to heal, grow strong, and keep the immune system going. Foods that work against you either are filled with harmful chemicals or are simply empty calories. If you can only eat so much, then you need to get the best bang for your buck!

This chapter is about hope. There are simple choices you can make to reap big dividends for your health. We'll look at what to seek out (nutrient-dense foods) and what to avoid (foods with toxins and foods lacking nutritional value).

EAT NUTRIENT-DENSE FOODS

Let food be thy medicine and medicine be thy food.
—Hippocrates

We often think of food as simply fuel, something to power us up and keep us going. We tend to forget our food equals the building blocks of what we're made of, what we're repaired with, what keeps us strong, and what keeps illness and may keep cancer away.

If we eat simply for fuel, we're only getting a small portion of what we need to survive. The same holds true if we're just counting grams of fat versus protein versus carbs. We may feel full, but our bodies are still wanting. It's as if we built a home out of flimsy wood. It may do the job temporarily, but over time your roof will come crashing down. Instead, we need to eat the most nutrient-dense foods we can. Look for fresh, organic, local, and raw. These foods have color, flavor, texture, aroma, life force, and enzymes. And they taste great.

If you can only eat so much in a day, you owe it to yourself to eat foods loaded with the building blocks you need for health. So always ask yourself before you eat, and before you shop, "How nutrient-dense is this food?" Here are simple guidelines to keep you on the right track.

- **Eat organic.** Organic foods are grown in a kinder, gentler way, without potentially harmful chemicals, pesticides, antibiotics, growth hormones, or genetic engineering, which were all designed for profit, not for our health. By going organic, you stay free of many of the dangers most nonorganic foods are laden with these days. In the old days we thought we could just rinse off our produce, but we can't wash off harmful substances that are engineered into foods or have already been absorbed by our foods. If our fruits, vegetables, and protein sources are getting bathed in chemicals, then sooner or later these chemicals find their way into our bodies too.
- **Eat a varied diet.** Just as a varied terrain helps your walking, the more varied your diet, the better your health. In simplest terms, you get different vitamins, minerals, and nutrients by eating fruits and

Beyond Organic

Check out biodynamic foods. It's a concept that's been around since the 1920s, invented by Dr. Rudolf Steiner. Biodynamics is defined as "a spiritual-ethical-ecological approach to agriculture, food production and nutrition." The farms work for sustainability, using everything they can from the farm and even fermenting the fertilizer to make better soil, and also use spiritual practices to bring greater love or *chi* to the soil. They believe in tending and treating the soil with great reverence and respect, and from there get great crops. We've been eating biodynamic greens from local organic farmers and can just feel the life force in them. There's something special about these foods that were grown with love and in balance with the soil. And barefoot walking on the soil of a biodynamic farm feels great. As a biodynamic farmer on Maui explained, "We don't raise plants, we raise soil." On that note, visit your local farm and if you can, pick your own greens. It's not just a learning experience but ear-to-ear grins for the whole family, and gets you more closely connected to the food you eat.

vegetables of all different colors and tastes. By eating foods that are sweet (sugars and starches), sour (citrus fruit and plain yogurt), astringent (beans, broccoli, turmeric), salty, pungent (horseradish, peppers, mustard), and bitter (green leafy vegetables, eggplant, and olives), you can help ensure you're getting a healthy balance of vitamins and nutrients in your diet.

- **Colors of the rainbow.** We're eating more colors of the rainbow in as many fruits and vegetables as we can, sampling all colors and flavors. If the colors and tastes of the rainbow are a natural pharmacy filled with amazing phytochemicals, vitamins, and nutrients, then wouldn't you want to eat more of this great stuff and less of the empty stuff?
- **Everything in moderation.** Shoot for balance. This means trying not to eat too much of any one food. Mix things up so you'll get

the nutrients you need naturally (from food, preferably not vitamin supplements).

- **Go raw.** Try eating more fresh raw vegetables and fruits and protein sources deemed safe for a raw diet. Those who propose eating only raw say raw foods boost your immune system, increase your health and recovery, and give you incredible energy. At this point, we've gone the whole nine yards and eat 90 percent raw. For others we recommend eating at least 50 percent raw, if not more.

- **Eat local.** Local foods tend to be the freshest, best-tasting, and kindest on the environment (they don't travel as far, so less fuel is burned). Food loses nutritional value over time: vitamins degrade, minerals leach out, and enzymes are destroyed. The more local your food, the more nutrient-dense it is. You also support the local economy. Look for a local food co-op or farmers' market, or seek out the "local" tag at your grocery store.

- **Get to know your grocer.** Learn about your foods by shopping at farmers' markets, local independent grocers, or local farms. Ask them about pesticides, their growing practices, what's in season, and even how to prepare something you've never tried before. A great farmer often becomes your new best friend.

- **Buy free-range omega-3 eggs.** When it comes to eggs, buy the good stuff. We look for free-range, organic eggs from happy chickens. Too many chickens cooped up in too small a place is both unsanitary and unhealthy (that's why caged hens need so many antibiotics). The wellness and happiness of the animals is just as essential for the animals' health as it is for your health. Happy chickens lay happy eggs and this does make a difference. Consider eating eggs high in omega-3, which may be better for the body and mind and help keep cholesterol levels down, especially if you're consuming a lot of egg yolks.

- **Know the difference: wild-caught vs. farm-raised fish and shrimp.** Stay away from farm-raised fish, as they've been shown to have high levels of toxins, and low levels of essential fish oils. According to a study published in *Science,* researchers found high levels of PCBs, dioxins, and other contaminants that pose a cancer risk in farm-raised fish as compared to wild-caught. Also, don't overdo it on fish because there is mercury even in wild-caught fish these days (not that any amount of mercury is truly safe). In case you've wondered, the bigger the fish, the greater the potential for mercury content. The same goes for radiation too, something that has just begun showing up in fish since the Fukushima reactor meltdown. The same dangers apply for shrimp too, from chemicals, pesticides, contaminants, and antibiotics. For farm-raised shrimp, a common practice is to pump antibiotics into the water to keep the shrimp from getting sick in overcrowded and dirty conditions. This is done everywhere, but in third-world countries they frequently use antibiotics that are banned in the United States. Wild-caught fish and shrimp may be expensive, but they're in your best interest. Ask your grocer or the restaurant server, and if you're unsure, pass in favor of something else.

- **Go complex.** The more complex your carbohydrates, the more nutrients they have and the better they are for your body. Look for darker-colored foods and grains. Opt for unprocessed oatmeal, whole grains, quinoa, and brown rice. Get even more bang for your buck by sprouting your grains. Grab a book or check online for the glycemic index of your favorite foods. Look for foods lower on the glycemic index to keep your mind and body happy and balanced throughout the day.

- **Less is more.** The fewer ingredients the better. If an ingredient on a food label is longer than eight letters, be careful!

- **Avoid empty calories.** Sugars, high-fructose corn syrup (more on this coming up), and fast-burning simple carbs do little good for your body. Whenever possible, take a pass on cake, white bread, sugary fruit juices, and packaged cereals. White foods are often bleached white and devoid of nutrients. Think of getting the maximum bang for your buck. If you're going to be out in nature, you want the best trail you can find, right? So if you're eating, you want the best food you can fuel yourself with too.

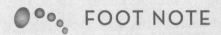 FOOT NOTE

When You're Going the Distance

We're not big fans of sweet drinks, and never of sports drinks. So when you're going the distance, what can you do to keep yourself fueled?

Look for foods that are high in natural fats, such as avocados, raw almonds and cashews (all nuts, for that matter), shredded coconut meat, and chia seeds. High-fat foods will burn slowly as you trek along or head on down the trails, instead of spiking and then crashing your blood sugar. What do we eat? Michael likes anything with shredded coconut in it or chia seeds for his real long-distance efforts, and Jessica likes trail mixes with raw cacao beans (or nibs), goji berries, and an assortment of raw seeds and nuts. We're also experimenting with making our own raw bars with the aforementioned ingredients along with raw oils, dates, and figs. It'll be a superfood party in a bar.

AVOID TOXINS

Most factory farms grow the same plant year after year, stripping all of the nutrients out of the soil (that's why our ancestors always rotated crops) and with the same nutritionally deficient but cost-effective fertilizer (again, why our ancestors used real fertilizer from animals). While nonorganic produce today often looks good, it's empty on the inside and can't give you what you need. Below is a list of red flags to help you make the right selection next time you go food shopping, hopefully at a local farmers' market.

- **Stay away from processed foods.** Processed foods, or foods that have been cooked, treated, or altered, may look like food, may taste like food, and may have the shiniest, fanciest wrappers, but they have no more nutritional value than eating multicolored cardboard.
- **Simplify your vocabulary.** If you don't know what you're reading on the label, it isn't natural. Now, that doesn't necessarily mean it's

harmful. But it's certainly not something our ancestors cooked with. If you can't pronounce it or define it, you might want to keep it out of your body. The fewer ingredients, the better!

- **Avoid high-fructose corn syrup like the plague.** High-fructose corn syrup (HFCS) and other added processed sugars have no place in food. Not only do they spike your blood sugar, they are one of the main reasons diabetes in the United States is at near-epidemic proportions today. Opt for organic honey, organic agave nectar (but not agave syrup, which is highly refined), or stevia leaves when possible.

- **No sports bars, meal replacement bars, or sports drinks.** The majority of these are too sweet and too synthetic to be any good for us. Many contain HFCS or other added sugars (more on this in a bit). They may be rocket fuel, but they can make you crash. Hydrate with water, not sports drinks. However, if you feel you need a sweet drink, then try nature's sports drink, coconut water. It's so naturally balanced with electrolytes (such as potassium and magnesium) that it's even been used in IVs for emergencies. Get the water unprocessed (never with additives) and straight from the coconut itself if you can find it—then you'll get to eat the meat too, an amazing fuel and true superfood! Mix it with wheatgrass for a true superdrink!

- **Shun preservatives.** Stay away from preservatives, additives, and artificial colors, flavors, and sweeteners. All those long names weren't found in your food in nature, so they likely don't belong in your diet today.

- **Just say no to fast food.** In Danny Dreyer's *ChiRunning*, he talks about foods that are low in *chi* or positive energy. We have to believe there's very little positive energy in fast foods, no matter how healthy they're touted to be.

- **Embrace microwave freedom.** Unplug the microwave, as we did. Study after study suggests not only that microwave radiation is harmful to our health (just another reason to go out, get grounded, and drain those ions) but chemically alters our food and destroys nutrients, producing tremendous amounts of free radicals in what we eat.

- **Go gluten free.** Keep the wheat glutens down. Two foods seem to make you crave more food when you eat them: sugar and gluten.

Additionally, many people are either sensitive to gluten or find it aggravates other food allergies. It's thought that gluten wasn't a natural part of our human diet to begin with, and if we didn't evolve to eat it, steer clear.

- **Steer clear of hidden MSG.** The free glutamic acid found in monosodium glutamate falls into the category of excito-toxins, neurotoxins that have the ability to overexcite cells to the point of death. Free glutamic acid is very inexpensive, makes foods taste great, and is extremely addictive. It's everywhere, even in restaurant and cafeteria food, yet is extremely harmful to our health. The Mayo Clinic and the FDA say an "unknown percentage of the population" is susceptible to dangerous reactions to free glutamic acid, reactions they call "MSG symptom complex." These include headaches; flushing and sweating; a sense of facial pressure or tightness; numbness, tingling, or burning in or around the mouth; heart palpitations; chest pain; shortness of breath; nausea; and weakness. Many people who have had mysterious chronic conditions found those problems went away when they removed free glutamic acid from their diets.

  Typically, we think of free glutamic acid as monosodium glutamate, something only found in Chinese foods. But free glutamic acid is found in thousands of everyday foods, including many protein drinks, meal replacement drinks, and infant formulas. Unfortunately, babies are far more sensitive because the blood-brain barrier hasn't fully developed yet. In our opinion, if your baby food has corn syrup or free glutamic acid, promptly throw it in the trash. Unfortunately, it is part of the production process and can be hidden within ingredients such as broth, casein, anything "hydrolyzed" or "autolyzed," vegetable protein extract, modified cornstarch, maltodextrin, soy protein isolate, whey protein concentrate, gelatin, yeast extract, malted barley, rice syrup or brown rice syrup, carrageenan, and even under the term "natural flavorings." So what's the answer? Look for the least-processed foods with only natural-sounding ingredients. Simple is beautiful. And if you experience problematic symptoms, see if they go away if you eliminate the food you just ate.

You don't have to follow all or perhaps any of these rules to stay healthy and happy for barefoot activities. But you really are what you eat. You want to be the healthiest you can be—for a lifetime.

Staying healthy isn't as simple as it used to be. Remember the days when the biggest food choice was whether to use butter or margarine? Over the last few decades, food has taken on a controversy of its own: Canola was good, then canola was bad. Fat was bad, but then not all fats were bad. Carbs were bad, but then some were not. Bread was good, but now gluten is bad.

To stay fueled and at your best, you need to understand more about how diet contributes to peak physical and mental performance.

DIETARY CAUTIONS: CORN SYRUP, CARBS, COKES, AND CANS

Have we had it backward about fat, carbs, and sugars all these years?

Tame the Sweet Tooth

In an interview recently, Michael was asked what advice he would give his five-year-old self if he met him today. Believe it or not, it wasn't "Take off your shoes." Instead his answer was "Stay away from sugar." Michael's struggled with tooth problems, GI challenges, and blood sugar issues for the better part of his life and is convinced it all began with a sweet tooth and processed foods.

Now there's a new study that just came out in the journal *Nature* that says we should regulate sugar the same way we regulate tobacco or alcohol because of its harmful effects on people, and in particular kids. Diabetes, virtually unheard of in the past in indigenous cultures, has been found to show itself twenty years after white sugar and flour are introduced to a people. In 1880 only 2.8 Americans out of 100,000 had diabetes. Today it's estimated that 1 out of 3 kids will get diabetes in their lifetimes and 1 out of 2 kids if they're a minority (likely because of the difficulty of getting higher-quality foods that have less sugar and corn syrup).

Adult and childhood obesity are at epidemic levels today, and this study contends it's due in large part to refined sugar. These days, it's commonplace to find food composed of 50 percent sugar or more (often hidden in the ingredients of processed foods). And the average American now consumes 150 pounds of added sugars a year or more (compared to 15 pounds in the 1800s). Many nutritionists call this a form of "nutritional suicide," as our bodies were never meant to function on such a fuel.

In 2012, New York City mayor Michael Bloomberg even banned supersized soft drinks in the city to save youth from the dangers of sugar and sweeteners, a move supported by former president Bill Clinton. Diabetes and obesity are two of the top killers in America today, and are growing at a disastrous rate—diabetes alone by an estimated 80 percent or more over the next decade.

Sugar short-circuits the body's endocrine system, destroying our ability to regulate our blood sugar and insulin levels. It also gets readily turned to fat and globs of LDL (the bad cholesterol), and it is highly addictive—some scientists say it's just as addictive as heroin or cocaine. MRI studies show that the more sugar you eat, the less your brain reacts to it, and therefore the more you need to get the same rush or kick.

So how do you kick the sugar addiction? Best way is to go cold turkey, though Michael admits it's quite challenging. Even a tiny bit of anything sweet, such as a piece of fruit, sets off a massive craving. If you can't quit entirely, work on eliminating all fruit juices and other sugary drinks (even nut milks can be high in sugar). Next remove all processed sugar. To do this, you'll have to become a supersleuth, deciphering all the names used for sugars on ingredient labels.

Overall, as you grow healthier and increasingly eat a more natural diet, you'll crave less sugar, shave off excess body fat, boost your energy levels, and create a more peaceful state of mind. You may even become one of the many diabetics who have successfully weaned themselves off of medication—always check with your doctor first. And, because sugar and sweeteners fuel cancer cells, many people have reported that cutting this fuel supply out of their diets played a role in overcoming the big C.

Sugar's Eco-Impact

Sugar, like so many other foods that are bad for our bodies, is also terrible for the planet.

A 2004 paper by the World Wildlife Foundation (WWF) found sugar may be responsible for more loss in biodiversity than any other crop ever, with giant forests chopped down for sugar plantations. Sugar cane production and the chemical fertilizers needed for it are the number one contributors to the incredibly rapid decline in both the Florida Everglades, where wading birds are down 90 percent, and the Great Barrier Reef, where coral close to the shore is down by as much as 60 percent. Fertilizers poison the soil and local water supplies and drain into the ocean. In addition to contributing to global warming, the fires used to burn the fields nearly annually release dangerous amounts of sulfur dioxide and CO_2 into the air. And those living near sugar processing plants are shown to have a marked increase in asthma and other lung conditions. Even the EPA isn't thrilled with the situation, with recent lawsuits such as in 2012 against American Sugar Refining Inc. (Baltimore Domino Sugar refinery) over emissions.

It's clear that if we want to improve the health of our planet and ourselves, reduce obesity, and shed pounds, we have to end our addiction to sugar.

High-Fructose Corn Syrup (HFCS)

The epidemic of diabetes and hypoglycemia in the United States kicked into high gear when corn-based sweeteners were promoted as an inexpensive alternative to sugar. Since then our health as a population appears to have taken a nosedive.

What exactly is high-fructose corn syrup? Corn syrup is made from mixing a type of corn typically used for livestock, ethanol, and other industrial products with acid. The result is an unnatural supersweet product. Not only does it taste much sweeter than table sugar (sucrose), it has an even more addictive quality to it. The more corn syrup you eat, the hungrier you become, just like with the excito-toxin in MSG.

Don't let the name *corn* fool you—it's anything but healthy. High-fructose corn syrup is banned in many countries, but it is all-pervasive in the United States. And it's not found only in sweet foods. Corn syrup may be disguised under many other names, such as insulin, glucose-fructose syrup, iso glucose, chicory, fruit fructose, crystalline fructose, and now corn sugar. Other corn-derived sweeteners to stay clear of include maltodextrin, dextrose, and maltitol.

How dangerous is HFCS? There are those who say that all sugars are the same, but a study at UCLA's Jonsson Comprehensive Cancer Center published in 2010 found that pancreatic cells could differentiate between fructose and conventional sugar and used the fuels accordingly. The cells use fructose to produce building blocks to produce new cancer cells.

Another powerful study in the *Journal of Pharmacology* illustrates the possibility that corn syrup is addictive and contributes to obesity. Princeton researchers gave one set of rats a mixture of either water mixed with sucrose (table sugar) at the concentration found in soft drinks, while another set of rats was fed a mixture with corn syrup at half the amount contained in popular soft drinks. The results were startling. The rats in the corn syrup group ballooned in size (48 percent more fat than those on a normal diet) and showed signs of metabolic syndrome, a set of risk factors that occur together and increase the risk for coronary artery disease, stroke, and type 2 diabetes. Symptoms include high amounts of visceral fat, particularly belly fat, and high levels of unhealthy triglycerides in their blood.

Oregon Health and Science University researchers found that not only does HFCS cause insulin resistance and induce obesity in lab animals, but it short-circuits the hypothalamus (which controls our appetite and our metabolic response to foods). When animals ate sucrose or table sugar, it did not induce hunger, yet when they ate fructose or corn syrup, it incited the brain to eat more.

One more study to hammer home this point. According to a commentary in the *American Journal of Clinical Nutrition*, between 1970 (when corn syrup was introduced) and 1990, HFCS use went up by a mind-blowing 1,000 percent:

"HFCS now represents more than 40 percent of caloric sweeteners added to foods and beverages and is the sole caloric sweetener in soft drinks in the United States."

Even popular sports drinks are filled with HFCS. We stopped using these "health drinks" a few years back because of this. When we tried drinking them again, they instantly made us feel ill. Yes, that's right, the sports drinks you thought were good for you and drank in copious quantities before, during, and after your workouts (after all, they're supposed to replenish your electrolytes and be good for your workouts and recovery) turn out to be the opposite. They spike your blood sugar levels, potentially tax your pancreas, don't produce the same insulin response, get turned directly into fat, and raise your triglyceride levels, thereby raising your risk for heart disease as well.

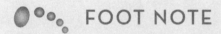 FOOT NOTE

Common Foods High in HFCS

- Regular soft drinks
- Fruit juice and fruit drinks that are not 100 percent juice
- Pancake syrups
- Ice pops
- Fruit-flavored yogurts
- Frozen yogurts
- Ketchup and BBQ sauces
- Jarred and canned pasta sauces
- Canned soups
- Canned fruit (if not in its own juice)
- Breakfast cereals

Note: Even foods labeled "natural" or "all natural" can be loaded with high-fructose corn syrup, according to an FDA memo to the Corn Refiners Organization in 2008. So even if it says "all natural," read the label.

Eliminating sweetened foods and sugary drinks can go a very long way to improving your health, but when you do want to use a little sweetener, look for the least processed one you can find.

Carbs

When it came to fueling physical activity, in the past the general rule was to eat carbs, carbs, and more carbs, with minimal fat. But today, that's all changing. We're finding the body was never designed to eat such a high-carb diet. Carbs raise blood sugar levels quickly, then crash, leaving you feeling empty. And quick-burning carbs that aren't used instantly are turned right back into unhealthy fat and LDL (the bad cholesterol).

Fats

In nature, humans ate more fat. Healthy fats such as monounsaturated fats (low in hydrogenated oils) are actually healthy for our bodies. These include monounsaturated fats found in nuts, avocados, and olive oil, and polyunsaturated fats such as in fish and flaxseed, which contain important omega-3 fatty acids. Among other benefits, these fats can actually help lower cholesterol levels, keep blood sugar levels balanced, and help with arthritis and even depression. The bad fats are saturated, most often found in meat sources and processed foods, and are responsible for raising cholesterol levels.

Fat is a slow-burning substance that is better than any rocket fuel (such as fancy sports-energy bars and drinks) when it comes to fueling the body for long distances. Additionally, it doesn't stimulate your appetite. When you're eating relatively more fat, you eat only when your body's hungry, not when it has an artificially induced sugar craving.

Beware of Palm Oil

Ever wonder, "Why is there palm oil in my peanut butter?" Recently food manufacturers have been switching over from partially hydrogenated oils to palm oil, touting its health benefits. However, the fat is anything but healthy. In fact, palm oil was removed from commercial popcorn more than ten years ago because of its high saturated fat content. It's common practice for companies to extract good fats to sell elsewhere, while replacing them with less expensive palm oil. Such is the case with most peanut butters, even those touted as organic!

Frequently used in meal replacement bars and sports bars, palm oil has another big drawback: it's extremely eco-unfriendly. Palm oil necessitates the slash-and-burn chopping down of rain forests in Southeast Asia.

Other names for palm oil are "palm fruit oil" and, unfortunately, "vegetable oil."

GMOs

Genetically modified organisms, or GMOs, are produced by taking genes from one plant or animal and inserting them in another. For example, some food crops such as corn and soybeans can be manipulated genetically to be resistant to pests. This is like science fiction coming true. And this type of genetic manipulation is anything but natural.

The concern is so significant that the European Union has taken the step of regulating GMOs, and many European nations such as France and Germany have banned their cultivation entirely. Concurrently, the United States has upped the use of GMOs, making it very difficult to keep genetically modified organisms out of the general food chain. And currently, genetically modified products do not have to be labeled, unless there is a significant nutritional difference or a known allergen from one food in another (such as a peanut protein in a soybean product).

There are no studies done on genetically modified organisms consumed by human subjects, so we don't know exactly what these things do to us. There need to be more studies, but what has been found in laboratory animals includes decreased growth, growth abnormalities, changes in development of vital organs, reduced immune responsiveness, gut structure and function changes, and even the potential for cancer.

Another major concern is allergies. Soy allergies are up and quite likely caused by genetically modified soy. It's very hard to avoid. However, that's minor compared to the deadly allergic reactions possible. For instance, if peanut genes are inserted into a food and a person with a peanut allergy consumes the GMO not realizing it, that person could become deathly ill.

Another very real risk is that of toxins transferring from a crop into a person. Some strains of corn have been genetically modified to produce *Bacillus thuringiensis* (Bt) toxins in order to resist pests, and studies have shown that 93 percent of pregnant women and 80 percent of unborn babies had this toxin in their bloodstream, presumably from the consumption of meat, milk, and eggs from livestock fed this corn. We don't know what this can do to babies, but one possibility is the Bt gene could turn back on in the gut of the baby, causing the gut to produce the pesticide it was producing in the crops. There's also the very real possibility of these genes latching onto bacteria and mutating in a way to produce "superbugs" that are resistant to antibiotics.

Furthermore, when you insert a gene from one organism into another crop, there's always the risk that new bacteria or diseases may be created. And by eating a living, changed organism, there is the very real possibility of growing something new (such as new types of cells or microorganisms) in your gut as well. There's just so much that's not known.

So the best advice is to avoid any foods you suspect may contain GMOs, look for "non-GMO" labels, and buy as close to organic as you can. If it's certified organic, it can't contain GMOs.

Processed Foods

If a food comes in a box or a can, is frozen, or has a long list of ingredients, chances are it's processed. Processed foods have been linked to a whole slew of diseases, from diabetes to heart disease, cancer, obesity, and much more.

Anytime something is done to food to alter it from its original state, that's a level of processing. A simple rule of thumb is to look for the least number of ingredients possible and to buy food that is closest to its original form. If the food label has names you can't pronounce, let alone know what they are, or if they have "artificial" anything, then it's best to steer clear. Even if a processed food is labeled "organic," then chances are there's little nutritional value left in it. Unfortunately, the food industry is promoting healthy eating in unhealthy ways. It is our job as consumers to be aware and educated, and to steer clear of deceptive marketing and packaging tactics.

Gluten

It appears that gluten can be very harmful. In a recent study published in the *Journal of the American Medical Association*, it was found that people with diagnosed, undiagnosed, or latent celiac disease or gluten sensitivity had a higher risk of death, mostly from cancer and heart disease. And gluten sensitivity can create inflammation throughout the body, affecting the brain, heart, joints, digestive tract, and more.

Michael found that he's sensitive to gluten and has been on a gluten-free diet for the last year. It's helped, and his stomach feels much better. Occasionally he's stuck eating something with gluten or eats it accidentally, and though it's not comfortable, he doesn't inflate nearly the way he used to.

Gluten sensitivity is classified as an autoimmune disease that creates inflammation throughout the body and can affect your brain, heart, joints, digestive tract, and more—and intensify diseases of those organs.

The best way to tell if you're sensitive to gluten is to go cold turkey for a month—no bread, no pizza, no baked goods, no soup mixes, or anything else that may contain gluten. After one month, sample something with gluten, and if you feel sick afterward, it's a sign you're sensitive to gluten. (Visit www.celiac .com for more details about foods that contain gluten.)

Chemicals in Cans

Many of us are aware of the dangers of BPA, a substance found in plastics such as those used in plastic water bottles, but few of us are aware that there's an even greater source of BPA: canned foods.

A 2007 survey by the Environmental Working Group found that the average food can has more than 200 times the government's traditional safety level for exposure to chemicals. Unfortunately, even though the dangers of BPA are known, there currently are no safety standards that limit the amount of BPA in canned foods.

A few food companies, such as Eden Foods and Trader Joe's, say their cans are BPA-free. Until more manufacturers make safer cans, you can work toward reducing the amount of canned food in your diet.

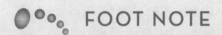 **FOOT NOTE**

A Few Thoughts on BPA

- Store food (particularly hot food) in glass or stainless steel containers, not in plastic containers.
- Never heat plastics in the microwave; don't put them in the dishwasher; don't use hot liquid in them.
- Replace canned foods with fresh foods (or even frozen) whenever possible.
- Use glass baby bottles or new plastic ones that are BPA-free, though some children may be allergic to all plastics.

Fluoride

Why are we talking about fluoride in a book on barefoot walking? Because fluoride is surprisingly detrimental to your health and to your bones. Early in 2011, the FDA finally started taking action on this by proposing a rollback in the amount of fluoride allowed in water, and a complete ban on the use of the pesticide sulfuryl fluoride, which leaves behind a fluoride residue on our food. The U.S. Department of Health and Human Services has chimed in, recommending a lower level of fluoride in drinking water.

While debate goes on in the United States, 97 percent of Europe doesn't use fluoride in drinking water; neither do many other countries worldwide.

Recent studies have shown just how dangerous it is. For one thing, people ingesting a moderate amount of fluoride are twice as likely to have hip fractures or other bone fractures. Drink lots of water, eat lots of nonorganic fruits and vegetables, and you're at even greater risk.

Fluoride has a host of health risks, including decreased brain function (particularly for kids), weakened teeth and bones, bone and thyroid cancer, cardiac dysfunction, inflammation, kidney stones, life-threatening anemia in pregnant women and their unborn children, and an increased risk of premature birth. In addition, fluoride is cumulative and builds up in the body.

We both stay away from fluoride. Regular bottled water won't do; you need to drink bottled spring water (with nothing added) or water filtered through reverse osmosis. Luckily, you can now find reverse osmosis water at many local supermarkets. Just remember to bring your refillable water containers (of course, stay away from plastic containers containing BPA).

OUR PATH TO RAWDOM

Just months before completing this book, Jessica sent us down an exciting path, the road toward raw foods. Michael had been 50 percent raw for over a year, but Jessica hadn't. In her words: "I *hate* salad! Salad is for rabbits." But then one fateful day, just after finishing a multiday detoxing fast, she declared, "I'm going raw! Well, at least ninety percent raw." Since Michael continues to be food-prep-challenged, that meant he was going fully raw too. We haven't looked back (though Jessica still turns her head when she smells a barbecue in the neighbor's yard). Here's how it all started.

Our Magic Bullet and Other Helpful Kitchen Gadgets

Though we both started to go organic when we moved to Boulder, Michael found himself eating lots of processed soy and tofu products. It wasn't too healthy, so with Jessica's cooking assistance, he began incorporating more fresh veggies. However, he was challenged by the need for extensive dental work (just say no to sugar, kids!) and struggled to get enough vegetables into his diet. That is, until Jessica's father presented him with a gift, a Magic Bullet. This high-speed mini-blender can turn just about anything into a soup, drink, or paste in sixty seconds or less.

After Jessica decided to go fully raw, we got a more powerful blender, the Vita-Mix. It's helped us make sprouted nut butters, nondairy milks, hummus, pâtés, raw soups, exquisite smoothies, and even raw chocolate balls and energy bars. To add yet another dimension to our meals, we bought sprouting jars and began sprouting seeds, nuts, and grains for some fantastic live foods!

What's next for us? We're delving into fermentation (pickling and making probiotic goodies) and picking up a dehydrator, which simulates sun drying by maintaining warm temperatures below 105–110 degrees, ensuring that the healthful enzymes in raw foods are not destroyed. This kitchen accouterment will allow us to make gourmet "breads," "crackers," "pizza," fancy desserts, and more, all in the raw!

Gone Raw!

There are some great reasons to go raw, and in our case raw vegan. First off, you eliminate almost all of the toxins from processed foods. So once you've passed through the detox phase, you immediately begin to feel better and look better. Second, you dramatically increase the nutritional value of your foods. You haven't cooked off all of the enzymes and nutrients that are destroyed once you heat things above 105–110 degrees Fahrenheit. And perhaps most important, you're eating live foods, meaning foods that still have living cells in them and are glowing with life force. You can feel the difference when you eat live foods. You feel vibrant and alive, and your eyes shine more brightly. When you start eating raw, it's as if you're eating the highest-powered, most energized food on the planet, and you feel high-powered and energized too!

We're still early on in our shift, and there are challenges ahead. It's not easy to go raw, and though we went cold turkey, you may need to wean yourself off gradually. Be kind to yourself, and set yourself up for success by putting the tools in place beforehand (a powerful blender such as a Vita-Mix, sprouting jars, and dehydrator are extremely useful and can be found in most raw kitchens). Make sure you also have a great source for organic seeds, nuts, fruits, and vegetables.

What have we found? Our energy levels are way up. The hours of sleep we require are way down. Food comas are completely gone. Our skin is more even-toned and glowing. Our muscle tone is leaner and our shape way better—even Michael lost body fat, then leveled out at perhaps the healthiest weight he's been at for years. Food cravings for processed food are gone. Our bodies' ability to tell us what we want is high. Our digestion is much better, and

◐°°₀ FOOT NOTE

Fermented Apple Cider Vinegar—The Age-Old Wonder Drug?

With all of the starches, sugars, and protein we're eating today, our bodies are more acidic than ever. To balance them and prevent harmful inflammatory processes, we need something that has an alkalizing affect on our bodies, such as vinegar. Raw apple cider vinegar (which hasn't been pasteurized), rich in potassium and enzymes, has been used as a medicinal substance since at least 5000 BC, employed to treat everything from arthritis to cholesterol, high blood pressure, sinus infections, sore throats, colds, flu, irregularity, overweight, bad breath, nail fungus, acne, age spots, cellulite, yeast infections, constipation, diarrhea, diabetes, and cancer, just to name a few. Michael swears by Bragg Organic Raw Unfiltered Apple Cider Vinegar and drinks two teaspoons with a little local raw honey three times a day. Jessica adds it to many raw recipes, including salads, hummus, dips, and pâtes.

there's no more bloating. Blood sugar levels are much, much better. And on the trails—wow, have our walking and running improved. Our energy levels and stamina are at all-time highs, powered by the life force in the foods that we eat.

Ferment for Life

Surviving without refrigerators for thousands of year, humans evolved to eat fermented foods and benefit from the probiotics, enzymes, and nutrition they contain. Today we're very familiar with fermented foods such as beer, wine, kombucha, yogurt, cheese, sauerkraut, miso, and more. It turns out fermented foods are fantastic for us.

Fermenting brings foods to life, adding friendly bacteria, antioxidants, detoxifying compounds, digestive enzymes, and more. A recent study in Korea found that fermenting soybeans and turning them into a paste helped reduce cholesterol levels, increase muscle, and even control diabetes.

When you ferment a food, you add nutrients and break the food down so more of the existing nutrients are bioavailable, or available for use by the human body. For instance, regular soy is difficult to digest, but ferment it and you unlock all of the available amino acids.

The list of possible fermented foods is nearly infinite. Almost anything can be fermented, and you can do it yourself at home. It's a fun science experiment, and with a little practice, you'll be making some delicious treats. A great place to start is *Wild Fermentation: The Flavor, Nutrition, and Craft of Live-Culture Foods*, by Sandor Ellix Katz.

Eat Life Force

Call it *chi*, *prana*, *mana*, or simply life force—there's an energy in every cell of our beings and in all living things, whether plant or animal. When we eat live foods, we take in this vital life force, a power that goes beyond calorie counting, the food pyramid, or any mechanical nutritional analysis. We all used to eat live foods thousands of years ago, and we were strong.

It wasn't until recently that we began breaking down foods into their elements, calling them a fat, a protein, a vitamin, or a mineral. Somewhere along the way we got lost and thought food intake could only be understood by chemistry and nothing else. Though science has its place, it has a long way to go. There's so much more to eating healthfully than what science currently tells us. Eating food is about consuming and recharging the body with life force and energy. It's not something you can measure on a calorimeter or break down in a lab, though you can see it with a microscope. Examine cells through a high-powered microscope, and you'll see they actually glow. That's what we want, foods that still radiate with life.

Live foods are foods that haven't been cooked, poisoned, dried, or altered in any way. They're straight from the farm, perhaps even picked by you. The minute you drink or eat them, your senses heighten, and it's like suddenly experiencing life in high-def. Check out *The Live Food Factor* and *Spiritual Nutrition* by Dr. Gabriel Cousins.

Take a Live Food Challenge

Go raw and go live for the next two months. Go 50 percent, 60 percent, or even 80 percent raw and live. To start, make sure at least half of your foods are live, uncooked, unprocessed, and fresh. For the other half, try to cut way back on the processed foods, and cut out as much sugar as you can.

These simple changes, with the boost of live foods, will make a dramatic difference in your health. You'll shed weight if you need to, gain energy, have more stable blood sugar levels, experience higher energy levels, and feel younger than ever before.

SUPERFOOD FAVORITES

There's lots of talk today about different "superfoods," foods that provide much more than just basic nutrition. These foods also tend to be some of the tastiest on the planet.

Truth be told, all fresh, organic foods are superfoods too, because they're still alive. The closer a food is to its source, the more vital nutrients and energy it has in it. Grow it yourself in your own organic garden, planter, or sprout jar, and it's truly a superfood extraordinaire.

While there are hundreds of superfoods out there, below are some of our favorites, many of which are very high in antioxidants, known for protecting the heart, preventing or reducing inflammation, and helping reverse the effects of aging:

- **Açai berries.** High in antioxidants, açai berries improve sleep, boost the immune system, help regulate cholesterol levels, may kill cancer cells, help detoxify the body, slow aging, and improve vision.
- **Avocado.** This humble fruit often gets a bad rap for fat, but it has monounsaturated fat, the good stuff. It helps stimulate the brain, has been shown to reduce blood pressure, potentially reduces belly fat, and, with the highest fiber content of any fruit, even helps reduce your cholesterol levels. Much to our surprise, the seed can be blended into smoothies, and since it is incredibly high in soluble fiber, it's fantastic for helping the heart.
- **Cacao beans.** Who needs a reason to love chocolate? Raw cacao beans are high in antioxidants, are great for stimulating the brain, make you feel good, can help you lose weight, have iron to help prevent anemia, are high in manganese to build red blood cells, and are high in magnesium to support the heart, prevent constipation, and reduce menstrual cramps.
- **Chia seeds.** Made famous by the Tarahumara Indians in the bestseller *Born to Run*, these easy-to-digest seeds are a complete source of protein, a fantastic supply of omega-3 fatty acids, and an amazing source of fiber. They help heartburn and indigestion and slow the release of carbohydrates into the blood, which is great for diabetics.
- **Coconut.** Contains easy-to-digest healthy fat (lauric acid), which helps balance blood sugar levels, boosts the immune system, has antibacterial qualities, and helps heal the gut (possibly helping with leaky gut syndrome). Young coconut meat is great for helping create breast milk, can boost thyroid function, and helps fight colon and breast cancer. Coconut water is nature's thirst quencher, naturally high in electrolytes; it also helps reduce the risk of kidney stones.

- **Goji berries.** Well known in Chinese medicine for their antiaging benefits, goji berries have one of the highest antioxidant contents of any food. These berries may also help stimulate the production of human growth hormone, boost the immune system, help protect the liver and kidneys, help improve circulation, and prevent fatigue.
- **Hemp seed.** Sometimes called "the most nutritionally complete food source in the world," hemp seed is a great source of protein for vegans. These seeds are rich in omega-3 fatty acids, boost the immune system, and may help fight eczema.
- **Kale.** This humble high-fiber green is very high in calcium, iron, potassium, manganese, vitamins A, C, B$_6$, K, and in phytochemicals. It's been shown to help prevent cancer, protect the eyes, and aid against diabetes, heart disease, and hypertension. Kale also has anti-inflammatory properties, helps lower cholesterol, and is a very powerful detoxifier. It even has high levels of omega-3 and omega-6 fatty acids.
- **Maca.** Perhaps the Viagra of nature, it stimulates the sex organs, increases fertility, and boosts the adrenal and endocrine systems, giving more energy. Maca helps fight depression and helps relieve symptoms of menopause.
- **Spirulina.** Rich in vitamins A, C, and E, B vitamins, calcium, and magnesium, known for its anticancer benefits, its energy-boosting benefits, antioxidants, and immune-system benefits, spirulina helps maintain heart health, control weight and aid digestion, and even help with PMS. (Other great sea veggies to consider are kelp and blue-green algae).
- **Turmeric.** This Indian spice (typically found in curry) is both nature's anti-inflammatory and an amazing cancer fighter. It contains curcumin, which has been shown to stop the growth of cancer cells. (Add these other great spices to your meals too: cinnamon, cloves, ginger, garlic, and rosemary.)
- **Wheatgrass.** Your blood's best friend, it increases red blood cell count, reduces blood pressure, eliminates toxins, balances body pH (like apple cider vinegar), fights tumors, stimulates the thyroid, restores fertility, and can even strengthens your gums when you gargle

with it. (Another great grass to look for is alfalfa—though technically it's a legume.)

The list could go on and on. The point is to eat fresh, live foods and a diversity of different fruits, vegetables, seeds, nuts, and berries. Each has its own unique helpful qualities and fantastic life force (when eaten raw) and can help you in special ways. Vary the diet, try new things, and discover your own superfoods!

Raw Honey: A Sweet Superfood

If you need something to satisfy your sweet tooth, raw honey from happy, local bees is our favorite option. Bees are little miracle creatures; get to know your local beekeeper or even consider raising your own bees.

Honey is something special. It's been shown to have antibacterial properties among its many health benefits—helping heal sore throats, preventing coughs, helping you sleep, reducing arthritis, lowering cholesterol, potentially reducing or preventing tumors, and even treating athlete's foot.

Super Veggies from the Sea

Jessica and Michael both eat lots of seaweed. We add it to soups and salads and use it to make wraps, or just eat it on its own as a snack. Jessica uses nori for wraps and wakame for soups and salads, while Michael eats dulse as a snack on its own.

Seaweed has been a staple food in Asia for countless centuries. Seaweed is one of the most nutrient-rich and potent foods in the world—some say up to sixty times more potent than its land-based counterparts. It also has some amazing health benefits. First, seaweed contains lignans, which help prevent cancer. It's also high in the B vitamin folate, which helps prevent colon cancer and may help fight birth defects. And it's high in iodine, which helps prevent cancer in areas with high radiation. Seaweed is also high in minerals such as magnesium and iron.

Add some sea veggies to your diet, and you can't go wrong. Each seaweed tastes different and has its own blend of nutrients, so try a bunch and see which you enjoy.

DRINK IT UP

Not all drinks are created equal. Many contain harmful sugars or sweeteners, others caffeine, a stimulant that's getting more and more bad attention lately. Others have little nutritional value but lots of chemical substitutes. We suggest you drink fruit smoothies, green smoothies, coconut water, and of course plain water, the greatest drink on earth.

Morning Smoothies to the Rescue

Want a great way to fuel yourself in the morning or get a midday boost? Try a raw smoothie. Done right, smoothies are a great way to get a lot of healthy nutrients and vital life force into you, without a caloric bomb.

We typically start our days with a smoothie that contains all organic ingredients and some superfoods: loads of kale, raw cacao beans, maca, goji berries, hulled hemp seeds, chia seeds, shredded coconut, fresh wheatgrass, a slice of ginger, and a dash of cinnamon. It varies from day to day—sometimes we add small amounts of local in-season fruit or sprouts that we've grown in the kitchen. What we do not do is load the smoothie up with empty calories— we use either plain water or coconut water (which is naturally sweet) as the base.

If you get creative with your smoothies, you can make magnificent living creations that will give you hours of energy (Michael's typically out on a three-to-four-hour hike on one morning smoothie) and keep you from crashing.

Green Supersmoothies

Want a midday pick-me-up packed with energy and tons of nutrition but not with calories? Try a green smoothie. Michael uses them to bring himself back from the dead when his blood sugar goes low. The more he supplements his afternoons with green smoothies, the more his blood sugar stabilizes.

They're simple: just toss your favorite organic leafy greens or sprouts and half of a banana into a high-speed blender, add some water, and voilà—a tasty, nutritious drink (add a stevia leaf for additional sweetness).

You'll be amazed at how these drinks make you feel the minute you drink one. In Michael's words, "I feel so alive!" And you will too.

Meal Replacement Formulas and Protein Powder

We believe in getting everything as close to the source as possible, but it's often hard to get enough protein into your diet if you're vegan or 100 percent raw and always on the go. One way is hemp protein; another is raw meal powders such as the Ultimate Meal, 19th Evolution, and those by Sunwarrior. High in protein and nutrients, they give you many more nutrients than you could pack in on your own.

We're not nutritionists, but anecdotally, we have found that many raw vegans don't need quite as much protein as other people—perhaps because what they get is more available to the body and doesn't need to be broken down or digested as much.

When in Doubt, Drink Water

Simply removing two small drinks from your diet a day (juice, soft drink, or other sugary concoction, typically about 200 calories each) reduces your caloric intake by more than 2,800 calories a week. That's significant because 3,500 calories equals a pound of fat.

So what do we recommend replacing sugary drinks with? You guessed it: water. Water is the best way to stay hydrated, well lubricated, and cool.

However, if you feel you absolutely *need* an energy drink for your workout, add chia seeds to your water. Not only do they give you slow-burning fuel (fat being much better than sugar) but once they soak up the water, they release it slowly in the body—it's like time-released water! So guzzling your chia water won't result in repeated trips to nearby trees or the desperate search for a lavatory.

Feel you need more calories in your drink? It's very unlikely you do, unless you're completely bonked. However, if you must, perhaps the best compromise is coconut water, without anything added, and preferably organic. Better still, buy the coconut, drain the juice, and then save the nutritious coconut meat for your meals.

Water Therapy

What's perhaps the simplest way to improve your health, other than barefoot walking?

Drinking water, and lots of it (at least four glasses), particularly first thing in the morning, is one of the easiest dietary changes you can make. It's a common practice in many Asian countries, where they've coined the term "water therapy." They say that drinking water first thing in the morning, at least forty-five minutes before eating or brushing your teeth, helps with digestion, diabetes, constipation, high blood pressure, arthritis, and excess weight.

Since 60 percent of the human body is water, it makes sense that we need to stay hydrated. This is especially important in the morning, when our bodies are filled with toxins after a night of processing food. Drinking plenty of water helps flush out these toxins.

Each morning, start with a couple of glasses of water; then work your way up to four. It's important to wait at least forty-five minutes before you have your first meal.

Michael's been doing this for quite a while. He found it challenging to consume that much in the beginning and admits he found himself making extra visits to the loo. The results are well worth it, though. He feels springier and more vibrant, and his blood sugar is under better control.

What kind of water should you drink? Experts disagree, but stay away from tap water. Your best bet? Spring water, or water filtered through a reverse osmosis system to which minerals have been re-added (you can find mineral drops at your local natural grocer). Whichever water you go with, bless your water and give it thanks. We write "love" on all of our water bottles and containers.

||||||||||||||||||||||||||||||||||||||||||||||||||||||||||||||||||||||||||||||||||||||||||||||||||||||||||||||||||||||||||||||||||||||||||||||||

EAT NATURE'S FOOD

The general rule when it comes to our diet is to try to eat as nutrient-dense and "natural" as possible. Not only is this difficult in our modern day and age, but it's quite the mental exercise. After all, what is "natural" anymore? The best you can do is keep asking yourself the tough questions: "Where did this come from? How was it made? What do all of these ingredients really mean?"

The closer you get to a food's original form, the better the food is for your body. It has more nutrients and fewer chemicals, so it's better for your body. The closer it was produced to where you are, the less transportation is involved, which is better for the earth. And the more organic it is, the better it is for the soil. Since we're running on the living, breathing skin of our planet and meeting it with the living, breathing, skin of our feet, there's nothing more important than the dirt.

PART IV

Discovering and Rediscovering the Joy of Barefoot Walking at Every Age

Man is most nearly himself when he achieves the seriousness of a child at play.

—Herodotus, Greek historian from 400 BC

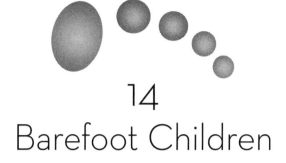

14
Barefoot Children

*If I had my life to live over, I would start barefoot earlier in the spring
and stay that way later into the fall. I would go to more dances. I
would ride more merry-go-rounds. I would pick more daisies.*
—Nadine Stair

We'd been hiking through a forest in Maui, on a trail that winds
through giant eucalyptus trees with a wide bed of thin fallen leaves and
dark coffee-colored clay beneath.

It was a forest we found quite spiritual for how it made us feel: it was both
closed in (it's a long way up to see the sky) and spacious, with layer upon layer of
lush growth all around, and more birds chirping than we could count.

On our first experience in this forest, called the Makawao Forest Reserve,
we heard a young child laughing and shrieking in the distance. We never saw
him, just heard his play. At times it was amusing; at times, admittedly, it was a
bit distracting.

Just toward the end of our hike, as we were returning to the car, we heard
him again, this time with a different tone. He was ahead of us on the twisty
trail, out of sight but within earshot.

"Thank you for this day. Thank you for this hike. Thank you for my family.
Thank you for my health. And thank you for everything." It was the boy, giving
a quiet prayer of thanks.

Awestruck, Michael picked up the pace, briskly leading us toward the parking lot, hoping to catch the boy and his mother before they drove off. He wanted

to give thanks to her for what she was instilling in her child. It was inspiring and gave us hope for future generations.

We could see them up ahead, a middle-aged woman with blond curly hair, clearly fit, and a five-year-old boy with long blond ringlets.

When we reached them, they were staring at our bare feet. We explained to the boy it helps us to feel the ground better and to connect with the earth.

That's all he needed to hear before he flung off his little running shoes! And his mother followed suit.

But we were in a parking area with sharp gravel—not exactly a kind and gentle place to start.

"Owww!" he squealed. But then his feet got used to the ground and he started running, laughing, and playing. There were no gingerly first steps, but an immediate sprint. He got it.

We spent the next half hour talking with his mother, an intuitive healer and massage therapist herself. She got it too, but not quite like her son. He never stopped running or playing on the gravel, laughing and giggling, as if he'd just ransacked a candy store.

Kids intuitively want to be out of their shoes. Children's small stature and light weight is an advantage and allows them to adapt much more quickly, which means less pressure on the feet. That's why this child didn't have any problem on the gravel after his first steps. It's why kids can be barefoot with their first steps, and stay barefoot afterward.

It's as if they've discovered a whole new world to play in. In this child's case, even though he'd just finished a hike, he was ready to go out and explore. We can't imagine he'll ever look at the world in the same way again, or want to have his shoes on while hiking. Months later we bumped into his mom, who delightedly reported, "He hasn't put his shoes back on since!"

How many times do parents tell their kids, "Put on your shoes! You're going to hurt yourself!" What if we rethink all that?

Children naturally love the feeling of going barefoot, running through the grass, playing on a beach, or running in soft dirt. Kenya, Ethiopia, and so many other third-world countries produce incredible runners who have infinitely fewer foot and running injuries—all because they started running barefoot as kids. Running barefoot may be what gives children those springs in their feet.

It's a shame that we force kids today into shoes. We stunt the development of their feet in shoes and make them feel it's unsafe to be barefoot. Study after study suggests how much stronger children's feet get, how much the bones and musculature of their entire bodies and even their nerve endings develop from walking and running barefoot.

A child who goes barefoot is building a strong, healthy body for a lifetime. He or she gains better balance, greater bone density, better joint strength, additional neural pathways, and even better blood flow and circulation. Barefoot activities also help build a body that will be injury-, fatigue-, and disease-resistant for years to come. Running, playing, and exploring barefoot help a child learn, grow, and be a natural kid again.

Even if your children have been in shoes all the way into their teen years, it's never too late to make substantial changes. Though their feet may be fully grown, they're still in the developmental years. Teenagers' feet likely haven't weakened and fully deformed from shoes the way adults' feet have. Moreover, teenagers still have growth hormones coursing through their veins to help them adapt to new stimuli.

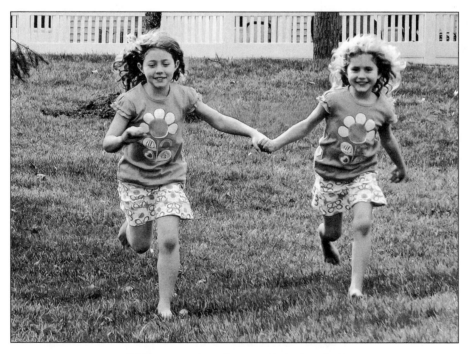

Children were born to run and play barefoot.

Let's learn how to help our kids develop their full physical potential—all by taking off their shoes or keeping them out of shoes to begin with.

NO RUNNING ON THE PLAYGROUND

Imagine a sign on a school playground that says "No Running on the Playground." (It exists in Howard County, Maryland.) Or the mother who asked, "But where will the children play?" when she heard a school was going to remove all the asphalt on the playground (from *Dirt! The Movie*). No wonder our kids are so challenged today. We're completely unplugging them from both nature and who they are.

In our effort to protect them, we're likely doing far more harm than good. So concludes Richard Louv, author of *Last Child in the Woods*, who says that by taking our kids out of nature, they're suffering from nature-deficit disorder. This describes a variety of symptoms, including lack of attention and focus, poor memory, poor impulse control, and anger management issues. He believes this is caused by being stuck indoors, in front of computers, TVs, and video games, and not having the time to play outdoors the way kids once did. He argues that nature-deficit disorder can be remedied by letting kids be outside and independent, playing in nature.

BAREFOOT BENEFITS FOR CHILDREN

Strong Toes Equal Strong Tots

Babies' feet have strong, healthy toes that are as nimble and dexterous as our fingers. There's a beautiful spread between the first and second toe, and each toe spreads out, perfect to act as a spring and launching pad for their newly discovered walking and running attempts. Keep kids out of shoes, and these feet stay in their natural shape—strong, wide, and with a powerful arch. Put them in shoes, however, and the toes get squashed together, the arch goes flat and weak, and the foot loses its spring-like character.

Studies show that if you start children barefoot (or keep them out of their shoes as much as possible), their feet get stronger, more supple, and more stable. Their feet stay warmer; they gain stronger connective tissues and muscles for their feet, ankles, knees, hips, and backs; and they have better posture than their shod counterparts.

Waking Up the Feet's "Eyes" to Better Feel the Earth

Touching the ground and thus waking up the nerve endings on the bottom of their feet, children become more aware of their surroundings and become wired to sense more. In essence, it's like waking up a new sense or talent. The earlier it's discovered and utilized, the more this awareness can be strengthened and grown. Consider this process to be somewhat like waking up the "eyes" on the bottom of your children's feet—helping them be better in touch with the earth, better balanced, more stable, able to run like the wind, and able to better feel the world around them.

Becoming King of the Hill

By giving kids a chance to be outside, to feel the ground, and to play and connect with nature in an unstructured way, we're giving them the greatest opportunity in the world to destress and be kids again. That in turn has an incredibly calming and empowering effect—especially for children with ADHD, with whom Michael has worked extensively, because he understands their frustrations.

Playing in the woods and feeling the ground or feeling nature gives kids a sense of being king of the hill. In today's world, we often rob our children of the opportunity to feel empowered. This makes children more fearful and takes away the self-esteem they need to overcome life's greatest hurdles. By letting them play free and feel the ground, you're giving children the chance to spread their wings, explore the world, let their imagination soar, and make decisions independently, helping them grow self-confident.

Habla "Coordination"

When a child feels and reads the ground, it's as if he or she is learning a foreign language. The brain grows new neural pathways and networks. The earlier we do it, the more neural pathways there are for learning even more new bodily "languages," developing memorization skills, and increasing sensory awareness. The better children are able to walk, run, or hike, the more capable and better balanced they will be at so many physical endeavors and activities.

Trigger Points and Reflexology

Studies have shown that stimulation from the ground is amazingly effective at reducing tension and aiding with relaxation. Like acupressure and reflexology, going barefoot has many health benefits, from lowering blood pressure to reducing anxiety and depression, and aiding the immune system—all great for our children.

By encouraging your child to go barefoot each day, you help your child recharge the mind and sync with the earth to put them back in the zone for focused, concentrated studies, anxiety-free.

FOOT NOTE

Barefoot in the Cold

In his book *Indian Running*, Peter Nabokov talks about the Navajo tradition of having kids roll around in the first or second snow of the year in order to build resistance to the cold and strengthen their immune systems. It turns out there's good reason for this. Although you don't want to risk your child getting frostbite, studies are showing that exposing your children's feet to the cold may help their bodies better adapt to the cold and regulate skin and internal temperatures.

Barefoot in the Heat

Who can forget those quick dashes across hot pavement on a hot summer's day? Or the hot swimming pool decks in the days before all kids wore flip-flops or Crocs?

Native peoples such as the Aborigines in Australia handle the most incredible desert heat barefoot, because they started walking on hot surfaces as children. Hot pavement's toasty, but only in the beginning. While hot pavement can burn children's feet if they are exposed to too much too soon, their feet adapt faster than adult feet.

While they'd like to let pain be their guide, kids often don't think ahead, and if they head out barefoot without a pair of shoes, they can get in trouble quickly. Best advice: monitor their early activities in the heat. Better yet, keep them outdoors year round. This way, as the temperatures climb, they'll acclimate gradually.

THE DANGER OF FOOTWEAR FOR KIDS

Since a child's foot is flexible, malleable, and growing, it's easy to do harm without realizing it. The foot will compress, bend, or mold to the shape of its footwear, all without complaint.

As foot expert Dr. Michael Nirenberg explains, "The downside of such a flexible foot is that if parents choose the wrong shoes or footwear for their children, they could create a deformity for their child." In essence, when we squeeze a child's foot into traditional footwear, we forever change the shape of the foot.

According to the late Dr. William Rossi, another leading podiatrist, due to footwear "foot defects and weakening begin at age three and progressively increase. Starting at age six, it is impossible to find five straight toes on shoe-wearing children."

Tight-fitting shoes and shoes with a strong inflare (the banana-shaped curve on shoes) force a child's big toe in, creating bunions, calluses, corns, and more by the time the child is an adult. It prevents the toes from working naturally and, since eighteen of the nineteen muscles of the foot are connected to the toes, greatly weakens the foot in the process. This is the beginning of adult plantar fasciitis and other weakened foot conditions.

In addition to being soft and flexible, a child's foot adapts incredibly well to its external environments. If a child is stuck in a shoe—or, even worse, in a shoe with arch support—the foot doesn't have to work, so the muscles, ligaments, tendons, and bones get weak and rigid and the foot loses circulation. Instead, if the child runs and plays barefoot on uneven surfaces and terrain, these same structures will quickly strengthen and gain flexibility and better circulation.

Shoes Can Harm Your Child's Feet

Researchers are weighing in on the damage shoes can cause when worn by children. In one study, scientists compared the feet of Americans who had been wearing shoes all their lives with Africans who had never worn shoes. The largest difference was in the big toe. Americans showed a surprising number of deformed big toes and bunions, caused, the researchers thought, by shoes curving inward—perhaps as a concession to style and to make feet seem more slender. Those pointy-toed shoes haven't done anyone a favor. The Africans' feet showed a straight big toe and no bunions.

The arch is the greatest natural shock absorber in the world. Researchers who examined 2,300 Indian children between the ages of four and thirteen found that children who grew up in shoes were more than three times as likely to have flat feet than those out of shoes. Their conclusion: shoes (particularly those with closed toes) negatively affected the growth of a normal arch. "We suggest that children should be encouraged to play unshod and that slippers and sandals are less harmful than closed-toe shoes," they said in their study, published in the *Journal of Bone and Joint Surgery.*

A Swiss study presented at the annual meeting of the American Academy of Orthopaedic Surgeons in 2009 found that about half of the 248 children surveyed were wearing outdoor shoes that were too small.

Note: This also means keeping a child out of socks, particularly tight-fitting ones, as much as possible. These socks will also bind the foot, force the toes together, and cause deformities of the foot as well as keep the foot sweaty and moist. In the winter, if warmth is necessary, seek soft-lined moccasins or booties. Uggs are now the fashion du jour, and with their roomy interior and soft, warm lining, there's no need for socks.

||||||||||||||||||||||||||||||||||||||||||||||||||||||||||||||||||||||||||||||||||||||||||||||||||||||||||||||||||||||||||||||||||||||||||

FOOTWEAR FOR CHILDREN

One of the most common questions we're asked at clinics and talks is what shoes to buy for children. While we have our favorites, such as Soft Star Shoes, it's easier to talk in terms of guidelines for your children's footwear choices.

Let us caution parents upfront: it's nearly impossible to find traditional shoes that will help more than harm.

Babies, toddlers, and young children don't like to be in shoes anyway. Ever notice kids tearing or kicking off their shoes and socks while riding in strollers at the mall? Many experts now believe putting pre-training shoes on babies in cribs causes discomfort and distress. We then compound the damage by double knotting and tying the shoes extra tight. In this case, baby does know best.

FOOT NOTE

The Canadian Paediatrics Society's Community Paediatrics Committee no longer accepts the old belief that a baby must wear shoes soon after birth. "Keeping a baby out of shoes in warm, dry conditions is a good idea because walking barefoot develops good toe gripping and muscular strength. Indeed, there is increasing evidence to suggest that wearing shoes in early childhood may be detrimental to the development of a normal longitudinal arch."

So let's talk about what can be done about it.

First, let's dispel some common myths about kids' footwear. Many of these myths are the same as for adults, which we've already discussed. But some myths are unique to children's footwear.

Myth: The sole of the shoe protects the foot. The truth: A good stiff sole actually eliminates the foot's ability to move freely, turning a beautiful, strong, resilient three-dimensional foot into a two-dimensional block of wood. This can do significant harm to a child's growth and development, not just of their feet but of their entire musculoskeletal system.

Chiropractors now know that the majority of problems in the back can be traced directly back to the feet; after all, it's our interface with the ground and how we learn to stand tall. If we've eliminated the foot's ability to move and flex and bend naturally, then we eliminate the rest of the body's ability to do so as well.

Myth: Shoes provide traction to keep a child from falling. The truth: Balance, not traction, is what keeps a child from falling. Balance comes from the child's ability to feel the ground. It's why there are so many nerve endings in their feet. When children can no longer feel the ground, they fall, no matter how much traction they have. And have you ever checked out a baby's toes? They grab for the ground like claws—that's more traction than they'll ever get from a shoe.

Feeling the ground is necessary to grow the brain's balance mechanism and ability to respond to sudden surprises underfoot. The brain can't build a strong balance and control mechanism if it doesn't have input—if, in essence, it's blindfolded.

Myth: Traction is safer than no traction. The truth: The average child takes approximately 20,000 steps a day. In a shoe with heavy traction, the shoe grabs on the ground and lurches to a halt with each step. Unfortunately, the child's toes do not. So the toes slam into the front of the shoe repeatedly—20,000 times per day. This crushes the toes and can do even more harm than stuffing them in a shoe that's too small.

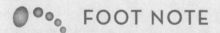 **FOOT NOTE**

Lynn T. Staheli, director of orthopedics at the Children's Hospital in Seattle, provides the following recommendations on proper footwear for young developing feet. The shoes should:

- Be flexible and allow free movement
- Be flat with no heel elevation
- Have a sole friction similar to the bare foot (no excess traction)
- Be made of soft leather or of similar construction
- Be lightweight

Dr. Staheli concludes that the shoes should not have arch supports or the stiff sides that were once deemed necessary to lend the foot support. Since the feet of young children are soft and pliable, abnormal pressure caused by stiff footwear may cause deformities such as flat feet.

Myth: Children's feet need support. The truth: Whether it's arch support, heel support, or ankle support, it's likely harmful rather than helpful. Support may help in the short term, but weakens the foot in the long term. Support in a child's shoe never gives the child's foot a chance to move or grow naturally. Instead it has to learn how to work with the support it was given, something it never would have had to do naturally.

A child's body is growing, adapting, and changing at an incredible rate. If we support the foot, the arch, or the heel, we begin to mess with the body's normal growth, strength, and flexibility. A heel support reduces the flexibility and strength of the Achilles tendon and can reduce its natural range of motion. An arch support weakens the arch (and changes the shape of the foot). And an ankle support weakens the very structure it was intended to protect.

Myth: Snug-fitting shoes are best. The truth: By now you know how bad this would be for the foot.

Myth: Extra growing room is the answer. Remember when you tried on shoes as a kid and your mom or the shoe salesperson would press on the front of the shoe to make sure there was a thumb's width of "growing room"? If there was, your shoes were pronounced "a perfect fit" and off you'd go wearing your new shoes. The truth: Traditional shoes for kids are a complete misfit to begin with. Buy them even larger and they're that much worse. Getting shoes that are too long (as most shoe stores recommend) puts the child's foot in the wrong part of the shoe. Instead of the shoe bending where the foot bends, it bends someplace else. Instead of the arch being where the arch belongs, it's in the wrong place too.

Myth: Shoes give necessary ankle support. The truth: Originally, the high top on baby's shoes may have been put there to keep the baby from pulling them off, because in this case, baby does know best. No support is the best support for a child's ankles and feet to grow strong and healthy.

Myth: Sneakers are better for active kids. The truth: Most sneakers are made by designer brands, not by those specializing in the movement of the foot. It's hard to find a sneaker that naturally fits the shape of the foot. A sneaker also doesn't flex naturally where the foot bends. Shoehorning a kid into a designer shoe weakens the foot and destroys its natural flexibility. Sneakers also have toe spring, which raises the child's toes when they should be naturally grabbing for the ground. Additionally, kids' sneakers are basically miniature versions of adult sneakers; where they're bad for adults, they're even worse for kids.

Myth: Heels add spring to the child's step. The truth: Even a slightly raised heel in a child's shoe is a big no-no. It's about scale. A one-half-inch lift for a toddler is like a two-inch heel for an adult. That means the average toddler's shoe or sneaker is the equivalent of a high heel.

Baby Those Baby Feet

It's a crime, but often babies are put in shoes months before they even take their first step. They're often called pre-trainers and are designed to help a child grow accustomed to shoes. This is wrong in so many ways.

Once a baby has begun to walk, you want to keep him or her out of shoes to promote natural foot strengthening and growth. A toddler's foot is both incredibly flexible and sensitive. By placing them in shoes, you reduce the flexibility of the foot by 80 to 90 percent. Imagine trying to type on a keyboard with tongue depressors attached to each finger! This completely destroys the child's natural movement (which is why they often walk like Frankenstein once we put them in shoes). In essence, instead of a foot that moves nimbly and feels the ground, they're forced to take pancake-like steps, with the feet hitting the ground flat.

Additionally, in a shoe a child's foot can perspire up to 50 percent more, leading to very unsanitary conditions. If the child's not in sneakers, then chances are they're in high tops, which fit snugly above the ankle, further trapping sweat and heat. Instead, children's feet need to breathe.

Footwear Guidelines for Kids

- **Infants:** Keep them out of shoes; there's never a need. If you're going outside, bundle them up, or keep on warm loose-fitting socks (socks you'd consider too big that aren't snug on the foot at all).
- **Toddlers:** Keep them out of shoes for their first steps and beyond. After all, they're called toddlers for a reason. If they're going outside to play, let them be barefoot unless it's an unsanitary or unsafe place. The more they're barefoot, the more they're going to be cut- and scratch-resistant anyway!
- **Early childhood years:** Yes, some places require shoes, such as schools. Consider very loose moccasin-type (soft-soled) shoes or huarache-type sandals like the Tarahumara wear, if the school will allow it. Many of these shoes can be custom designed by the children in their favorite colors, in school colors, or with plenty of bling to keep them in fashion. And keep the kids out of shoes at all other times. No matter what shoes you use, make sure they fit like a loose-fitting sock, not a snug shoe.
- **Preteen and teen years:** Choose soft-soled thin and light shoes, shoes that let the toes move independently, and shoes that have plenty of room, not just in front but at the sides. Encourage teens to be barefoot as much as possible because their feet are still growing. Still stay away from traditional shoes and watch out for those heels. At this point, look at the adult guidelines as well. For some sports your preteens or teens may need a traditional shoe (such as for soccer) so do the best you can to get the flattest, lightest, widest shoe you can and get them out of shoes the minute they're not playing soccer. Ideally, we would get the entire team to practice playing soccer barefoot. After all, many of the world's best soccer players, such as those in Brazil and throughout the rest of Latin America, grew up playing barefoot!

PLAYTIME BAREFOOT ACTIVITIES

Imagine finger painting with your toes. That's the kind of fun you can have while introducing your children to "barefoot time" every day.

When your children are young, work to build the dexterity and strength of their feet by encouraging barefoot time each day. This can go beyond barefoot running and walking time to include barefoot games, and even art and dexterity exercises with the feet.

Here are some examples of activities children can try with their toes. However, anything they can do with their fingers, they can try with their toes. Well-known painters without hands paint with their toes, and pilots have even flown airplanes hands-free, so quite literally the sky's the limit.

Exercises
- **Art with feet.** A variation on finger painting. Use a paintbrush grasped in the toes like the famous armless artist Simona Atzori. Or try using the feet to mold something out of clay or Play-Doh (fantastically messy but a ton of fun).
- **Games for feet.** Play pickup games with the feet, such as picking up golf balls. For a more advanced version, use feet to pick up and build things with Legos. Another variation: throwing things with the feet, such as Frisbees or even sticks, like the kick-stick racing once popular with Native American children.
- **Exploratory exercises.** Present blindfolded children with different objects to touch with their feet to try to identify them. For a fun-tastic outdoor activity, have children go into a backyard or playground blindfolded (do this in a safe location with supervision) and have them describe the surfaces they're touching with their feet.
- **Activities that strengthen the feet.** Sign your children up for gymnastics, modern dance, children's yoga, and circus arts. They'll exercise their brains and their feet.
- **Follow-the-leader (dexterity exercises).** Play follow-the-leader barefoot where you must step exactly where the leader has stepped (over grass, safe obstacles, and other tactile surfaces). Our kid-at-heart

friend Paul Weppler submitted this game: Kids throw down six-inch-diameter pieces of carpet over an obstacle course. They then try jumping barefoot from one piece of carpet to the next without touching the ground. Slacklining is also perfect for kids (see description of slacklining in chapter 11).

- **Corn mazes.** If you get the chance, take your family to a giant corn maze in the fall for an a-*maze*-ing barefoot experience. The difference between a labyrinth and a corn maze is there's no way to get lost in a labyrinth; through a series of twists and turns it guides you to the center, and then back out. However, in a corn maze, there are always fun dead ends, blind turns, and false paths.

There's nothing more natural than a child dancing barefoot through the grass. It doesn't just strengthen their feet but sets them up for a lifetime of vigorous health. It keeps their senses awake, helps build stronger bones, muscles, ligaments, and tendons, gives them greater balance, and kindles a special bond with nature.

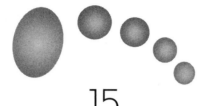

15
Barefoot Seniors Turn Back the Clock

My grandmother started walking five miles a day when she was sixty.
She's ninety-three today and we don't know where the heck she is.
—Ellen DeGeneres

Jack Burden is a dear friend of ours who describes himself as more than a friend—he's a "pain-in-the-butt" parental figure. At eighty-seven he served as best man at our wedding, and we've since found that he lives up to that role in other ways, for often he does in fact know best.

We've never pushed him to go barefoot. However, he uses a grounding pad, and he gets the benefits of being grounded and of following guidance from the universe. But as he describes in crotchety fashion, "Darn it, with my old sensitive feet I can feel a crumb on the floor! There's no way you're gonna get me to walk barefoot."

However, do you know how he keeps in shape? Barefoot exercises and barefoot time spent on a home mini-trampoline. He uses it every day to get the blood flowing and, in his words, "keep the lymphatic fluid pumping and get everything back to the heart." At least ten to twelve minutes a day, every day.

He has great balance and walks with purpose in his step; even at his age, it's hard to keep up with him. A big part of that is his barefoot tramp time. He's working on his feet, his core (stabilizing muscles), his balance, and coordination, all by going barefoot.

Do we wish he'd give barefoot walking a try? Sure. But he is, in typical Jack fashion, doing it his way and still reaping the rewards in many ways. He's also converted to a fairly minimalist shoe that's flat (no high heel or high toes), has a wide forefoot to give his toes and bunions room to breathe, and has no arch support so his feet can stay strong. And maybe it's from the trampoline, but boy does he have a bounce in his step!

Want the secret to eternal health? Take your shoes off.

Whether you're an avid walker, new to walking as an exercise, or struggling to stay on your feet, taking off your shoes can help. Any time spent barefoot helps regenerate nerves, stimulate bone growth, increase circulation, and lay down new bone. Add the benefits of strengthening your heart and lungs while decreasing blood pressure, and you've found the fountain of youth in your feet.

Seniors can reap incredible benefits with barefoot living. But age also presents its own set of challenges. That's why it's even more essential for this demographic to start slowly, because recovering from overdoing it takes even more time. But no matter your age, no matter how soft your feet, you can and should go barefoot and strive to walk unassisted. You may eventually kick off your shoes for life.

USE IT OR LOSE IT

When it comes to your body, you have to respect that same principle we've mentioned before: use it or lose it. If you don't use your body, well, nature's not so kind. Whether it's a bone or joint, a muscle, your cardiovascular strength, or anything else, if you use it, it gets stronger, and if not, it weakens.

As Dr. Henry S. Lodge states in *Younger Next Year*, you can get healthier and fitter at almost any age. Both mind and body can regenerate at any age if properly stimulated. Use your body by going barefoot, and you will feel the ground and wake up your nervous system, vestibular system, vision, and balance; it will stimulate new brain cell growth and create new maps in your mind—all while sharpening your senses in the process.

As neuroplastician Dr. Michael Merzenich reminds us, you're never too old to start, and you can gain back losses, at least when it comes to the mind. No matter what your age, if you start working out or using your body more, it gets stronger. The human body can wake up. Who cares how many candles are on your next birthday cake.

Dr. Lodge and his coauthor Chris Crowley talk about how we must become full-time athletes once we pass the age of sixty. You need to commit to your health in order to stay young, healthy, and fit, or to get back to the fitness you had.

Now, Michael's not past the age of sixty, but having broken his hip, he understands a bit about this philosophy and why you or your grandmother might not be so excited about physical activity.

As Michael says: "Doctors told me I couldn't, shouldn't, and wouldn't be able to run again. They advised *against* exercise, rather than doing *more* of it.

"But this isn't the first time I've heard this warning. Ever since my first serious injury, a broken femur, tibia, and patella (upper and lower leg and knee) at the age of ten, I've been told time after time that if I work out, I'll risk injury and just make things worse. I was also diagnosed with an arthritic knee at the age of twelve and told to back off. And yet by working out, the arthritis, along with every other condition or challenge, has magically gone away. Some people call me a 'medical miracle.' But I'm not. I've just committed to working out to recover and build my strength."

So the advice for you older readers and for your parents and grandparents is to commit to working out daily, strengthen what you have, challenge yourself, and see yourself get stronger *at any age*.

BAREFOOT BENEFITS FOR SENIORS

I walk for four hours per day while many other elderly people remain seated for this time. Their legs are tired and my legs also are getting tired by walking. By nightfall, my legs have gotten healthier whilst their legs have actually got weaker.

—Fauja Singh, who took up running at the age of eighty-one and at the age of one hundred set nine records, from the 100 meters to the marathon

In the PBS special *The Art of Aging: The Limitless Potential of the Brain*, Ryohei Omiya demonstrates you can reverse the effects of aging on the brain starting at any age.

In 2004, Ryohei set the national record in Japan for the 100+ age group in the 60-meter dash (28 seconds). The record still holds today. He joked, "It was more like walking than running." However, at a younger age, Ryohei had struggled to be mobile. At eighty-five, he suffered a stroke. Four years later, when his wife died, he stopped being active and began to show signs of mild dementia.

"He stayed in his room all day. He sort of drowsed with his mouth open. We [Ryohei's family] all just got the feeling that his health was failing. At the time he leaned on me to walk and he didn't walk far, not even a hundred meters. We were afraid he might slip too," shared Hiroki Omiya, Ryohei's daughter-in-law.

In an effort to improve Ryohei's health, Ryohei's family began taking him out walking to get some exercise. Remarkably, as his activity levels increased, his interest in life returned, and at ninety-nine, Ryohei began running again!

Exercise for Your Brain

Until 1998, there was no hard evidence that the brain cells known as neurons could regenerate. The accepted assumption was that nerve cells regenerate in all parts of the body except for the brain and spinal cord. We also thought 100,000 neurons (out of 100 billion) died on a daily basis and could never be restored.

Thanks to the work of Dr. Peter Eriksson, a researcher in the Department of Clinical Neuroscience at Sahlgrenska University Hospital in Sweden, we now know that neurons regenerate even in the brains of the elderly. New brain cells are formed whenever you stimulate the brain, and challenging and different stimuli help the most.

Hundreds of studies point to the rejuvenating benefits of exercise. Just think—your brain doesn't have to get weaker, but instead can grow stronger.

Going barefoot literally wakes up your mind. In *The Brain That Changes Itself*, Dr. Norman Doidge writes:

> If we went barefoot, our brains would receive many different kinds of input as we went over uneven surfaces. Shoes are a relatively flat platform that spreads out the stimuli, and the surfaces we walk on are increasingly artificial and perfectly flat. This leads us to de-differentiate the [brain] maps for the soles of our feet and limit how touch guides our foot control.

Then we may start to use canes, walkers, or crutches or rely on other senses to steady ourselves. By resorting to these compensations instead of exercising our failing brain systems, we hasten their decline.

By learning how to coordinate your body and gain balance by going barefoot, you're creating additional neural pathways in your brain and throughout the nervous system. In essence, going barefoot is helping grow stronger minds, wake up the mind-body connection, and rewire our brains.

Feeling the ground for the first time is like learning a foreign language or playing a new musical instrument. It requires the brain to process information in a novel way, with new dimensions and sensations never perceived before. This dramatically helps stimulate the mind, forcing it to relearn how to learn.

Just standing on a cobblestone mat (more on this soon) helps begin to rewire the mind. However, imagine walking on uneven surfaces and how much that would stimulate your mind. A good barefoot walk on a trail would be like reading a Braille novel with your feet, giving incredible stimulus to help wake up the brain.

Diabetes Control

"[People with diabetes] should be closer to the ground and exercising their feet to increase blood flow and muscle development," Dr. Ray McClanahan of the Northwest Foot and Ankle Clinic observes.

"The problem is," he says, "some of these folks not only have a circulation issue, but the bigger issue of neuropathy, where they can't feel anything. If the diabetic person has lost what we call protective threshold, their nerves will not alert them to possible skin and bone damage. We test this with a monofilament wire in the clinic. If they can't feel it, they won't feel sensory warnings, and will damage their own tissues."

Diabetics with foot neuropathy are challenged because they can't feel their feet and won't know when enough is enough. Instead of building skin thickness, they may instead be wearing the skin thin, creating sores that can be deadly for diabetics.

"There is no question in my mind that all diabetic people would benefit from wearing footwear that is foot shaped—flat, and wide at the ends of the toes," according to Dr. McClanahan. "Interestingly, most therapeutic footwear dispensed to people with diabetes has heel elevation, toe-spring, and tapered toe boxes. Often called 'extra depth' shoes, these do not take into account the need for the toes to spread, thus curtailing circulation to the toes, and squeezing the intermetatarsal nerves, at exactly the point where nature intends them to branch into their respective toes."

He goes on, "With advanced diabetic neuropathy, the diabetic patient also loses muscle tone in the muscles furthest from the core of the body, the intrinsic flexors. So their toes become hammered, their fat pad moves too far forward, and they ulcerate under their metatarsal heads. Elevated heels and toe spring hasten this muscle weakness, yet are included in nearly every therapeutic shoe option for diabetic people."

Early diabetics, without neurologic damage, may do well with a more minimal shoe, which may allow them to exercise more comfortably and naturally, he suggests. One powerful possibility is that someone with diabetes may feel comfortable in a minimal shoe and thus exercise more, shed weight, and get the diabetes under better control.

While we can't recommend it, we've heard many stories of people starting barefoot in a controlled environment, such as a cobblestone mat in their house, where they can keep a safe eye on their feet, regain blood flow, and improve nerve sensitivity to the feet, even with advanced neuropathy. Check with your doctor before attempting this, and never try this outdoors, but perhaps it's right for you.

⬤°°₀ FOOT NOTE

Diabetes Complications

Does anyone wear right-sized shoes? A 2006 study of 440 veterans with an average age of sixty-seven found that only 25 percent of them wore appropriately sized shoes. The study was published in the *Journal of the American Podiatric Medical Association*.

But even more shocking is that more than half of the veterans (mostly men) had diabetes; 7 percent had serious foot ulcers that would be slow to heal. Diabetes presents a serious risk to feet. Complications from foot ulcers or loss of sensation, known as neuropathy, caused by diabetes can create serious health issues. Many of the foot problems for these veterans were caused by their poorly fitting shoes, not necessarily by their diabetes.

In fact, people with diabetes are fifteen to forty-six times more likely to suffer an amputation. In patients without diabetes, poorly fitted shoes may make existing foot conditions worse.

"Since many people with diabetes can't feel whether their shoes are too tight or too loose, footwear that fits correctly is extremely important. Getting these patients fitted by experienced professionals should be a top priority," said American Podiatric Medical Association president Dr. David Schofield.

Dr. Bernhard Zipfel, researcher and podiatrist, notes that while the APMA justifiably instructs people with diabetes who have lost protective sensation not to go barefoot, "they, however, unfortunately also do not actively encourage outdoor barefoot walking for healthy individuals. This flies in the face of the increasing scientific evidence . . . that most of the commercially available footwear is not good for the feet."

Balance

The most important key to fitness in seniors is balance. Why? If you're balanced, you can climb stairs, walk, or even run without the fear of falling and breaking a hip—one of the most serious injuries seniors face.

Going barefoot and feeling the ground is one of the best ways in the world to gain balance. When you're in a shoe, you can't feel the ground, and you're literally walking blind without any input as to what's beneath you. Ever tried standing on one foot? Perhaps it wasn't too tough. Now try doing it with your eyes closed. We all tend to teeter pretty quickly with the loss of just this one sense. The difference is as dramatic when going barefoot versus wearing a shoe.

○°°°₈ FOOT NOTE

Our friend Dr. Bill Weber, a highly acclaimed author and expert on Colorado flora, began walking barefoot after the age of ninety. Until that point he was using a walker or, on his best days, two walking poles. Now he's doing laps around the neighborhood barefoot and has traveled to Antarctica to celebrate his newfound "freedom" on two legs. In a sense he's reversed the effects of aging by going barefoot.

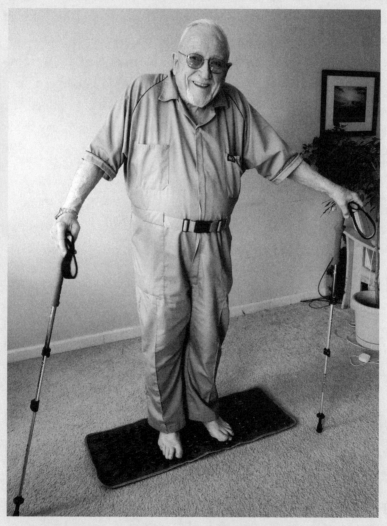

Bill Weber wakes up his feet on a cobblestone mat. Just weeks after this photo was taken, he was out and about without his walking sticks.

Gaining or regaining balance is not as simple as taking off your shoes. In fact, studies show that if you just get out of your shoes, you'll initially have *less* balance than before. This makes sense because your muscles are weak and shoe-dependent, and you haven't done the mental training to learn to stabilize yourself.

Instead, as long as you're still quite mobile, slowly start incorporating barefoot time into your routine. The goal is to wake up nerve endings on the bottom of your feet. Start with a little time standing barefoot. Then begin walking barefoot on a cobblestone mat to wake up the dormant nerve endings. (Note: If your mobility is already compromised, seek assistance from a friend, family member, or medical professional, depending on your needs.)

Once you're comfortable spending time barefoot, you can start incorporating balance exercises. The next step would be to do one-legged standing exercises. You can begin these by holding on to a wall, a railing, or someone standing next to you. At first, spend a minute or two each day barefoot, just practicing standing first on one leg and then on the other.

FOOT NOTE

Arthritis and Barefoot Walking

Walking barefoot may be better for people with osteoarthritis by reducing the load on the hips and knees. Consider this: Grandma is likely wearing big clunky shoes, and yet she still leans heavily on her walker to get around. Imagine if Grandma were to dump the walker and her shoes.

A 2006 study in the journal *Arthritis and Rheumatism* suggests that the design of modern shoes may predispose people to develop osteoarthritis. At the least, shoes make this type of arthritis worse.

So what should Grandma wear? Specialized footwear (low, flat, and flexible) has been shown to take the load off already painful knees, according to a study published online in the journal *Arthritis and Rheumatism.*

Building Strong Bones

If you're not getting weight-bearing exercise or stressing your muscles, you lose bone. One of the leading reasons our bones get brittle is because we're not exercising or using our muscles enough. This can devolve into a vicious circle: if you're worried about falling and breaking a hip, you may exercise less or move less in general. With the "use it or lose it" principle, if you do less, you lose what you have, in this case bone density, making you more prone to breaking a hip.

As you're working on balance, you can begin building stronger bones. Better balance helps prevent falls, and staying mobile helps your bones get strong. The two work hand in hand. Not only that, but if your bones are stronger, chances are you can handle a trip or fall without a serious injury. It doesn't matter how much calcium and vitamin D supplementation you take—if you don't do weight-bearing exercises, you lose bone density and develop that dreaded brittle-bone disorder called osteoporosis.

According to Dr. Gary Null, author of *Be a Healthy Woman*, "Not only is weight training safe, it is important for preventing osteoporosis. As muscles are pulled directly against the bone, with gravity working against it, calcium is driven back into the bones. It also stimulates the manufacture of new bone. This adds up to a decrease in the effects of osteoporosis by 50 to 80 percent." This is significant news. Additionally, studies are showing that arthritic joints can regain mobility through exercise.

Going barefoot and gaining stability, coordination, and balance helps you gain the freedom you need to break this cycle of bone loss. Doing balance exercises barefoot, walking barefoot, or even light jogging barefoot can help you keep the bones you have, grow them stronger, and help prevent the dreaded hip-breaking fall.

Gaining Cardiovascular Strength

No matter your age, if you keep your heart and lungs healthy, it increases the quality of your life. This is why authors Lodge and Crowley advocate becoming a full-time athlete, working out six days a week, after sixty. If you can keep active with walking or doing other aerobic activities, you greatly increase the quality of your life in almost every respect. This is largely due to the endorphins and other chemicals released in the brain during cardiovascular workouts. These natural "happy chemicals" improve mood, possess anti-inflammatory qualities, boost the immune system, and do much more as well.

Walking and other types of aerobic exercise have been shown to greatly reduce symptoms of tension, anxiety, and depression. They strengthen the heart and lungs, increase blood flow, and help the body eliminate toxins (all of which helps you feel better). As fitness guru Jack LaLanne said, "There are plenty of excuses, but there is no real reason you can't exercise every day." He did up until his death at age ninety-six.

Cardio exercises also serve to keep body fat and obesity down. This can have a significant effect on the health of seniors, as keeping weight off the joints allows you to continue to be active and gain mobility and fitness even if you're frail or arthritic.

One particularly efficient way to be aerobic yet kind to your joints is exercising in the water, such as doing water aerobics, aqua jogging, or even walking a loop in the pool. Lots of seniors have discovered the healing power of water (maybe the real "fountain of youth") in swimming pools at the Y and in water aerobics classes with like-minded seniors in wellness centers throughout the country. Although some seniors wear water shoes to grip the bottom as they walk and cavort together in classes (and prevent them from slipping on the pool deck and in the locker room), they're still getting many of the benefits of going barefoot, particularly if their shoes are wide.

Stronger Core

When you go without shoes, you use your core (your stomach and back muscles) to keep you balanced. This has particular importance for freedom, mobility, and remaining pain-free as a senior. Many seniors suffer from back pain, which is often traced back to an earlier injury or trauma, and then exacerbated by inactivity, an unhealthy lifestyle, deteriorating posture, and a weak back.

When you strengthen your core, you help protect and strengthen your back, take your guarded muscles out of spasm, and make them more pain-free. This is the theory behind the practice of Pilates. Founder Joseph Pilates was able to keep his back strong and healthy like a twenty-year-old well into his eighties.

Grounding Effect

Touching the ground barefoot doesn't just feel good, it *is* good for you. It helps drain off any excess electrical charge you're carrying on your skin and sync you with the vibrational frequency of the earth. Studies have shown far-reaching health benefits, including reduced inflammation, reduced effects of arthritis, decreased free radicals, added boost to the immune system, and greater amounts of natural cancer-fighting agents in the body. That, coupled with the antianxiety and antidepressant effects, makes getting grounded almost a must as part of staying healthy at any age, but especially as you grow older.

Reflexology

Reflexology is the practice of massaging or relieving tension, improving circulation, and helping return the natural function to all parts of the body by stimulating pressure points or zones on the hands, the ears, and in particular on the feet.

When you go barefoot, you stimulate all of the reflex points on the bottom of your feet, helping reduce tension, improve body function, reduce inflammation, and much more. Studies are suggesting reflexology not only strengthens your immune system but can even help fight cancer.

In a pilot study, Oregon Research Institute scientists engaged men and women aged sixty to eighty-eight in a cobblestone mat walking activity for eight weeks. At the end of the trial, the walking participants experienced improvements in psychophysical well-being, reductions in daily sleepiness and pain, significant improvement in perceptions of control over falls, and reduced blood pressure—a classic reflexology response.

FOOTWEAR FOR SENIORS

The answer to the footwear question is simple: choose moccasin-like footwear, low to the ground, with flexible soles and no high heels. If the flexible sole is too much, begin with a hard sole (please work down to a thinner sole, though, to wake up the nerve endings on the bottom of your feet—this is essential for your entire body's health, as well as for your mind), but the key is to be low to the ground. Again, you want a wide toe box to allow the toes to wake up, move, and spread for balance.

Studies are showing that an uneven or bumpy footbed inside your shoe can wake up nerve endings too. While such a footbed would not get you closer to the ground (and therefore not aid with stability), it may be a way to safely wake up nerve endings in your feet.

○°°₀ FOOT NOTE

Wrong Shoe, Big Pain

Pressure from ill-fitting shoes can be a pain in the . . . foot. A 2005 study found that most older people (men and women ages sixty-two to ninety-six) wore shoes narrower than their feet. Women were especially at risk with shorter, narrow shoes, according to the Australian researchers.

They also found that wearing shoes markedly narrower than the foot was associated with corns on the toes, bunions, and foot pain. Wearing shoes with heels higher than about an inch was also associated with bunions and plantar calluses in women.

The study concluded that incorrectly fitting footwear is common in older people and is strongly associated with foot deformity and pain. Therefore, choose shoes by how they feel, not by the size marked on the box (see chapter 19 for more on footwear selection).

RESUSCITATE YOUR FEET

It's never too late to go barefoot, and the health benefits can change your life. Better balance, increased strength and mobility, more freedom, better mental abilities, a potentially stronger immune system—the benefits of going barefoot as a senior are too great to be ignored.

Overall, going barefoot gives you greater health and freedom. Who says you have to sit around or stay in shoes as you age? Instead, why not get younger, this year, next year, and the ones thereafter, all by shedding your shoes?

PART V

Dancing with Nature

In early days we were close to nature. We judged time, weather conditions, and many things by the elements—the good earth, the blue sky, the flying of geese, and the changing winds. We looked to these for guidance and answers. Our prayers and thanksgiving were said to the four winds—to the East, from whence the new day was born; to the South, which sent the warm breeze which gave a feeling of comfort; to the West, which ended the day and brought rest; and to the North, the Mother of winter whose sharp air awakened a time of preparation for the long days ahead. We lived by God's hand through nature and evaluated the changing winds to tell us or warn us of what was ahead.

—Unknown speaker addressing the National Congress
of American Indians in the mid 1960s

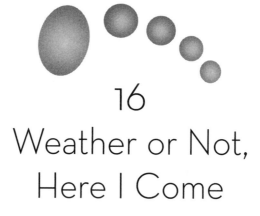

16
Weather or Not,
Here I Come

*Sunshine is delicious, rain is refreshing, wind braces us up, snow is
exhilarating; there is really no such thing as bad weather,
only different kinds of good weather.*

—John Ruskin

Jessica says: "As a teenager, I developed cold feet. No matter how thick
my wool socks were, my feet were constantly freezing in my winter boots if
I stood outside too long. And if you shook my hand, you'd shudder at the chill
my cold hand would send up your arm.

"My circulation only worsened as I entered my twenties, to the point where
I kept my gloves on when I shook someone's hand, or at least I apologized pro-
fusely for the embarrassingly cold shock. I felt like a cold-blooded animal and
hoped strangers didn't find my cold hands representative of a heartless person. I
wanted to say to them, 'I'm warm on the inside!'

"As for my feet, if I ever went skiing or snowboarding, no amount of
air-activated warmers seemed to last very long. You could count on me to head
back to the lodge before anyone else as I struggled to rub life back into my
numb, stiff toes. In my late twenties, there were a few scary moments when I
wondered if I'd gone too far. I'd flick my blanched toes with my fingertips and
feel nothing.

"I began to wonder if I had Raynaud's disease, a condition in which blood vessels and capillaries constrict, limiting blood circulation due to an overreaction to cold temperatures or stress. This may have been the case, but starting barefoot training at this time opened up the valves and the blood began flowing freely again.

"At the end of my first winter barefoot, there was snow outside our back door one morning. Michael was outside with the dogs, and I stood barefoot on the landing waiting for the happy scampering crew to charge their way up the stairs and through the door. After they were all in, I looked down at my feet. I was standing on a mix of snow and ice and it hadn't even registered. The surface felt cold, but my feet maintained their warmth. My feet were liberated!"

Michael says, "Last year on book tour, Jessica sent me to Phoenix and Scottsdale to conduct several talks and clinics.

"I'd just flown from our new home in Taos, where it had been warm, but it was nothing compared to the heat I received in Arizona. My first hike was over 100 degrees, from 104 to 108 to be exact, at least according to the thermometer in my car as it wilted in the desert.

"I went hiking among a giant expanse of saguaro cactuses, sand, stone, and shrubs, not far from town but protected by jagged dry mountains obscuring the city's skyscrapers.

"It was silent, magical, vast, and hot. Out on the trails, with undulating hills, wavy air, and cactus everywhere, you could barely find any sign of human life, nor any water, as far as the eye could see.

"And did I mention it was hot?

"If the air is over 100 degrees and the sun is shining bright, then by noon (or if you're in Phoenix 8:00 a.m.) the ground has been soaking up the rays and is *warmer* than the air. The darker the ground, the hotter it gets. In this case, I was walking over dark gray rock and ancient lava that'd been pounded into pebbles from the flooding that occurs during the wild summer monsoons.

"I can only guess at the temperature on the ground. But it felt great underfoot. I'd been building stamina in Taos, and always liked the heat on my skin. I felt an energy from it, along with a warmth and power that seemed to radiate up through my legs and my entire body.

"To be safe, I brought my 'hand weights' with me, and a bit before the car I put them back on. I didn't know how much my feet could take, not just because of the egg-cooking temperatures on the trail, but because the pebbles were very coarse underfoot." The more your skin is softened by the terrain, the more susceptible it is to the heat.

Like it or not, the roads aren't always smooth, the trails aren't always soft, and it's not always spring. Let's look at the major challenging conditions out there, from heat to cold and rain to snow; from different road conditions, trail conditions, and potential hazards to watch out for—and the gear to best prepare you for a rocky road ahead.

HOW COLD OR HOT IS IT?

Air temperatures can be quite deceiving. Even though it may be a pleasant, sunny 60-degree day, that doesn't guarantee that the surfaces you walk on, whether man-made or natural, are going to be just as warm and pleasant. If the 60-degree day is a fluke in the dead of winter, chances are likely the ground is still holding on to a freezing temperature.

Not all surfaces are created equal; for instance, denser surfaces are slower to cool and slower to heat. So there are quite a number of factors to consider when you're gauging ground temperature, such as the temperature of previous days, humidity levels, and surface material.

Ground temperature has a much bigger impact on your feet than air temperature, so forget about weather reports and pay the most attention to how your feet feel. Different surfaces (ice, snow, cement, asphalt, mud, brush) drain away different amounts of heat from your feet. For example, wet snow takes away more heat than dry snow, and wet mud sucks away heat even faster than moist snow. Wet blacktop also takes away more heat than dry blacktop.

Pavement and cement are slow to cool off. Cement seems to hold its temperature better, but once it's cold, due to both color and density, it's far colder than the blacktop. If you've had a good cold spell, or the cold has set in for the season, even on a warmer winter's day the ground temperature may be far colder than the air.

Different surfaces also hold different amounts of heat. For example, pavement, ice, and wet conditions can be deceiving, particularly depending on recent sunlight. Sometimes the ice next to the bright-colored sidewalk is warmer than the sidewalk itself. Blacktop, even if wet, may be warmer than a lighter colored surface. And if there's snowmelt in your path, the wet surface may be warmer than the dry one you're treading on.

Hot surfaces can be tricky as well. On any given day, pavement and cement are likely two very different temperatures, and trails far different from both. Cement heats up gradually over time, then cools off gradually as well, while pavement or blacktop heats up fast, then quickly sheds its heat. Trails are another story entirely, depending on the dirt, dryness, color, and rock beneath. Make note of this and walk with attention so you don't get burned. Extreme conditions are never to be taken casually.

WALKING IN HEAT: CONCRETE ADVICE

Because you can't always choose where or when to walk, it's best to prepare for as many conditions as possible. If you're walking in the summertime, unless you do it around dawn, chances are you'll have some days when the asphalt is baking hot. But not to worry—a little hot tarmac can actually be a good thing. No other condition helps temper and strengthen your feet like hot stone.

Humans may have adapted naturally to this in the past. According to evolutionary biologists, we first started walking bipedally, or erect on our two feet, in the hot African savannah. This may explain why our feet are able to adapt so well to the heat. It strengthens our skin, increases padding, increases circulation, aids foot strength, and more.

Adapting to the Hot Stuff

First and foremost, heat stimulates pad growth more than anything else. This additional padding in turn helps you handle the heat and rough surfaces. In essence, you're growing stronger "shoes" in the summer. This will benefit you in all conditions year round.

Walking in heat also increases circulation to your feet. Your body adapts and increases capillaries and blood flow to your feet to help keep your feet cool and strong, and for recovery and healing. After an invigorating walk in the heat, or even in the cold, your feet will remain hot at night. This isn't because they're burning, but because of the extra blood your body's pumping to your feet to rebuild and grow your padding stronger.

This increased blood flow will help keep your feet cool in the summer and help keep your feet warmer in the winter too. And there's another tremendous benefit. Increased blood flow means shorter recovery times, both for normal recovery from a hard workout and in case you overdo it. Increased blood flow helps ligaments, tendons, and even bones heal faster. This can help with injuries that have never fully healed in a shoe because you couldn't get enough blood flow.

FOOT NOTE

Always bring your shoes with you. When your feet feel too hot, don't think twice—put them on. In fact, put your shoes on before your feet feel too hot and before they feel too cold, because by the time they feel too hot or too cold, you've likely gone too far or done too much.

Although hot conditions are ideal for pad development, they can be quite dangerous too. Heading out in the heat before you're ready could leave you badly burned, with blistered feet that look like pepperoni pizza.

Whether you're a beginner or expert, once spring rolls around, you want to baby your feet into the heat. While heat may stimulate growth and improve circulation, it requires significant time for feet to recover in between sessions of walking on hot surfaces.

Transitioning into Hot Weather

One of the best ways to transition to the heat is to alternate between hot and cool surfaces on your walk, such as between a blacktop road and a light-colored cement sidewalk. You can do this for 100 feet to 100 yards at a time, or however long your feet can handle letting the heat be your guide. Never push too much or too far. If your feet start cooking, head back onto the cool stuff. By alternating, you let your feet cool down between efforts. It's the long steady heat that'll cook them.

Always look for routes where you can find shade if necessary. Road temperatures can easily be 10 to 20 degrees cooler or more in the shade, not to mention the air being cooler as well. Look for routes that offer protection if you need it. You might spot trees along the side of the road, a way back through the trees on a trail, or even the shade of nearby buildings. Shade's another way to extend your walk and keep you safe.

The worst thing you can do is go out in the heat two days in a row. While your feet are growing stronger, the day after a hot walk your feet have temporarily lost their resistance to the heat. Your skin's now soft, your padding mush, and you'll burn yourself extraordinarily fast.

Five Safety Tips for the Heat

1. Start with short distances (100 feet to 100 yards).
2. Alternate between hot and cool surfaces (10 to 20 feet at a time).
3. Listen to your body. If your feet feel hot, *stop* or get on the cool stuff.
4. Never head out where there isn't shade to hide.
5. Never do two days in a row in the heat.

Once the heat hits, follow these weekly steps to keep from cooking your feet:

- Week 1: When it gets hot, skip the long midday walks for a week or so, and instead go out for short walks in small doses. Walk ten feet on pavement; then hop onto the grass to cool off. Repeat two or three times and call it good. This helps temper your feet and keeps you close to home. Always walk with "hand weights" and never think twice about putting those shoes back on.

- Week 2: Venture out for short distances and walk just five to ten minutes at most.
- Week 3 and after: Gradually walk longer in the heat and add one long walk a week for the first month or two.

Water, Water, How Much Water

When it comes to hydration, think safety first. Most of us don't drink enough water during the day. Train yourself to understand how your body reacts with proper hydration and how you feel when you're dehydrated. Drink fluids at three particular times: first thing in the morning to flush out your system, before each walk or workout to keep well hydrated, and at the end of the day so that your muscles have a chance to fully recover and replenish overnight.

Always play it safe. No matter what, bring some water in a hydration pack (not in a water bottle held in one hand) when you're just starting out and getting to know your body in the heat. If you start to wonder if you made a smart decision, get yourself home, to the shade, or to a cool car, fast.

Pack Light

When the going gets hot and you need to carry water along with you, look for a hydration belt or hydration pack that doesn't affect your stride (Amphipod provides some ergonomic options). Use a pack that fits well and has good support for your hips and waist. The lower you can get the weight, the less work for your upper body. The lower your center of mass, the better it is for your stride. A hydration belt may work well too, but just make sure it doesn't affect your stride, arm movement, shoulders, or back. You don't want your pack throwing off your form, for example, causing you to lean to one side, bend forward at the waist, or hunch.

Go with the lightest pack that meets your needs. Think light so your body can move most naturally.

Singing in the Rain

Remember what a joy it was to be a child, dancing in the rain, stomping in the puddles, and laughing until your sides hurt while getting drenched in a good downpour?

Well, playing in the rain, as long as you stay warm enough, can actually stimulate your immune system, increase your circulation, and give you plenty of those "laughter drugs" or endorphins.

Walking barefoot in the rain also gives you a heaping dose of vitamin G. Water is an excellent conductor of electricity; the more moisture in a surface the better it conducts. So we drain positive ions even faster in the rain. This same phenomenon explains why a shower can feel so good, and swimming in the ocean is so incredibly refreshing; the combination of water and electrolytes (a fancy word for salts), which conducts electricity, is even better.

"Is it bad for my foot padding?" you may ask. No, it's not bad, and it won't wear away the skin. However, if you're out in the rain and your pads get soft, then either stop or keep going in the wet stuff, but not the dry. If your skin looks prune-like, you don't want to go onto a dry coarse surface; that's where you'll wear stuff off.

But walking in the rain? Highly recommended. It's not just good for the body but makes you feel like a kid again.

WALKING IN COLD: GET INVIGORATED

The cold isn't what you think, and neither are your feet.

In a shoe, you rely on your footwear to support your body weight, so your feet don't have to work very hard, and thus the body doesn't pump much blood flow to them. Instead it shunts or redirects blood to where it needs it more, and your feet get cold. Out of a shoe, your feet have to do the job of supporting your body weight, so your feet get extra blood flow, so much blood flow that a few minutes in the cold fully barefoot can keep your feet toasty and warm for the rest of the day or night when you get back inside.

The more time you spend barefoot in the cold, the more your body adapts and the better your circulation. The trick is, you need to start with very short amounts to give the body a chance to adapt.

We wouldn't recommend going to the point of getting numb, and for now, only walk barefoot when the temperature of the ground is above freezing. Below freezing, you run the risk of frostbite or damaging your tissues. If it's early in the day after a night of freezing temperatures, rest assured that the ground is still frozen. Some signs to look for are frost, ice, frozen puddles, or heavy condensation in the air when you exhale.

There are two ways to get into cold-weather walking. First and easiest, keep up the barefoot walking as the weather gets colder and your feet will naturally adapt. If there's a really cold spell, just throw on a pair of cheap, disposable thin socks (preferably made of natural fibers) to take the edge off until your feet warm up.

Second, start in with real short distances, and then go back to your shoes. Open and insert some disposable air-activated (not preferred) or reusable (preferred) heat packs into your shoes, and let them warm your shoes as you walk. By the time you need to throw your shoes back on, the air inside will be warm and cozy. Remember, your shoes only hold the air temperature of your feet. In other words, if your feet are cold, then your shoes will be cold, unless you have an external heat source, such as a hot pack.

Walk for at least five to ten minutes in your shoes or inside on a treadmill before slipping off your shoes in the cold. Then spend a few minutes, but no more than ten minutes, out of the shoes before putting them back on. If your toes get numb or tingly, get them back into the shoes. If you warm up well and feel comfortable, you can repeat this once or twice; then head for home and get warm.

Last, never do two days in a row of cold-weather barefoot walking until you've fully acclimated (usually about a month). This gives your feet a chance to rest, recover, and grow back stronger.

Hot Tips for the Cold

1. **Stay on your toes.** There are four reasons why staying on your toes keeps your feet warm:
   a. It works your foot more; therefore the body must deliver more warm blood to the foot.

b. It leaves less contact area with the cold ground.

c. It focuses more weight on a smaller area of your foot, giving you greater traction and allowing you to grip with your toes.

d. It keeps you from slipping and falling backward. Never walk flat-footed or on your heels on ice or you will slip, slide, and fall.

2. **Dress for the North Pole.** Make sure you're extra bundled up to keep the rest of your body warm; even consider two hats for your head. In the cold weather, Michael likes to wear a puffed-up purple coat that makes him look like Barney the dinosaur. The trick is to always keep the rest of your body extra warm. This makes it very easy for the body to take extra blood and pump it to the feet.

Socks Take the Edge Off

A cheap pair of very thin socks can be your best friend for getting into barefoot walking in the wintertime. They take just a bit of the edge or bite out of the cold and protect you in the most bare-bones fashion from the elements.

No, they won't last long, and since we're very much into sustainable non-petroleum-derived products, we recommend natural fibers, but at a couple of dollars a pair, socks are an efficient way to get started. They're much better than minimalist footwear since they still give you tactile sensation off the ground, and if you buy them loose (consider bumping up a size) they won't constrict your toes. And since they're natural materials, you'll still get some of the same earthing benefits as you'll get fully barefoot. However, stick to white socks. When colored socks get wet, the dye can seep into our skin.

Snow

Unless you have years of experience in cold-weather walking under your belt, we don't recommend walking barefoot in the snow. You may have seen YouTube videos of us running barefoot in the snow. But running in the snow is much

⬤ °°°₀ FOOT NOTE

The warmer your hands, the warmer your feet, as your body doesn't have to concern itself with keeping your hands warm.

Always wear gloves. On extra cold days, take along a couple of hand warmers. There are $1 or $2 packets you can pick up at a sports store or supermarket (or preferably find eco-friendly, reusable packs such as Wonder Warmers). Open the packages before they are needed, as they take up to twenty minutes to warm up. Once the warmers are exposed to oxygen, they begin to heat up and warm your hands. You can reuse them if you place them in air-free zipper bags and keep them in your freezer.

easier than walking, because you get your body temperature higher. It's much harder to do this while walking.

So stay out of the fluffy stuff, at least for now. And if temptation gets the better of you, save it for the last snows of the season. A good spring snow isn't that cold because below the snow the ground is usually well above freezing. In those cases it's like standing in soft, squishy cotton candy, rather than an ice dip in the Arctic.

Watch for these signs of frostbite: gradual numbness and loss of touch, a tingling or burning sensation, feeling as if your hands or feet are wood, associated pain that then goes away (as the frostbite progresses), change in the color of your hands or feet from pinkish red to blanched white or white-purple (or, far worse, black).

If you think you have frostbite, get inside *now*. Warm things up under 104–105-degree water if you got cold fast. Don't go too hot, because you won't be able to tell what's scalding and what's not. The general rule among winter emergency specialists is this: freeze fast, thaw fast; freeze slow, thaw slow (an example of a slow freeze would be on a multiday expedition).

Emergency medical attention is always a smart option.

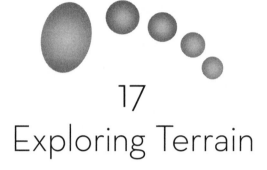

17
Exploring Terrain

*To me a lush carpet of pine needles or spongy grass is more welcome
than the most luxurious Persian rug.*
—Helen Keller

After climbing a sacred hill on Maui (described in chapter 5), Jessica
continued her exploration down the other side of the hill. "I wasn't ready
for the adventure with our new friend David to end," she says. "I was still on
cloud nine, living the high from 'being the mountain goat.' So at the bottom
of the hill I wandered off to investigate an interesting land formation set between two hills—not steep enough to be considered a valley, but more like a
U-shaped, natural half-pipe kids would use for skateboarding. I walked up one
side and let gravity and forward momentum carry me up the other side, switching back and forth, yelping with childlike glee. It may sound difficult, but it was
relatively easy—for my feet were sticking to the walls of this half-pipe.

"When I finally ran out of breath, I knelt down to examine this new
awesome surface that I had never barefoot walked on before. It was a colorful
mélange of clay that resembled an assortment of Play-Doh modeling compounds smushed together. The clay ranged from purplish gray to orange-red
to yellow. After the rain, it was wet and soft (and therefore grippy for my bare
feet).

"To further my investigation I began scraping it up with the tops of my fin-
gernails. Before I knew it, I was smearing it on top of my feet. It just felt like the

natural thing to do. And the cool dampness of the clay felt soothing on my feet too.

"The ground became my clay palette: a glob of gray, a swoosh of yellow, dabs of orange. I painted a sun and its beaming rays on a gray backdrop, all on my bare foot. The painting stayed with me until we trekked to a raging waterfall later in the day. I was disappointed to watch it wash away, but nothing in life is permanent.

"A few weeks later, Michael and I brought a film crew back to this special half-pipe with the purpose of filming a fun barefoot montage. It hadn't rained recently, so the clay was dry and brittle and

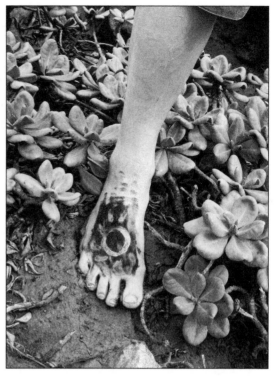

Jessica's cheerful foot adorned by nature's paint and lots of love.

more challenging to walk on. Sadly, I wasn't able to use the clay as paint either. It just goes to show you never know what to expect. The same path you've walked for decades in a shoe will be a completely new adventure when you walk it barefoot, and a new adventure yet again the next time you walk it without shoes. When you walk barefoot, you realize the terrain is ever changing. You'll be forever aware and never bored. Just be present and enjoy the moment, because it may never come again."

If the world were flat, fully paved, and always 70 degrees, it'd truly be a dull place indeed—and a poor place for a foot that thrives on challenge and change. Fortunately, different conditions, temperatures, and surfaces abound. As barefooters, we're truly three-dimensional, since we can feel far more than in shoes. This makes varying conditions much more interesting—and challenging.

In this section we'll examine different surfaces and discuss what to avoid and what to seek out. We'll also look at the ups and downs of uphills, downhills, and mountain trails.

THE BENEFITS OF EXPLORING TERRAIN

When you feel the ground, you're truly all-terrain. You sense and adjust to conditions instantly. Landing on the ball of your foot allows you to instantly change your step or lift back up if you need to, in order to avoid rocks, glass, or other obstacles. This is much harder in a shoe, and when you're tired in a shoe, you're likely to trip and stumble over the humblest of obstacles.

When you try out new trails and surfaces, you further wake up your feet, legs—and mind. You force your body to find new ways to adapt, balance, and carry you forward. In essence, each new surface is like learning a new language. We'll outline some fun, unexpected terrain options in a bit, but it's important that you practice the ape walk, a special walking technique for tricky surfaces, before diving in.

EXERCISE

The Ape Walk

What do you do when you hit a surface your pads, feet, and technique aren't ready for, such as an unexpected gravel trail, sharp stones, or a sidewalk that's needed repaving since the 1950s? It's simple—lower your heels, bend at the knees, drop your arms, and do the ape walk. When you begin trails or rough surfaces, you may find some surfaces particularly challenging. This could be your first trail, or first rocky one, or even a bridge or other unusual surface.

This technique not only allows you to traverse the most challenging of surfaces but also, by helping you do the tough stuff, contributes to building stronger feet and padding in the process. The next time you're on gravel or something particularly challenging, rather than put on the shoes, use it as a chance to experiment and build your strongest pads ever. While maintaining proper walking form, relax the feet, bend the knees, and squat down low to show off your best ape impression. You'll feel your quads burn in no time.

Walk with your legs bent 10 to 15 degrees (you'll be squatting down six to eight inches). Let your arms lightly swing back and forth as if you're an ape. Try not to let your torso and head swing from side to side by tightening your core as much as you can. Imagine you're an ape, strutting your stuff for your clan. Now where's that banana?

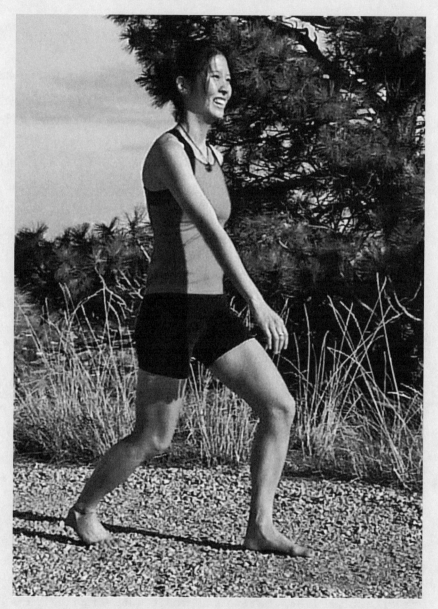

Dropping down low and doing the ape walk is a great way to handle challenging terrain.

NAVIGATE THE ROADS LESS TRAVELED

Let's explore some of the roads less traveled and discuss how to walk on them.

Smooth Cement Sidewalks and Bike Paths

This is the easiest surface for beginners, but not a favorite over the long haul. The smoothness makes them easy, and the surface gives tremendous feedback. It helps you feel the ground, learn to stride light, and work on your form. However, cement paths have several major challenges.

First, they're likely the hardest surface you'll ever walk on—and completely unforgiving. Second, they're perfectly flat and therefore unnatural. There are no undulations, imperfections, or changes on the surface that give your feet a chance to rest and recover, flex, and receive proper blood flow. In nature, we never walk on perfectly flat surfaces. Surfaces change, sloping one way, then another, getting rough, getting smooth, getting soft, then hard again. These constant changes allow your feet to recover.

On the trails, if you overwork muscles on the smooth stuff, don't worry—you'll work different muscles on the rough stuff. If you fatigue muscles on a flat stretch, don't worry—the hilly stuff up ahead will shake them loose.

On a perfectly flat cement path, however, the chance of an overuse injury goes up infinitely because you work your feet and legs in the exact same way, step after step, mile after mile.

BIKE PATH SAFETY

Runners and cyclists often go whizzing by on paved paths. Particularly in the beginning, however, you'll be walking quite slowly. Staying far to the side keeps you out of harm's way. There's quite a bit of debate as to which side of a path is safest. Michael prefers the left so he can keep an eye on cyclists and they don't sneak up from behind. Often the rule is dictated by what others are doing. Check your local parks department to see if there's a rule, and if not, choose whichever side feels safest to you.

Keep your MP3 player and cell phone off so that you're more aware of what's going on around you. If you have your dog with you on a path, keep Fido on a very short leash and as far to the side as possible. Stay alert in both directions.

Be visible. Wearing bright colors on a bike path always helps, as does wearing reflective gear at night. Some clothing, such as IllumiNite, turns your entire outfit into reflective gear at night. Also wear a blinky at night (a red or orange blinking light you can clip onto your belt, pack, or jacket collar) and consider a headlamp or waist lamp, such as GoMotion. The lower the headlight source, the less shadows will disrupt your vision.

Asphalt or Blacktop Paths

These paths tend to be far kinder and more forgiving than the smooth cement ones. Yes, they're not quite as smooth, and therefore a bit more challenging if you're just getting into the barefoot game. However, once your feet toughen up a bit, chances are you'll come to like these surfaces.

Asphalt is a combination of steam-rolled rocks and oil, and that combination adds far more spring to your step. The oil acts as a rubbery surface, making the ground softer and more forgiving. Additionally, it's not pancake flat. There are always imperfections and undulations in asphalt. This helps keep your feet and legs fresh and helps prevent overuse injuries.

Asphalt heats up fast. So you'll have to watch yourself in the summer, particularly in southern climes and at high altitude. Pavement is not only hot to the touch but may even have patches of melted asphalt or rubberlike crack fillings that have turned to hot oily goop; you'll want to avoid these.

Compared to cement, asphalt (which is less dense) cools and heats much more quickly. In the winter, this means asphalt is better to walk on in the daytime and more challenging at night, as it will warm up quickly with the sun, then shed heat quickly at night. If you hit the path after dark, head for the cement.

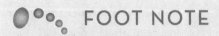 FOOT NOTE

The Grass Is Not Always Greener

Believe it or not, some grass is very sharp and can stick into your feet. If you're in sharp or dry grass, it's best to do a shuffle with your feet, meaning only raise your feet an inch off the ground and let your toes lead the way. Your toes move the grass forward so that it's not sticking up directly underfoot. This shuffle lets you get through the sharp stuff without getting pricked.

New England Roads

If you live in parts of the Northeast or somewhere else that's pedestrian-unfriendly and doesn't have sidewalks or shoulders on the roads, be careful. To be safe, walk on the left rather than right side of the road in order to see what's coming and get out of harm's way if need be.

But these roads have an added dimension of danger: road debris. Often littered with glass, broken plastic, or even sharp wires, walking here (even with thickened pads) is asking for trouble. Best to find someplace else to walk, such as a local park, a nature preserve, or the local track if you're out of options.

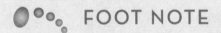 FOOT NOTE

Left or Right, Which Is Right?

The rules are clear when it comes to walking on the road. Always walk on the left side so that you can see oncoming traffic and oncoming traffic can best see you. Be careful and on alert if you're walking on any roads. Also be aware that there's camber (a sloping) on the edge of the road. If you're constantly walking on the sloped left side of the road, you'll likely suffer an overuse injury over time. This means either mixing things up on a very quiet (or closed) road or sticking to bike paths, sidewalks, nature, or your local park.

Running Tracks

There are many types of tracks out there today. The most important thing to watch for is overuse injuries. A running track is a perfectly flat surface, which nature never intended, and if you're walking in only one direction, you're more than doubling your chance of an overuse injury. So whichever track you end up walking on, alternate directions and walk half of your laps in one direction, and half in the other. This is exceptionally important, as the tighter turns, particularly on the inner laps, put significant strain on your stabilizer muscles and all of the joints of your feet. If you walk continuously in one direction lap after lap, or workout after workout, you're inviting a substantial overuse injury. So mix things up; better yet, alternate between the track in both directions, plus the infield, and perhaps any paths around the area as well.

Pay close attention to your body on rubber-coated tracks too. These are fun and springy but give you less feedback for your feet. It's difficult to keep from landing hard, and as with all tracks, the perfectly flat surface makes it even easier to create an overuse injury. They are also squirmy underfoot, which can cause shin splints.

Dirt Roads

Ahhh, the joy of getting off the hard stuff and onto something more natural. If you can find a good dirt road, you've found a friend for life. They're softer than pavement, have more natural undulations (which help prevent overuse injuries), and help build pads.

Of course, there are different types of dirt and consistencies, but that's half

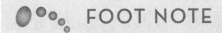 **FOOT NOTE**

What's Your Walk Score?

WalkScore.com rates the walkability of a city or a neighborhood. If you're looking to move or relocate and want to see how walkable an area is (or how little you'll have to drive) simply type in an address and hit enter. A high rating means almost everything you need is within walking distance. A low score means you need to drive everywhere.

the fun. Some are rock hard, others as soft as a beach. Some are sun-baked and cracked in the summer; others have dry, sharp angulations from muddy vehicles and footprints that dry incredibly hard. Still others become washboard-like from vehicles. The most challenging dirt roads are gravel filled.

All dirt roads help promote pad development. Watch for ice hidden in the dirt in the winter, and for sharp dried mud and clay and potentially thorns (in the Southwest) in the summer. Dried mud can be the best at strengthening and toughening your entire foot, including the soft belly of your arch, which if you have a high arch rarely meets flat pavement. However, this also means you have to start light, as the skin and muscles around your arch and soft spots of the foot won't be ready for this. Do too much too quickly and you'll not only scuff up the bottom of your feet but spectacularly bruise them as well.

Gravel Roads

Although we can adapt to anything, gravel roads are a pain. The rock on them isn't natural. It's mechanically ground-up granite, with jagged points. These rocks don't move when you hit them, but stick straight up underfoot. They're hard and sharp.

Yet there's almost no better surface (except perhaps jagged dried mud) for building your pads and foot strength fast. Just start incredibly slowly. Consider walking 100 yards or less your first time; then call it quits. If you can master gravel, you can walk on just about anything.

City Sidewalks

Oddly enough, New York City's sidewalks are among our favorite surfaces. They're incredibly smooth, worn down by millions of feet treading along year after year; and they're not too hard. Perhaps best of all, the curbs tend to be smooth metal surfaces. This means you can walk on sidewalks, the edge of the road, or almost anywhere else you need to (just be careful of cars and other vehicles). It's very smooth and one of the fastest walking surfaces available.

HITTING THE TRAILS

When it comes to barefoot walking, trails are what we were born to enjoy.

From a reflexology point of view, nothing stimulates your feet, and thereby everything in your entire body, more than walking on trails. You'll touch and stimulate each and every nerve ending of your foot, helping reduce blood pressure, relax your mind, and improve your overall health.

There are an unlimited number of types of trails, each with its own unique characteristics, traits, and challenges. One mile you're walking on the soft stuff, the next dried sharp clay, the next bounding over rocks. This can be quite enjoyable. It keeps things from getting boring, gives your feet (and mind) a great workout, and keeps you from becoming fatigued.

Dirt Trails

After a few weeks on the roads or bike paths, it's time to hit the trails. Each dirt trail has its own feel, energy, and minerals to it, and you'll quickly find ones you resonate with. Watch your form on the dirt; it's easy to go back to old habits as you start into them. Just try to stay light and keep from hitting your heels. It's also fun to watch your footprints as you go, or see them on your return journey. Pay attention to whether there could be rocks hiding under the dirt. If it seems likely, tread extra lightly. Soon enough your feet will gain eyes and find the obstacles for you.

Rocky Trails

This is heads-up walking at its finest. Make sure to walk with your eyes scanning the horizon, anywhere from six to eight feet in front of you and beyond. Over time, you'll learn to see what's coming ahead and what's beneath your feet simultaneously. This is important because you'll find yourself moving from rock to rock in rhythm with the trail.

●●°°。 FOOT NOTE

Happy Trails to You

What is proper hiking etiquette for passing or letting someone pass—especially if you are going downhill and someone is working his or her way uphill?

Sometimes contentious, this issue does have a general rule: the uphill walker/hiker has the right of way, but all rules are meant to be broken. If you're heading uphill and the approaching hiker, runner, cyclist, or horse appears to need the right of way, give it to them. If you see someone struggling as he or she approaches, give that person the right of way as well.

The right of way for uphills may have developed out of the assumption that the uphill hiker has gotten into a rhythm and we don't want to break it. No matter who technically has the right of way, if you can yield to help others, then go for it.

Technically, you're also supposed to get off the trail on the downside of the slope, but very few people know this, or remember this. It's much more important to give the person, cyclist, or horse plenty of room to pass.

This rule is about courtesy and compassion. And it doesn't hurt to smile and say, "Happy trails!"

Walking through rocks can be a meditative experience. There's something stimulating, yet relaxing about it. It's incredibly powerful for quieting the mind. Why? Because when the mind's completely focused on picking your steps, there's no room for stray thoughts to enter.

Things to watch out for: loose rocks, gravel, and big rocks with lips.

After the feet tire, you're incredibly susceptible to tripping on such uneven surfaces. At times like these, consider putting on your shoes and walking your way back out of there.

Lava Rock

There's a type of lava rock in Hawaii called *a'a*, which is what the first European settlers probably yelled out in pain if they tried to walk on it barefoot.

It's hard and coarse, and yes, it can be quite sharp. For an experienced foot it doesn't feel too bad (and for kids who grow up on the islands, it's a piece of cake), but it still requires intense concentration. Michael loves the lava both for the meditative experience and for the energy he feels through his feet. He feels there's no better way to strengthen the feet—it forces each muscle and joint in the foot to work, grow strong, and gain flexibility, all while taking in the energy of the earth.

Pine Needle Trails

Pine needle trails are one of our favorites, because they feel so good, though you'll quickly learn why they're called pine *needles*. When you're walking on a well-trodden path they seem to stay at bay, but if you're in virgin forest, particularly on soft ground, they may nip you from time to time. They're not a big deal, nothing more than a little ouch. But overall, this is a really fun surface to walk on, and if you're not careful, you may find yourself running among the pine needles as well.

Wood Chip Trails

Wood chip trails take a special sense of trust in the beginning. We were recently out on a trail that had been closed due to fallen trees. The trail had been reopened and all of the fallen trees had been converted into wood chips. The wood chips compress and are surprisingly cushy underfoot. Mulch in a city park, however, is to be avoided. You never know what may be hiding there.

Sandy Beaches

Beaches are universally fun places to walk. However, watch out for a few things. First, don't start into your barefoot practice on your vacation to Florida by walking on the beach. Instead, you want to start on the hardest surface you can to learn proper posture and form before you hit the soft stuff. Walking on the beach is more challenging than it seems and can stress and strain muscles before they're ready (good soft sand is like a weight-training workout).

Second, beaches have a lot of camber. It's rare to find a beach at low tide that's flat. That means if you walk in one direction down the beach, which strains your IT band, ankle, and hip on one side, make sure you walk back the other way as well. Realize that if you have weak hips or stabilizing muscles, this exceptional workout can easily become too much. If you feel your muscles working too hard or tweaks of pain as you walk on the tilted surface, rest and recover, or get yourself to flatter ground. Listen to your gut and always follow the two-question rule ("Should I stop? Should I stop?") as mentioned in chapter 8.

Third, beaches are a great way to scuff off all of the strong skin you've worked so hard to gain. A good beach is like the greatest loofah sponge in the world. So try staying on either the wet sand or the dry sand, without meandering back and forth. As a general rule if your feet are wet, keep them wet, and if they're dry, keep them dry. Traversing back and forth wears skin off the most.

Additionally, keep your beach walks to every two to three days, both for the skin on your feet and to give your muscles a chance to rest and recover.

If you're lucky enough to live by the beach, you're lucky enough—so the saying goes. As you build up to barefoot walking, this surface may become your sole daily workout. Enjoy your strolls along the beach. Watch the birds and the waves. Enjoy the sunrises and sunsets, the ebb and flow of the tides. Many of us who don't live near a beach are quite envious indeed.

TAKE A HIKE

Want to connect with nature, breathe fresh air, and get away from it all? Then take a hike, barefoot. Even in the most congested of cities, a short drive can get you out into the country, to a state park, or a national park, and get you onto the trails.

Be prepared to be amazed. A barefoot hike will awaken your senses. As you quiet the mind, you leave room for your brain to open up to all of your other senses. You become a connoisseur of the trail and what's beneath your feet. Some barefoot hikers liken the experience to wine tasting in the wilderness. Or as we describe our favorite trail, mossy and damp with globs of mud and just a hint of pine.

Not sure where to go? Look for a local hiking club, for a chapter of the Sierra Club, or for a group on Meetup.com. There's almost always a group around with your same skill level, and there are even barefoot hiking groups as well. A quick Google search online found dozens of groups and this website too: www .barefooters.org/hikers.

UPS AND DOWNS OF HILLS

Uphills strengthen your feet. You can begin walking barefoot up a neighborhood hill during the second month of our walking plan, then walk back down in your shoes. Walk slightly on your toes if you can, to help strengthen things fast and grab with your toes. The uphill motion puts lots of pressure on your skin, which helps build your pads.

Uphill walking is a strength trainer and foot conditioner as well. However, start slowly, as your calf muscles may be quite weak, and the dorsiflexors on your toes (muscles that pull your toes up) are likely weak if not dormant. When you walk up hills, your dorsiflexors help keep your toes up to prevent stubbing them. This action quickly becomes natural, particularly if you accidentally stub one or two. However, these muscles and the associated ligaments are likely atrophied if you've been shod your entire life.

What Goes Up...

A common question at clinics and talks is whether you can stay light when walking downhill barefoot. You never want to brake with your heels, but stay light on the front of your foot, which helps absorb the shock and keeps you better balanced. The best technique for downhills, whether on road or trail, is to stand tall, keep your arms up, and lean back slightly, letting gravity slow you down. Keep your core tight, and never bend forward at the waist.

You'll find on the trails, whether downhill or not, that the times you slip and slide are when you're on your heels. Furthermore, heels were never designed as brakes. When you keep pressure on your toes, you help maintain traction. Keep your arms down and relaxed.

Downhills require you to decelerate with each step. You will be taking faster, shorter steps (that's gravity working). Picture yourself taking itsy-bitsy steps. This is how you go down hills. Fortunately, if you're keeping your strides short, there's little impact or force on your joints. Your muscles, however, are getting the workout of a lifetime, because downhills require your muscles to lengthen as they contract, rather than shorten; this is known as eccentric muscle contraction.

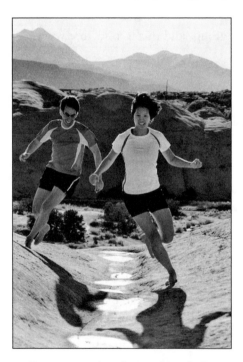

Once you go barefoot and touch the earth, you gain a childlike awe for the world and an agility you never knew you had. It's pure joy as Jessica and Michael skip on slickrock in Moab, Utah.

Every step you take on a downhill is an eccentric muscle contraction. This is more than double the work the muscle has to do on the flats, and a reason it's particularly important to get into downhills slowly. Rest assured you're going to have delayed-onset muscle soreness (DOMS) after your first few downhill workouts. So it's essential for the first few months that you do downhills only once or a maximum of twice a week, and never two sessions in a row.

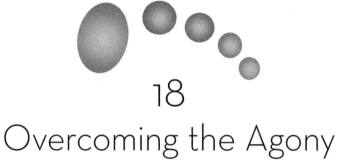

18
Overcoming the Agony of the Feet*

When our feet hurt, we hurt all over.

—Socrates

t's rare that we really hurt our feet, or even badly stub a toe. In six years Michael has cut himself only a few times, with no substantial trips or falls, though he admits to pushing things at times. However, he's never been hurt while barefoot walking; these incidents only occurred while running *and* trying to catch Jessica. "Maybe I'll learn," he says wryly.

He adds, "One spring on tour, I smacked a tree root hard with my foot running through the woods while trying to keep up with Jessica. More recently, I cartwheeled accidentally on a steep grassy slope, *also* trying to keep up with Jessica while we were filming our movie.

"Both of these incidents occurred as I was pushing it, not staying mindful, not staying present, and thinking more about keeping up with Jessica—and with the camera. They were the universe's way of keeping me in check, letting me know again and again no harm will come if I stay present, but if I don't, then to expect reminders. When I leave ego alone, I never seem to get hurt."

* Michael Sandler and Jessica Lee are not trained medical advisors. Advice given here is gleaned from the athletic world's experts on sports medicine and Michael's professional athletic experience. Consult your own doctor and seek emergency medical attention when needed.

If you experience pain of any kind while walking, be smart enough to stop walking, get home fast, and apply first aid. Life's little boo-boos and some bigger overuse injuries can happen when we don't heed the warnings. This is time to throw aside pride and call for help or a ride home if necessary. Michael used to keep a few dollars under his cap for bus fare if necessary.

Understanding injuries and their potential causes and solutions can help you get and stay healthy—and recover in the event of an injury. In this chapter we'll look at many of the common challenges facing walkers, whether in or out of shoes. Expect to toss more than a few myths and common misconceptions about barefoot walking and foot injuries by the wayside.

People often ask us whether we worry about getting injured when walking barefoot. To them we respond that the greater risk is getting injured in a shoe. In a shoe or out, accidents sometimes happen—you walk too far, you do too much, you accidentally step on something sharper than your pads, or you smack something with your toe. While accidents do happen, the far greater risk to our health is not being active and sitting on a couch.

Can you get hurt walking barefoot? Yes. But most injuries are avoidable. Follow these simple rules of the road and you're well on your way.

Top Ten Reminders for Avoiding Injuries

1. Go slow.
2. Let your skin be your guide.
3. Build foot strength.
4. Focus on form.
5. Leave the tunes behind.
6. Get loose.
7. Get aligned.
8. Go fully bare.
9. Learn to rest.
10. When in doubt, see your doc.

Although there's no way to cover every conceivable injury or pain, here we'll cover the basics. A caveat here: when in doubt, always see a doctor (preferably a barefoot-friendly one).

That said, here's what works best for us and other barefooters (and maybe for you too).

FIRST, THE FIRST AID

Walking is man's best medicine.
—Hippocrates

Cuts

The most common worry in the beginning classes we teach is getting cut by broken glass, sharp rocks, and other jagged objects. The truth is that serious cuts are among the *least* common injuries. In the beginning your eyes are glued to the ground. And once you're aware of your surroundings and have toughened up your feet, you'll avoid most sharp objects and be relatively shielded from the rest.

Michael used to pack New-Skin liquid bandage with him in case of a minor boo-boo. If he had a nick or scratch, typically on the top of the foot from brushing a rock on the trail, he would paint it over and continue. These days, he takes a more natural approach—in the great outdoors, he simply covers anything superficial with dirt or mud, and the bleeding instantly stops. We're not sure how Western medicine would feel about this, so we can't recommend it. Nevertheless, this is what Michael does unless he's in a city. A key point: If you do suffer a serious cut, the first thing to do is stop your activity if at all possible. Consider your session done for the day; your only job is to attend to the injury. If the cut is deep, do not seal it up until you've let the blood push out the dirt, bacteria, and other sources of infection. Let the wound bleed until it's clean.

If it's a deep puncture wound, consider seeking medical help. You may need your doctor to completely clean it out and possibly administer a tetanus shot to prevent infection (update your tetanus booster every ten years). But if you can't remember when you had a shot and it's been more than five years, you'll likely be offered a booster anyway.

Once you've cleaned the wound as best you can on the spot with clean water, put on your shoes (assuming you brought them along as "hand weights"), get home, and clean the wound thoroughly with hydrogen peroxide, iodine, Betadine, or another sanitizing solution. If it's small, leave it uncovered to breathe. If not, cover the cut with a bandage or breathable wound-care strips. Before you go out again, use products such as Nexcare's New-Skin to seal and protect the cut. Don't even think of walking barefoot unless the cut is sealed or protected. Never go out with an open wound.

Cracks

Skin cracks can be common when you begin walking barefoot, particularly if you're in a dry climate or it's winter. Cracks typically occur on your heels, around the side of your big toes, or anywhere where the strong skin on the bottom of your foot meets the weaker skin on the sides.

Cracks occur for many reasons: changes in climate (from warm and moist conditions in the summer to cold and dry in the winter), dehydration, too much time at the beach (salty conditions), a hereditary predisposition, a foot fungus, or other skin conditions.

Podiatrists such as Dr. Ray McClanahan recommend using a foot fungal product such as Lamisil to help kill fungus and alleviate the condition. Homeopaths may recommend products such as tea tree oil, a natural disinfectant.

No matter the reason for the crack, the best way to prevent skin cracks is to be vigilant by keeping your feet moisturized with beeswax each night before you go to bed. There are many products you can use, but our personal favorite may be Waxelene, followed by Climb On! Use these products at night so that your feet aren't too soft during the day.

On that note, while you want to moisturize your skin, you do not want to *soften* your skin. Stay clear of products that suggest they'll soften your skin. Soft skin is weak skin and won't serve you well underfoot. Instead, moisturize and let that skin grow strong. (Note: Anything you apply to your skin is absorbed into your body. Our advice is to avoid chemicals, petroleums, or any products you wouldn't choose to eat. If you wouldn't want to ingest it, then you shouldn't put it on your skin.)

Infections

Another fear for beginners is that they'll step in something nasty and get an infection through a cut or crack. To reduce the odds, try this:

- Walk awarefoot so you don't step in anything bad. For example, in a park, beware of dog deposits; in the woods, keep an eye out for other animal droppings. Stay away from stagnating pools of water (especially in hot, moist climates). Avoid unsanitary areas—or if you can't, put on your shoes until you're clear of them.
- Always keep a sanitizer such as hydrogen peroxide, apple cider vinegar, or a towel with soapy water waiting by your door. You may have stepped in something disgusting without even realizing it. And even if you were running in a beautiful wooded area, you might have picked up unwanted passengers such as ticks. Rather than track the remnants of your day's adventures through your front door, make a habit of thoroughly examining and washing your feet and legs as soon as you arrive home.

The moment your feet feel raw, end your walk. This rule actually applies across the board, but it's especially pertinent to ensuring your feet aren't susceptible to penetration. If your feet get soft, tender, or raw, you're liable to get cut and leave yourself open to infection.

Blisters

Blisters are a common condition if you wear shoes. They're caused by friction between your skin and another surface. They're quite uncommon when walking barefoot if you start slowly. If you've started in too fast, they can occur, but that's why you carry your "hand weights" (shoes) with you, so when you start to feel your skin getting warm or sensitive, you can put your shoes back on and head for home. There's always warning; never wait for a blister to form. Blisters and barefoot walking never need go hand in hand.

First Aid Kit

No matter how mindful you are and how much attention you pay to the road or trail, accidents still happen. That's the nature of being human.

Keep the following in your barefoot first aid kit:

- **Band-Aids.** You'll never know when you need them, and more likely they'll be there for your walking partner who developed a blister while wearing shoes.
- **New-Skin or superglue.** Either of these can quickly seal a small cut or scrape, though New-Skin is preferred as it is medically approved (superglue was originally used by medics in the Vietnam War). If you break the skin, you can put a bit of New-Skin on it quickly, before it really starts to bleed. (Note: Don't cover a puncture wound this way, unless you plan on peeling back the glue the minute you get home.) All cuts should be cleaned out, and this is especially important for puncture wounds.
- **Coban.** Bring a little of this self-adhering bandaging with you. You can use this to protect a nick or scrape, or for dozens of other purposes. You never know when this will come in handy.
- **Safety pin and tweezers.** Catching a piece of glass is a rare event, but catching a tiny thorn is not quite as rare. Either way, having a safety pin and tweezers helps you remove the offending object quickly, before it becomes any more than a mild nuisance.

COMMON ACHES, PAINS, AND INJURIES FROM THE BOTTOM UP

If you're active, you run the risk of a boo-boo now and again, particularly if you're in a shoe. But that shouldn't stop you. Instead, learn the basics about the challenges and how to overcome them, and when in doubt see your doc.

FOOT AND ANKLE CHALLENGES

Plantar Fasciitis or Pain on the Bottom of the Foot

Causes: The plantar fascia is a band of connective tissue that runs along the bottom of the foot from the base of your toes to your heel. A big sign you have plantar fasciitis is pain on the bottom of your foot or heel with your first few morning steps. (If you've ever wondered how to pronounce this painful condition, it's "planter fash-ee-eye-tis," or simply "ah-yeeeeee" first thing in the morning.) This inflammation on the bottom of the foot is a common problem caused by weak muscles and a confined foot.

Weak muscles are a common condition in a foot that's been inhibited in a shoe or where there's too much arch support obstructing the foot's natural spring-like movement. When muscles are weak or atrophied or don't have room to move, the plantar fascia is forced to do the supportive work of the foot. Since this tissue was never designed for such a job, it can quickly become inflamed.

In our shoe testing experiences, it's quite common for us to put on a shoe that inhibits the foot and almost instantly we feel it pulling on our plantar fascia, even with our superstrong feet.

Solution: Barefoot walking can help strengthen the feet and chase your plantar fasciitis away. However, you have to start slowly and never go barefoot if you experience acute pain. If you've just recovered from acute pain, start first with a week or two of Golf Ball Grabs before you start walking barefoot. When you begin, start with only twenty yards.

The slow and gradual building up of Michael's own foot muscles—and the creation of an arch where he virtually had none before—put the support work back on the muscles where it belonged, allowing his plantar fascia tissue to heal. Doing too much too quickly can make this condition worse.

Heel Spurs

Causes: Unchecked plantar fasciitis, which continues to worsen, may often lead to heel spurs. Heel striking is also considered a leading culprit by the latest research. Heel spurs are calcium deposits or bony scar tissue caused by excess pulling by the plantar fascia on its attachment to the heel. It's thought that heel spurs develop as a protective skeletal response to stress or microfractures to protect the heel from further impact.

Some people with this condition often feel like they must have bruised their heel or hit a rock, though they can't remember any initial blunt impact. That's often an early indicator that you're doing damage. Unfortunately, it's incredibly painful. It's called a spur because it digs in, like the spurs on a cowboy's boots, with each step.

Solution: Strengthen the feet, get off the heels, work out the knots, and allow time for the inflammation to subside. By walking barefoot on the forefoot, you take pressure off the plantar fascia and arch, reducing the pull on your heel. You'll want to begin slowly and ice frequently. Also, massage frequently or roll the foot over a golf ball or other small ball such as a Foot Rubz ball. Don't roll over the spur itself, but over the plantar fascia to stretch it out and take tension off of the spur. Bone doesn't change overnight, so realize that even after your feet have strengthened, it could be many months or longer before the pain disappears. Focus on exercises that don't irritate your heel. Use support in between strength training exercises. Physical therapy, ultrasound, acupuncture, mudpacks, and other anti-inflammatory and scar-tissue-reducing measures may also be helpful in reducing the spur.

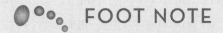 FOOT NOTE

How to Ice Your Feet

For faster recovery, use ice to cool down your feet after a workout and to prevent inflammation.

Use ice for five to ten minutes after a workout on your feet and any sore joints. However, if it's really hot outside or it's been a long walk, ice for up to twenty minutes. Look for Mueller or other adjustable cold/hot pack wraps. You simply keep them in the freezer until you need them (they're reusable). Then strap the pack around your foot or leg with the Velcro wrap—easy. Or improvise with a bag of frozen peas and an Ace bandage. Prop your legs up a wall or tree and rotate the ice packs between any parts that need them. Then go for the mud. A little bit of calcium bentonite clay or mud painted on any parts that need it will go a long way toward reducing inflammation and kick-starting the healing process.

Pain on Top of the Foot or on Top of the Big Toe

Causes: This is one of the most common challenges when transitioning into barefoot walking. Typically it's tendonitis, though it could be a stress fracture. If early warning signs aren't heeded, tendonitis can lead to stress fractures of the metatarsals. If you rest and the pain doesn't go away, or if it gets worse during a workout, rather than better, you likely have a stress fracture. Always check possible fractures out with a doc.

Both problems can also be caused by feet that are rotated to the sides—typically a long-term condition caused by motion control shoes, oversupportive shoes, or hip strength and flexibility imbalances. Also watch for small aches, pains, or fatigue that causes you to change your stride—another common situation that can lead to injury.

Both tendonitis and stress fractures have the same cause: doing too much too fast, misalignment, or poor form. Pain on the top of the foot from stress fractures or tendonitis is the most common condition when you transition too quickly in your minimalist shoes. It's very hard, though not impossible, to do this when you're fully barefoot and let your skin be your guide. Foot and toe pain can also be caused by walking on tired feet (which causes sloppy form), walking with a weighted pack without building up to it, or hopping into treadmill walking too quickly. In short, if the muscles aren't ready, they'll pull on the tendons, causing inflammation, and then begin to pull on the bones.

Solution: Back off, rest, ice after workouts, wear shoes with a bit less flexibility to rest your feet, and work to stretch your toes and legs out; tightness throughout the legs and hips at this time can exacerbate the condition. Additionally, keep walking every other day (or less) on uneven surfaces rather than on concrete or asphalt, to keep up the blood flow in your feet to expedite healing. Tread lightly and go slower than a turtle's shadow. The condition usually subsides within four to six weeks, though tendonitis can last up to eight weeks. After you've healed, restart slowly, focus on form, and let your skin guide you.

Stubbed Toe

Causes: Be careful in the house. This is the most dangerous place of them all, and where you're most likely to stub a toe or slam into something; we both have. Stubbing toes is not very likely outside when going barefoot; however, you can stub a toe if you hit a rock hard on the trails. If this is the case, it may cause bruising of the toe, or in a severe case (again unlikely) could cause a fracture, which may mean a trip to the doc.

Solution: Keep your home free of debris on the floor and try to be mindful when you walk (this is hard when the phone's ringing or someone's making a racket in the background). Hit a rock a few times outside and you become much more aware and careful of what's going on down by your feet, and far less likely to continue hitting them.

Bunions

Causes: No matter what you've been told, bunions are not normal or hereditary, except perhaps for the choices in your shoes. Certainly you can have the same feet that your mother had, and there may be a genetic predisposition for them looking that way, but look at your footwear first.

Why? Because the foot is both adapting and trying to protect itself. If the toes are squashed against the inside of the shoe day in and day out, the foot fights back. It creates a bony callus, or protrusion, over the side of the foot to try to give the toes and forefoot room to breathe.

Solution: Unsquash your feet. Take them out of shoes every chance you get. And to retrain your feet, wear products such as Correct Toes, which help keep your toes apart.

Calluses (aka Corns)

Causes: Both calluses and corns are a thickening and hardening of the skin, created to protect our feet from our shoes. Out of a shoe we tend to develop a nice even covering of smooth, thickened skin over the entire surface of the foot that contacts the ground. However, in a shoe, we develop irritations caused by the material, or seams, or the ways our toes are crammed or forced together. To protect the foot, our skin builds a barrier, a thickened area of skin, called a corn (typically circular) or callus. Corns are actually a type of callus. The main difference between the two is that corns are more circular in nature, hence the name (like a kernel of corn).

Solution: If these are irritating, they can be sanded down or softened with various solutions applied overnight (from tea tree oil to apple cider vinegar, lemon juice, and more) and then removed. Alternatively, they can be left alone if they're not irritating you out of a shoe, and over time they will naturally diminish or peel away. They won't recur outside of the offending shoe, since there's no pressure or friction to create them.

Hammer Toes

Causes: Hammer toes are toes that point up and back down like a tent. They look like little hammers, each one aimed down at the ground, and typically with a bony callus on each joint.

When crushed in a shoe, or when you're stuck sliding around in a shoe, your toes are forced to point down and grab into the sole. Over time this extreme grabbing causes the toe to become gnarled and grow bony calluses on

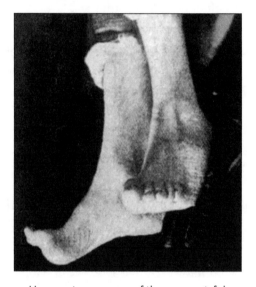

Hammer toes are one of the many painful
consequences of wearing ill-fitting shoes.

the top. This condition continues to worsen, with less flexibility or ability to straighten out, until the toes are almost frozen in the position of little hammers. At that point many believe surgery is required to break the toes, insert wires, and straighten them out again. Not so fast. With Michael's weak feet and narrow shoes, his toes once resembled little hammers working their way toward surgery. But that was years ago. Once out of shoes, they once again became straight as arrows.

Solution: Stop trying to shoehorn your tootsies into an ill-fitting shoe. Get into a wider shoe or out of the shoes altogether. Make sure your feet don't slide in the shoes, causing your toes to grab. Let your toes relax and spread. Give them the room they need to be toes again.

Neuromas or Pinched Nerves

Causes: A neuroma is an inflamed, squashed nerve in your foot. These nerves tend to get *very* upset and can cause excruciating pain. Many people who have them believe, or have been told, it's because of the shape or weakness of the foot. Often they're told they have one toe that's longer than the rest (typically Morton's neuroma) and that's the reason for their woes.

Of course you'll pinch nerves in your feet when you're wearing shoes that are too tight. When the foot is half the width it's supposed to be and the metatarsals are stacked on top of each other, it makes sense that nerves will get angry.

Solution: Not surgery to correct the feet, but giving the nerves room to breathe, helping retrain the foot to relax, and giving the foot time (out of a shoe) to recover. Using Correct Toes in small increments often helps as well.

Toe Fractures or Impact Fractures

Causes: Hitting your toes or forefoot into a rock when walking unaware or in footwear that prohibits you from fully feeling the ground.

Solution: If you think you've broken a bone or bones in your toe or foot, see your doctor, particularly if you experience swelling. Chances are you'll need weeks of rest, unless it's your smallest toe. If it's your small toe, the medical professionals may tell you there's nothing you can do, so let pain be your guide. For either type of toe injury, work on walking more awarefoot, in or out of a shoe.

Bruised or Bloodied Nails

Causes: If you've hit a rock really hard, you may have damaged a nail or soft tissue beneath the nail.

Solution: If you're in severe pain or there's swelling under the toe, this is the time to see a doctor. Either way, you may have to wait it out, and there's a chance your nail will fall off. The doctor may relieve the pressure by drilling a small hole in your nail (don't try this at home).

Ingrown Toenails

Causes: Ingrown toenails are a common condition in walkers from too-tight shoes. They're typically caused by a toe that's squashed in a shoe and pressed up against the side of the shoe. Without anywhere to go, the toenail grows into the toe rather than out.

Solution: The answer is simple and it doesn't involve minor bathroom surgery. Simply get out of your shoes and your nails won't be squashed into the sides of your toes. Now, you may need to see a podiatrist at first to clean things up to begin with, but once you're out of shoes, as long as there's no infection, this condition should take care of itself.

Foot Fungus

Causes: Feet trapped in a dark, sweaty, unbreathable place get stinky and diseased.

Solution: Nail fungus can't survive in oxygen. Get your toes out of shoes and get the fungus under control with antifungal medications or homeopathic remedies (soaking in organic raw apple cider vinegar is said to work wonders). You'll need to trim the excess nail and sand it down (see a podiatrist for this) to allow the remedy to reach the nail bed and expose the fungus to oxygen. Unfortunately, curing fungal nails takes time and diligence. Throw your infected shoes away and choose new shoes that allow your feet to breathe better. If you're dealing with athlete's foot, which is a scaling, flaking, itchy rash, typically on the sole or soft spots of your foot or in between your toes, try honey.

Foot Fatigue

Causes: Even when you gradually introduce barefoot walking, there'll be times when your feet get tired or sore.

Solution: In the beginning our bodies are sometimes unpredictable. If your feet are tired, rest is best. If your feet are sore, particularly if there's an acute sore spot, ice your feet for ten to twenty minutes after a workout; then elevate your feet (prop them up against a wall) to quickly reduce the inflammation. If they're still in acute pain, ice on and off for twenty minutes at a time and grab the mud. We like to paint our feet with a mixture of calcium bentonite clay, sea salt, and apple cider vinegar, which draws out inflammation and promotes healing. Topical creams and ointments such as Topricin that include arnica (*Arnica montana*) as a main ingredient may also help reduce inflammation.

Though you may be tempted, do not use a heating pad or soak your feet in a hot bath. In cases with acute inflammation, heat can make inflammation worse. If there's still pain, consider a visit to a doctor. Once acute pain subsides, work to loosen things up with stretches (using a tennis ball, golf ball, or other foot stretching device) and do your best to determine what happened, or the source of the pain.

Ankle Strains and Sprains

Causes: Shoes grab, lurch, and roll. This is the number one acute injury in a shoe. Fortunately, it's far less of a problem when you're barefoot and are closer to the ground and can feel the ground. It'd be very difficult (though not impossible) to twist an ankle under such circumstances.

Solution: If you've sprained or strained an ankle and are in a lot of pain, or if it's changed color or bruised (particularly below the ankle), get to a doctor and make sure you haven't torn or broken anything. If the doctor tells you it's a sprained ankle that will never fully heal, he or she is operating in the old paradigm. In a shoe, that diagnosis may be right, but out of a shoe, your foot will develop additional vasculature and additional blood flow to the area so it can heal and grow strong. So even if you've been told you have permanently weak ankles, rest assured this can be changed.

Pain Around and Just Above the Ankles

Causes: Typically soreness or mild tendonitis is caused by weak stabilizing muscles and instability around the ankles. This is common if you start into barefoot activities too quickly. It can also occur if you're wearing too heavy a shoe and the muscles around and above the ankles aren't used to carrying the weight (something they were never designed to do). This may also occur if you've been barefoot over the summer or using the most minimal of footwear, then suddenly change to more substantial footwear for the winter.

Solution: Pain goes away quickly with rest. Use a foam roll on your legs to reduce muscle tension. Try resting for a few days. Consider foot and calf massage to help increase blood flow. Then build back more slowly. Work on balance and stability exercises too. Once you're more stable, these problems should go away. If they're mild, ice after workouts, and never work out these muscles two days in a row. (If the problem's from heavy footwear, back off from the big boots, rest, then try to find lighter solutions.)

LOWER LEG CHALLENGES

Shin Splints

Causes: Shin splints are an insidious problem. You rest, they feel better. You're active again, the pain returns. Shin splints are caused by a rotational or shearing force along the lower leg as your leg wants to go one way and your shoe forces it to go another. No matter how much you rest, the pain returns as soon as you're back in your offending shoe.

Solution: Walk barefoot and lightly, preferably up on your forefoot. The less time in a shoe, the less the rotational force. Of course, rest and ice if it's just begun, and never start barefoot walking if you're in acute pain. However, if you're starting into more minimal shoes and the pain's just started, hop out of your shoes and walk a block or two barefoot. Chances are it'll take your shins out of spasm, relax tight muscles, and help strengthen and tone weakened ones. A bit of barefoot walking after a walk in shoes can help hit the reset button for your shins and other tweaks, aches, and pains.

Tight Calves and Achilles Tendonitis

Causes: This is the number one short-term problem when starting barefoot walking or developing a forefoot stride. We were intended in nature to be barefoot, but if we've spent a lifetime in a shoe, our calves and Achilles tendons are now shortened and weak. Walking barefoot or on your forefoot is like doing fifty calf raises each minute. Without preparation this action will quickly aggravate ill-prepared calves and Achilles tendons.

Solution: If your calves or Achilles tendons are sore, take time to let them rest before you go again, which may be a week or two. During this time focus on cross-training to keep healing blood flowing to the affected area until the pain is completely gone.

In cases of long-term Achilles tendonitis, several new studies suggest muscle

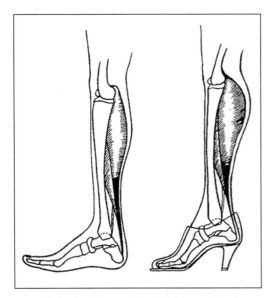

High heels shorten the Achilles tendon by up to 50 percent, leading to painful results. Note the black area is shorter on the right with high heels.

retraining is necessary to rehabilitate the Achilles tendon. Also, work on rolling out your calves and Achilles tendons with a foam roll, and consider hiring a knowledgeable deep tissue massage therapist to work out the knots and get things loose. Acupuncture can also help. However, only after things have loosened up should you ease back in, starting with a minute or two of walking to begin.

Warning: If you ever experience a snakebite-like feeling at the base of your Achilles tendon or calf, stop immediately. You're being warned of an imminent tear to your Achilles tendon. Ice, rest, and don't begin again until it feels better—typically at least two to three weeks.

KNEE AND UPPER LEG CHALLENGES

Patellar Tendonitis or Pain Just Beneath the Knee

Causes: A common problem in a shoe, though less so when barefoot. When you're walking in a shoe, you likely drive force straight up through the knee, which can lead to tendonitis in the patellar tendon—the tendon connecting the lower leg to the knee. When you are barefoot, the condition can be caused by introducing new terrain, challenges, speed, or duration too quickly, and in particular steep uphills and downhills. It can also be caused by introducing weight training too quickly.

Solution: The key is rest, stretching, changing your form, and being kinder to your body. Work on rolling out the quadriceps with a foam roll to relieve the

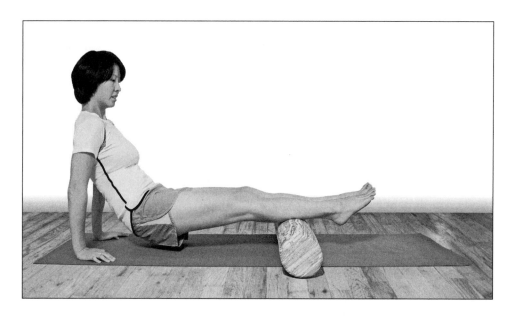

Gently roll your calves and Achilles tendon over a foam roll, looking for tight spots. When you find a spot, remain there for one to two minutes until it loosens up.

tension (also massages of the quad and hamstring will help), and rest. Once the pain has subsided, build back more slowly, introduce new terrain and challenges with greater care, and walk with shorter strides.

Chondromalacia

Causes: You may have heard of "runner's knee," which is pain felt inside or beneath the knee. Walkers get the same condition. It can be caused by walking in high-heeled dress shoes or high-heeled athletic shoes. These shoes lean you forward, pulling on your hamstrings and putting pressure on your knees. This pain can also be caused by increasing time, duration, or intensity too quickly, or by swinging your arms to the sides or walking asymmetrically. A grinding knee is a common problem in a shoe, where force is driven up through the knee, but very uncommon when barefoot.

Solution: Just as with patellar tendonitis, back way off, get out of your fashion footwear, strengthen imbalances, use a foam roll, keep your arms moving forward, and build back slowly. Watch your form, and be careful you're not bending forward at the waist, that you're staying light and tall on your forefoot, and that your feet aren't pointing out to the sides.

Tight Hamstrings and Hamstring Pulls

Causes: Tight hamstrings typically come from time spent in a high-heeled athletic or dress shoe. By bending you forward at the waist, that type of footwear forces you to walk in a constant stretch.

Solution: Work on getting your pelvis level, and, of course, get out of those high-heeled shoes. Above all else, don't walk with intensity until your hamstrings are loosened up. Of course, never, ever, stretch tight hamstrings when they're cold before any activity. It's a perfect way to help them tighten up more and get them to pull or tear on your walks.

Leg Length Discrepancies

Causes: Many people are born with an undiagnosed leg length discrepancy (LLD)—one leg is longer than the other. If you were never in shoes, this would never be a problem because the body would feel the ground and find a way to get balance. However, in a shoe, that becomes darn near impossible. According to an article published in *Podiatry Today*, leg length discrepancies "occur in 60 to 90 percent of the population." With both walking and running, a leg length discrepancy causes you to drop your hip, rotate your pelvis, and move asymmetrically, a leading cause of injury. While most leg length discrepancies are small, some may be more than an inch or greater due to traumatic injury or surgery.

Solution: Gradually work into getting balanced by walking on your forefoot and feeling the ground through barefoot walking. Walking on your forefoot or up on your toes gives you an "independent suspension," helping you get both legs (and thereby your hip and pelvis) level without a heel lift. Road camber can help too.

Road Camber to the Rescue

Road camber is the gentle downward slope on the side of a road designed to drain rainwater. It's also the perfect tool to help you overcome a leg length discrepancy. Camber training helps you learn to hold your body in position with your core and compensate for leg length discrepancy by adjusting how high or low you land on your foot.

On a quiet road or cambered bike path, begin by walking close to the side to compensate for your longer leg. Go to the left side if your left leg is longer, the right side if your right leg is longer. Walk on your forefoot (consider it your independent suspension), which allows you to make minute adjustments. As you grow stronger and more aware, you can start venturing more toward the middle of the road, though keep an eye out for traffic.

HIP AND UPPER BODY CHALLENGES

Hip Issues

Causes: Many problems are associated with the hips—tightness, inflammation, tendonitis, grinding, popping, and more. Imbalanced hip strength and tight hips often get you in big trouble. Other tight muscles such as your hamstrings, glutes, and quads can pull directly on your hips. Hip challenges can also come from leg length discrepancies.

Solution: Do away with high-heeled athletic shoes. They're terrible for the hips. Work to reduce tension on your hips, glutes, and upper legs by stretching out all muscles in the area, in particular your hip flexors and glutes by using a tennis ball or RunBare ball. Work on proper form and make sure you're not wearing an oversupportive shoe that's rolling your feet or legs to the outside. Also, watch how you sit.

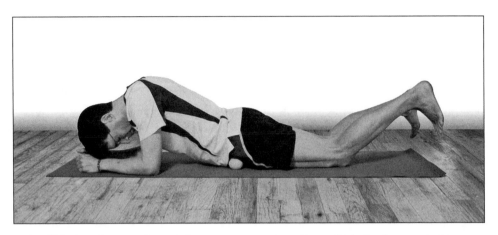

You'll find a tight rope of muscle between your groin and inner thigh. Resting on a ball here will greatly help loosen this up, helping relieve tension on your back and increasing fluidity and efficiency in your stride.

Side Stitches

Causes: A side stitch—a stabbing pain in the side of your gut, typically just below the ribs—is caused by weak abdominal muscles or a weak core. Stitches are not to be confused with stomachaches; they don't have anything to do with what you ate for breakfast or lunch. They often occur if you increase duration or intensity too quickly, are walking on very uneven surfaces that you're not used to (where you really have to tighten your core to keep balanced or from wobbling all over the place), or from carrying something in one hand, throwing you off balance. They can also occur when you begin walking up long hills or any other strenuous movement that causes you to have labored breathing.

Solution: When a stitch occurs, stop for a minute, get yourself back in proper position, and try again, but more slowly. If it's still there, massage the area gently to get blood flow to return, then head for home, as you've done more than enough. After resting for a day, work on engaging your core throughout the day, whether in the kitchen, driving, at work, sitting down, or walking around. Start doing core exercises and consider Pilates classes, which can work wonders.

Stomachaches

Causes: Overeating or a new diet before or during a walk; in severe cases, dehydration or overheating.

Solution: Look at what you ate and drank—and when—before you walked. If you build up to things slowly, you can walk sooner after eating. But you have to introduce this slowly, or you'll feel sick to your stomach. Stay away from experimenting with new foods right before exercising, and don't ingest sports bars or sports drinks; they're almost all glorified candy or science experiments and can greatly upset your stomach.

Sore Back

Causes: Typically caused by a high-heeled shoe, causing you to rotate your pelvis forward, thereby straining your back. It can also occur from overextending the leg with each stride and hitting your heels hard into the ground. It may result from your core being very weak as well.

Solution: Work on making your pelvis level, and never walk in high-heeled shoes. Get tall, engage the core, take shorter steps, and stay more on your toes, or at the very least roll gently off your heels. Seek a flexible, thin shoe so you can land extra lightly. Also watch how you sit.

Lower Back Relief in a Chair

Want to save your back, work your core, and be more comfortable at work? Try sitting on a balance ball, or placing a balance disk on your chair. They help you sit upright while taking pressure off of your lower back. Simply sit tall with your legs firmly planted on the ground and your core engaged. The surprising result: you will sit without pain and gain better posture in the process.

Neck Problems

Causes: Tends to be caused by cocking your head to one side, holding tension in your upper back and/or shoulders, wearing heavy shoes, walking with improper form, or a weak core and neck. Can also be caused by walking asymmetrically, such as carrying an MP3 player in one hand or trying to use your cell phone as you walk.

Solution: As with back challenges, work on proper form and symmetry and core strength (use this as an opportunity to try Pilates). Additionally, make sure you're walking relaxed (focus on light and easy movement) and that you're not carrying tension, especially in your shoulders. A great way to do this is to bring your arms above your head into a *W* and then drop them down by your sides. This relaxes your shoulders and prevents you from shrugging. If you have trouble releasing the tension, consider a massage therapist, acupuncturist, chiropractor, or even Feldenkrais specialist to help you loosen the tension that's built up in your body and become stuck in your back and neck. This is a great opportunity to have someone videotape you or have you walk in front of a mirror in a dance studio and see how upright, erect, and symmetrically you walk.

Breathing Issues or Shortness of Breath

Causes: If you've been leading a sedentary life, you may just be out of shape, and if you've never worked out aerobically, you may not know how to comfortably breathe at speed. However, breathing issues may also be caused by a weak core, bending forward too much, rolling in your shoulders (narrowing your chest rather than raising it up and spreading your shoulders wide), tightening up rather than relaxing, or building up speed too quickly. Of course, it can also occur from walking in heavy shoes or trying to push things too much. It can also be caused by holding fear or tension in your lungs, or by being afraid to take deep breaths—both of which are common in our fast-paced society. Last, it can also be due to poor air quality or heat, asthma, or other conditions that should be checked out with a doc.

Solution: What to do? Generally this is quite typical as you start getting back into shape. However, if there's any doubt when it comes to the heart and lungs, check it out. When you're just getting back into shape, you need to concentrate on making your breathing a conscious movement. Focus on slow, controlled, relaxed deep breaths. Let your breathing be your guide; if you're getting winded, slow down.

Overall, the secret to staying healthy and walking barefoot for a lifetime is to listen to your body and build up slowly. Trust your intuition; work on balance, symmetry, flexibility, and core strength; and above all else, focus on your form. If you're walking symmetrically with near-perfect form, not only will you learn to float along, but you're likely to stay injury-free.

PART VI

If You Really Must Wear Something on Your Feet

Smile, breathe, and go slowly.

—Thich Nhat Hanh

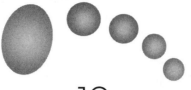

19
Minimalist Footwear— Uncensored

Jessica says: "I remember the day Michael fell in love with Taos. It was the day I brought him to Taos Pueblo, the longest-inhabited village in North America that still claims residents. Today it's home to more than one thousand Pueblo Native Americans who continue to preserve the living and cultural traditions practiced ten centuries ago.

"There we met Robert Mirabal, considered a Native American Renaissance man. He's a Grammy Award–winning musician, composer, painter, master craftsman, poet, actor, screenwriter, horseman, farmer (saving heirloom seeds), and a bright beacon of light. When you embrace your calling, magic happens. Robert makes traditional Native American running moccasins, exactly the kind Michael had been searching for over the last five years."

We do wear footwear from time to time, and when we do, we love moccasins like Robert's. The best moccasins give your feet the freedom to move naturally and allow you to feel the ground, all while still providing protection from the elements. Like with us, once you start barefoot walking, your choice of footwear will be dramatically different. This chapter examines the good, the bad, and the best.

A MINIMALIST SHOE VERSUS THE MOCCASIN

A few years ago no one had ever heard of minimalist shoes, or shoes that let your feet move more naturally, closer to barefoot. And yet in 2010, more than 200 million pairs were sold, and they're expected to sell half a billion pairs in successive years.

Why? Because this trend is catching on.

In 2008 there were perhaps two or three minimalist shoe models. Now there are dozens if not hundreds of different models being manufactured by start-up companies such as Altra, Feelmax, Lems, Luna Sandals, Soft Star Shoes, Tread Light Gear, Xero Shoes, and ZEMgear as well as nearly every major mainstream manufacturer.

We recently gave a talk at a running specialty store. There on the wall were shoes labeled as "minimalist" or "most minimalist" or "lightest minimalist." What surprised us wasn't the sheer number of minimalist shoes, but the fact they were anything but minimal. To Michael, some were like ski boots; they all sported an inch or two of rubber underfoot, with the vast majority promoting heel striking.

Whether the shoe's designed for heel striking, midfoot striking, or even something else, there's nothing minimalist about taking you farther away from the ground. The term *minimalist* is relative too. After all, a car is minimalist compared to an SUV but not compared to a scooter. Something can be minimalist only in comparison to something else, which is why the term's so confusing or misleading. So we came up with a better term: *moccasin-like*.

If you think of an ancient moccasin, there's not much to it. It's more like a leather sock than anything else, without any rubber, any support or structure, along with a wide forefoot and a loose attachment. In other words, the ancient moccasin allowed the foot to move unencumbered while providing minimal protection. So the more moccasin-like the shoe, the more naturally you'll move and the better it is for you.

Says Dr. William Rossi, "Ironically, the closest we have ever come to an 'ideal' shoe was the original lightweight, soft-sole, heel-less, simple moccasin, which dates back more than fourteen thousand years. It consisted of a piece of crudely tanned but soft leather wrapped around the foot and held on with rawhide thongs. Presto! Custom fit, perfect in biomechanical function, and no encumbrances to the foot or gait."

Michael's Checklist for Selecting a Moccasin-like Shoe

When you look at minimalist footwear, ask yourself, "How moccasin-like is it?" Specifically answer these questions:

- ☐ Do they give my toes room to spread?
- ☐ Is there three-dimensional flexibility to the shoe?
- ☐ Can my feet truly feel the ground?
- ☐ Are my toes sitting flat, rather than pointing up toward the sky?
- ☐ Does the shoe allow my arch to move freely, like a natural spring?
- ☐ Is the sole flat and close to the ground?
- ☐ Does the shoe have a uniform bottom or pattern on it, rather than grooves and different treads to try to guide my feet?

The more questions you can answer yes to, the more likely your footwear will work with you, rather than against you. If they don't have these attributes, then you have something that's maximal, rather than minimal. Unfortunately, in today's world, marketing hype often trumps science. And that's what was on this shoe wall.

Beware of the hype and judge for yourself. If there's a hunk of rubber under your foot, is it really minimalist, or just marketing?

FOR THE TIMES YOU MUST WEAR SHOES

Sometimes you'll need or still want to wear shoes. Here are a few instances:

- **Transitioning to barefoot walking.** Even after your first few months, in between barefoot sessions you may not be ready for a zero-arch shoe. Consider using shoes with incrementally less arch support to wean yourself into footwear freedom. Think of arch support as training wheels. As your feet grow stronger, you'll need shoes less and less until you remove them entirely.

- **For challenging terrain.** Even for the most experienced barefoot walker, some surfaces such as gravel, snow and ice, meltingly hot pavement, or perhaps rough roads may require shoes. Have your shoes (aka "hand weights") along in case the going gets rough.

- **To prevent infections.** If you're walking in a third-world country where parasites abound, or anywhere sanitation, standing water, or sewage may be a problem, and especially if you have a cut or an open wound, wear your shoes.

- **In public.** Unless you're trying to make a statement, bring footwear along for grocery stores, restaurants, or other places where people may balk at bare feet. Michael's choices for public footwear are moccasins or Japanese tatami-mat sandals without a rubber sole, which let his feet breathe and toes spread and rest upon a more natural surface. Jessica chooses flip-flops made of recycled materials, though she's always on the hunt for a more eco-friendly solution.

- **At work.** Consider flexible shoes that are easy to kick off under your desk if you sit at work. Some shoe companies make casual minimalist shoes that may be work-appropriate.

- **At school.** While studies show that children are best left unshod, convincing your school administrators or your child's PE teacher may be an uphill battle. Find good natural footwear for class (Soft Star Shoes and Tread Light Gear both accommodate kids' sizes, and Feelmax shoes look more like traditional shoes) and more protective shoes for field activities where spiked shoes are involved.

I Can't Go Barefoot at Work!

Very few people can go barefoot at work. If you can, you're exceptionally lucky. For the vast majority of us, we have to do the best we can.

Consider wearing a minimalist shoe. Some products look like traditional shoes but are more minimalist and let the foot move more freely.

If you work in the armed forces, in factories, or in the shipping industry (such as UPS or FedEx), you're likely sporting a boot to meet safety regulations. This often makes sense. If you're in the field, you could step on something sharp, dangerous, or worse. And if you're in a factory, a steel-toed boot really can protect you if you drop something on your foot. If you're in the military, consider the Nike Special Field Boot. It's not perfect, but it's much better than a traditional boot.

In these cases, the best thing (and a very important point) is to work on your foot strength and toe spread when you're not at work or are off-duty. Strengthen your feet by walking without shoes whenever possible. When it comes time to pick out a new boot, choose one with ample room in the toe box and with the least heel possible.

- **If you have a foot problem.** Whether because of nature, nurture, or too many surgeries in the past, some feet may never fully take to barefoot walking. However, barefoot walking and feeling the ground are still fantastic for your health. If your feet have seen extra woes, wake them extra slowly both in and out of shoes. Make a slower transition to natural, less supportive shoes.

DON'T TRUST THE SHOE HYPE

You may be constantly barraged by footwear propaganda and marketing hype. How can you separate hoopla from hype?

Here's false propaganda to watch out for:

- "Pronation, or rolling the foot downward or inward is bad, and if you pronate you *must* use motion control or stability shoes." Not true, particularly over time. You may just need to strengthen your foot.
- "If you get sore knees, you need more cushioning." False. Cushioning makes you hit harder and causes sorer knees.
- "Materials in most shoes compress so fast they lose their cushioning almost overnight." Not true. You want to feel the ground. Even with hundreds of miles on your shoes, they're likely still too cushioned.
- "Shoes must be replaced every 300 to 400 miles." False. The older the shoe, the less structure the shoe still has and therefore the more naturally your foot moves and feels the ground, and the *less* likely you'll suffer an injury. So dig out those comfortable old shoes and put 'em back on (unless the sole of the shoe is worn unevenly).
- "Shoes with a thinner sole don't last." False. While there's less cushion, the shoe still lasts for hundreds of miles as long as you walk with good form and don't drag or shuffle your feet.
- "Shoe store video analysis or force plate analysis reveals all." We wish this were true, but it depends on the analyst and the test. For instance, standing on a force plate reveals little or nothing, as your dynamics will completely change after you start moving.
- "A properly fitting shoe cures all." If only this were the case, but it's much more than fit. Today's shoes have high heels, toe spring, heavy cushioning, and more. Even if your foot fits the shoe well, it's still likely to hurt you.
- "Shoes should fit snugly." False. Snug shoes don't allow your feet to expand when they contact the ground, putting more force on a smaller area of the foot while decreasing stability. If your toes can't spread, your foot is in trouble.
- "Your arch height determines the amount of support you need." False. Many people ask, "What shoe is good for a *high* or *low* arch?" However, the better question to ask is, "How much support do I need for a *weak* or *strong* arch?" Just because someone has a high arch, it does not mean you give them a big arch support. When you go barefoot, your arches naturally get stronger and taller—and you need less arch support.

Eventually, more muscle fills in the area below your arch, and over the course of years you may end up with a flat, extra-strong foot. There's no right or wrong arch height, or one height that needs support more than another. It's arch *strength* that needs to be taken into account.

NATURAL FOOTWEAR

The goal of minimalist or natural footwear is to allow you the most natural stride possible. No shoe is perfect, but some are far better than others. With new shoes coming on the market almost daily, use this guide to weigh the plusses and minuses of your selection.

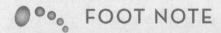 FOOT NOTE

Do Those Toning Shoes Work?

Just before we went to press, both Skechers and Reebok settled lawsuits against them for false health claims. You've likely seen the shoes that claim to tone you while you walk—they're nearly as big as boots, and not nearly as safe. You'll work more muscle groups, the manufacturers say. Well, they don't work more groups of muscles, but they do strain your muscles in different ways, which is why you may be sore in the beginning. Toning shoes have a rockered bottom to force you to roll up and over a hump under the foot, or in essence, fight up and over the shoe. Changing your stride to something less natural is a dangerous game because your body is a chain of muscles, ligaments, tendons, and bones, and affecting any one part of the chain affects every other part as well. And if you look at the thickness of their unstable, rocker-style soles, you could seriously twist an ankle, especially in an aerobics class. We do not recommend these shoes.

A more natural way to tone, and a far better way, is to go barefoot and work all the muscles of the body, and it's free!

Michael's Checklist for Selecting a Minimalist Shoe

☐ **Light weight.** Any weight on your foot changes the dynamic of the stride, and the heavier the shoe, the more your stride changes. Weight can cause your heel to drop first, or put undue stress and strain on the shins, which were never designed to carry weight in the first place. A good minimalist shoe is exceptionally lightweight, no more than six to eight ounces (170–227 grams) or less per shoe. Unfortunately, this takes out of the running many shoes (over 95 percent) that claim to give you a more natural stride.

◐°°°₀ FOOT NOTE

At a hundred strides a minute, in a pair of eight-ounce shoes you're lifting a pound per stride, a hundred pounds a minute, or three tons an hour. Double the weight of the shoe for a supportive trainer, and you're carrying six tons of weight on your feet, legs, and back per hour. That's the weight of a good-sized elephant. No wonder joints crumble!

☐ **Low to the ground.** The number one acute walking injury is ankle sprains, and there's no better way to lose stability than being high up off the ground such as in a well-cushioned shoe. You gain greater stability and feel of the ground as you get lower. Ideally, shoes should be less than half an inch off the ground.

☐ **No heel lift.** Even if the shoe is close to the ground, if it's not flat, it's trouble. Ideally, consider shoes with less than 2 to 4 mm discrepancy between heel height and toe. Anything more can substantially affect your safety.

☐ **Little or no toe spring.** When you are barefoot, your toes sit flat on the ground and grab for propulsion. But shoes that curve the front of the foot up eliminate the use of your toes. Consider shoes with little or no toe spring or curve up. True flats or shoes without a curve in front are best for a more natural stride, stronger and healthier feet, and better stability and propulsion.

☐ **Wide toe box.** Reject narrow and tapered shoes, even if they meet all other criteria. Feet do not come to a point at the center and your third toe is

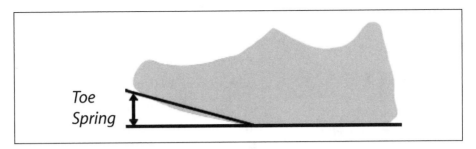

Toe spring, the upward curve at the front of your shoe, eliminates the use of your toes, taking you off balance and weakening your feet. Steer clear and choose shoes that are flat.

never the longest. Your foot naturally expands with each stride, both as a spring and for stability. Most minimalist shoes are still designed in the old paradigm, with a narrow, unnaturally shaped, center-pointed toe box that does not allow your toes to spread or grab. This forces more weight onto a smaller area, which leads to overuse injuries such as tendonitis and stress fractures, and also creates a very unstable platform on which to land. Other minimalist shoes are too narrow in the midsection, which manufacturers do on purpose to build in hidden arch support. As you lace up these shoes, it pulls the material by your arch tight, restricting the movement of your arch.

☐ **No arch support.** Your foot can't move naturally if the arch is propped up. Ideally, you want zero support for your shoe's arch. Any more than that keeps your arch weak. However, if you've been locked in a traditional shoe for years,

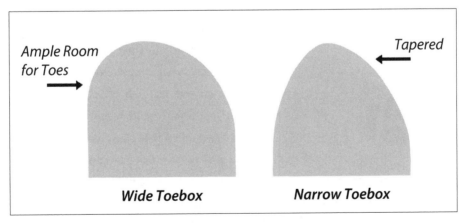

To keep your feet healthy, give your toes room to spread in a wide toe box that doesn't taper to a point.

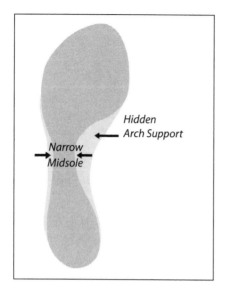

An hourglass-shaped sole with a narrow midsole may be hiding arch support and preventing your foot from moving naturally.

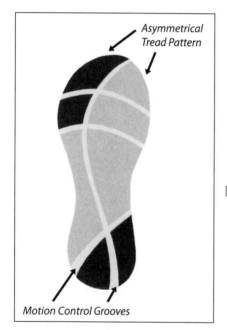

Color-coded rubber and a groove or channel down the sole of a shoe are telltale signs of unwanted motion control.

you may want to wean off slowly, at least in between barefoot workouts.

☐ **No motion control.** The majority of shoes today are designed to move or guide your foot from one place to another through your stride. This guidance completely negates the foot's desire to naturally go where it wants. Avoid shoes with asymmetrical soles, including grooves, channels, pods, or pockets. Often these are color-coded, to make them easy to spot. Another obvious indicator is a notch on the heel of the shoe. That's where motion control begins. While these features may look cosmetic from a distance, they force your foot to follow the shoe.

☐ **Look for a straight shoe.** Most shoes, even minimalist ones, are built on a curved last. This may look cute or stylish, but this curve, called inflare, pushes your toes inward in the shoe. When you flip a shoe over, it's easy to spot this banana-shaped curve. Steer clear of these shoes, as they cram your toes against the side, leading to bunions, hammer toes, and neuromas. Your shoe should be nearly straight, like your foot.

☐ **Look for a fully flexible sole.** Most shoes have grooves or flex lines to determine where they want your feet to bend. However, you want your foot to bend everywhere, both up and down and side to side. So look for a thin, floppy sole that can bend and twist any way it wants to. The more flexible the sole, the lighter and more naturally you'll walk.

☐ **Stay away from heavy cushioning.** The shoe may appear to be the most comfortable you've ever been in, but it's likely a heavily cushioned clunker. Instead of protecting your feet, these comfortable shoes are likely going to hurt you. You'd never catch a baseball with a boxing glove, so why would you try to walk while wearing the equivalent of a cushy ski boot? Get the least cushioning you can.

- ☐ **Make sure they're breathable.** Feet sweat. Not only do nonbreathable shoes allow fungi and bacteria to quickly set up shop, but they soak your pads and wear away your skin. Hot shoes are a terrible way to maintain the toughened skin you've worked so hard to build. Hot feet also swell, which can lead to a whole host of health problems. In the summer, get a light-colored shoe too, which keeps the foot cooler.

- ☐ **Slip on.** Can the shoes slide on and off easily or fold up for easy transport? The more convenient your shoes, the more you'll use them when the going gets tough, and stow them away when things ease up.

- ☐ **Green.** Whenever possible, look for eco-friendly shoes that are constructed with natural or recycled materials, less materials overall, and are preferably locally made. Always vote with your dollars. Also consider supporting the "little guys"—the smaller, less-conventional shoe manufacturers need our support and have more on the line. They tend to be the most innovative and the most receptive to new ideas, and they are likely to drive future trends.

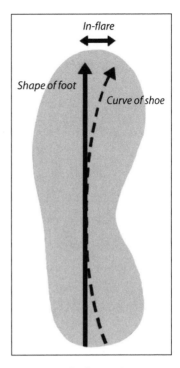

Beware of inflare—a banana-shaped shoe. This unnatural curve contorts the foot and forces toes inward, often leading to bunions and other painful deformities.

🦶 FOOT NOTE

You can test the flexibility of a shoe by putting your hand in the shoe and trying to move your hand around like a puppet. If the shoe flexes to the shape of your hand, you're in good shape. If not, the puppet's dead—move on.

☐ **Consider Huaraches.** Try a modern take on the original sandals of the Tarahumara, such as those by Luna Sandals and Xero Shoes. They let your feet move more naturally and breathe.

HOW TO WEAR MINIMALIST FOOTWEAR

Few barefoot walkers will be barefoot 100 percent of the time. Personally, we're about 95 percent barefoot in the warmer months, and perhaps 50 percent barefoot through the winter. No matter how much or little you wear shoes, consider the following.

To Sock or Not to Sock?

Avoid wearing socks inside shoes if at all possible. Once you've been going barefoot, your feet generate much more heat. And even if you haven't been going barefoot, your feet have to work more in minimalist footwear, so you tend to pump more warm blood to the feet, rather than less. Unless it's too cold, stay out of socks to keep your feet closer to the ground, to keep your feet from sliding around (which could create a whole host of problems and challenges), and to keep your feet from getting hot, wet, and sweaty. As barefoot walkers, we abhor moisture, and even in wicking socks, this is hard to avoid.

Now, there is one consideration for socks: the cold. If your feet can't get warm, then by all means put on some socks. Try to find the thinnest socks that work for you. It's not the thickness of socks that determines how warm they are; it's actually trapped air that keeps your feet warm. If there's no trapped air, there's no warmth. Also look for looser socks that allow the toes to wiggle and maintain a more natural shape. Another reason why looser is better: tight socks reduce blood flow to the feet, causing them to get cold. We recommend wool socks over synthetics because wool stays warm even if it gets wet (look for organic, humanely grown, mulesing-free wool, typically *not* from Australia). Properly fitting socks can be a lifesaver, or at least a toe-saver!

If it's really cold and socks aren't enough, try inserting a flat insulated footbed into your shoe to keep the heat in. We think the product Toasty Feet works wonders.

How About Insoles, Orthotics, and Footbeds?

For some people, there is a time and a place for insoles and orthotics, particularly if there is a true foot condition or past foot surgery. For those who wear them and are getting into barefoot walking, insoles may be an excellent recovery tool or device to wear in between your barefoot walks as you gradually build up your feet.

As for the traditional footbeds you find in all but the most minimalist shoes, remove them. Footbeds typically add 2 mm or more to the height of your foot in an effort to give you extra cushioning and arch support—two things you're trying to avoid. So unless you temporarily need the support, pull the insoles out of your shoes.

Laces

While they may be a necessary evil, avoid shoelaces whenever possible. They unevenly distribute force or bind your feet. If you're going to lace up, keep them loose, but not quite to the point where your feet slide around. Consider switching to a wide flat lace that will stay in place (as long as they don't get twisted) and won't dig into your foot. Better yet, look for shoes with alternative binding systems (such as Velcro or a drawstring) or no laces at all.

Sizing

When it comes to barefoot walking, no longer do you want a snug, tight-fitting shoe. Instead, you want something roomy that allows your toes to spread.

Especially for women, whose shoes tend to be incredibly snug in the front, you want to get a shoe that's wide enough for completely unencumbered movement of the toes. This may mean choosing the men's model in the correct size, or even bumping up a half to a full size to accommodate your toes.

Typically, feet change size when you go barefoot as well. On average, feet gain one-half to one full shoe size as they get stronger and revert to a more natural shape. Make sure you choose a shoe that allows your toes to curl as well as spread, and if you're looking at a glove-like shoe, choose one that's not too tight across the instep, unrestrictive for the toes, and allows your toes to lift up as well as curl down.

HAPPY FEET

Become your own expert when it comes to footwear. Go to your closet and to the store. Look at each shoe, top to bottom, front to back, and inside and out. Check out the soles, their thickness, and any grooves on the bottom. What is the shoe trying to get you to do? Slide your hand in, feel around, and look at the flexibility or lack thereof throughout the entire shoe. Twist it from side to side too. Will it allow your foot to move in all directions? Is the toe box (or toe pocket) flat? How about the heel? And is there any hidden arch support? Look at every aspect of the shoe and ask yourself, "Why did they do that, and what does it mean for me?"

Don't buy the marketing hype; instead, trust a combination of your deductive reasoning and your intuition. You'll know if the bells and whistles are indeed helpful, useless, or even potentially harmful. Be wary of footwear that uses buzzwords such as "barefoot technology" or "barefoot-like shoes" yet is inches up off the ground, rockered, or lugged. A design may be touted as encouraging "natural movement" yet do just the opposite.

Ultimately, ask yourself, "How moccasin-like is this shoe?" If it seems pretty close, it may be worth a try. If not, give it a pass. The key is keeping it simple.

There's a time and a place for shoes. Choose wisely, and they can be a lot of fun, or if nothing else, they can give you freedom and protection when you need them. Ultimately, shoes are neither supportive nor corrective but serve only to cover or protect.

And remember, no matter what shoes you get, you can—and should—always slip them off at the first chance you get!

PART VII

The Final Step

When we walk upon Mother Earth, we always plant our feet carefully
because we know the faces of our future generations are looking up
at us from beneath the ground. We never forget them.

—Oren Lyons, Onondaga Nation

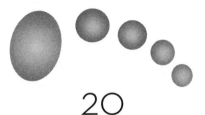

20
Leading by Your Footprints

We shall not cease from exploration and the end of all our
exploring will be to arrive where we started . . .
and know the place for the first time.
—T. S. Eliot

Are you enjoying your time in the woods? Have your health and well-being taken a giant leap forward? Do you want to explore and take the next step?

Then now may be the time to try barefoot running.

BAREFOOT RUNNING, ANYONE?

You needn't be an experienced marathoner to get into barefoot running, just someone who desires to jog instead of walk, or move a bit faster and farther across the terrain. And here's the kicker: at a certain speed, jogging is lighter, easier, and more energy efficient than walking at that same speed.

Personally, we find there's a time for walking and a time for jogging. At times we find ourselves walking, then suddenly breaking into a trot. Other times we head out for a run and soon find ourselves on a relaxing hike. Simply put, walk when you are inspired to walk; run when you are inspired to run.

Barefoot running helps take your bone density, strength, and fitness to an entirely new level. It gives you even greater balance, stamina, and energy for your entire day. So if you'd like to try barefoot running, give it a try. We recommend our book *Barefoot Running: How to Run Light and Free by Getting in Touch with the Earth*, and our DVD, *Barefoot Running*. No matter what you do, start slowly, even if you're a barefoot walking guru, because barefoot running will ask more of your feet, your legs, your calves, and your entire body.

Keep Exploring

Want to explore with your two feet, but you're not into running?

Consider signing up for charity events, big walks, long walks, or even epic adventures (cross-country, anyone?). Volunteer with the Sierra Club, the Nature Conservancy, or other groups that maintain trails or plant trees. You could travel to an exotic location, experience a new part of the world, and connect with the earth barefoot. (We plan to learn from the Native Americans, Aborigines, Maori, and other indigenous peoples about connecting with the earth and living harmoniously with nature.)

Or you could go on a barefoot retreat, such as the ones we're holding through RunBare. The next step is up to you, but once you've gone barefoot, you're now footloose and fancy free. Once you've freed your feet, it's time to explore the world, live a bit more, and get out and play!

BEYOND BAREFOOT

We used to think of barefoot walking and barefoot running simply in terms of their healing benefits, both spiritual and physical. But the more time we spent with our bare feet on the earth, the quieter we grew and the more we looked and listened to the world around us. Soon we began to see, hear, and even *feel* Mother Earth's story. Before we realized it, we had gone beyond the barefoot experience and started living the earth experience.

The more we connect with Mother Earth, the more we find ourselves wanting to care for her. For the soil beneath our feet is of far greater importance now, as our awareness of, understanding of, and concern for the earth grows. We could write hundreds of books on the benefits of connecting with the earth, but in the end, the most convincing arguments are the ones experienced firsthand by living the earth experience. Walking barefoot, hiking barefoot, running barefoot, or simply sitting or lying on the ground—it doesn't matter *how* you connect. The earth always greets you. We need only show up, pay attention, and be human.

Being human, however, comes with important responsibilities, specifically becoming a steward of the earth. She gives us life, nourishes us, shelters us, and protects us. Even with advances in science and technology, our health, happiness, and abundance are still inextricably interwoven with the earth. The survival of our children and of future generations depends on our caretaking. Though taking on this responsibility may seem daunting at first, once we realize that living green really means taking better care of ourselves, the right choices become natural. For to take better care of ourselves means to take better care of Mother Earth.

STEWARDS OF THE EARTH

A nation that destroys its soils destroys itself.
Forests are the lungs of our land, purifying the air
and giving fresh strength to our people.
—Franklin D. Roosevelt

Everything matters. Every decision we make is an opportunity to either help or hurt the planet. The challenge is, it's often hard to see the effects of our actions, and harder still to know what to do. And that's why we need to educate ourselves. We need to read books, scour the Web, watch documentaries (take a look at those we list in the resources section), and listen to our intuition. If something feels wrong, check it out.

Through our actions, large and small, we can all make positive changes on the planet. Below are ten changes we've made in our own lives. Though we don't have all the answers, we know every little bit helps.

Earth-Saving Choices

First, we buy used. We've sworn off buying anything new for the house, except for cleaning supplies and toiletries. This greatly reduces our carbon footprint and the amount of natural resources we use.

Second, we avoid big-box stores with their huge eco-footprints, and buy locally whenever possible. This helps the local economy, reduces fuel spent on shipping, and, when it comes to eating, means fresher, more nutritious food.

Third, we look for natural materials. Plastics are made from oil, as are most synthetic materials. We're trying to cut out as much plastic as we can, saying "no thanks" to plastic bags, and even toting reusable containers and utensils with us to restaurants. We also buy in bulk or with the least packaging possible. And we avoid bottled water, produced by an industry that uses 17 million gallons of oil annually and produces a whopping 3 gallons of CO_2 per 1 gallon of water, for a total of 2.5 million tons of greenhouse gases annually. All of this plastic either ends up in landfills or directly contaminates our water and soil.

Fourth, we buy used or organic clothing. We try to buy only used clothing due to the huge eco-footprint of textile manufacturing. More and more, we steer clear of synthetic materials or high-tech fibers, which are heavily processed, made almost 100 percent of oil, and contain carcinogenic materials and allergens. Even natural fibers have their impacts, such as bamboo, which is highly chemically processed, and nonorganic cotton, which is responsible for 25 percent of all pesticides used on the planet. So if we have to buy new, we look for organic cotton and hemp. However, organic or not, it still takes 1,800 gallons of water to make one new pair of denim blue jeans and 400 gallons just to make a single cotton T-shirt.

Fifth, we're electricity misers. Burning coal is essentially burning the earth; strip mining for coal reduces mountains to rubble and destroys the soil. So we've switched to energy-efficient lightbulbs, gone back to our laptops over desktops (and shutting them down rather than putting them on standby), use fewer lights at night (which also helps our bodies wind down for a better night's sleep), and unplug everything we can before turning in for the night. We even hang-dry our clothes whenever possible. Our next step is to return to an Earthship, where we'll be running on solar, wind, and geothermal power again.

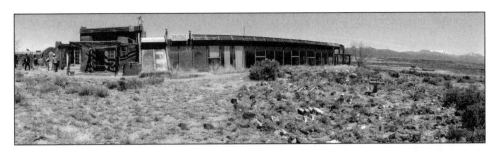

Futuristic homes built into the earth are one way to reduce our eco-footprint. The north side of the building (not shown here) is covered by earth.

Sixth, we've gone off natural gas. It was hard to justify when we discovered how much water, air, and soil was being poisoned through hydraulic fracturing (aka fracking—the pumping of up to 596 different toxic chemicals plus water into the ground to fracture the earth and release gas).

Seventh, we conserve all the water we can. We started by using www.water footprint.org to gain a better understanding of our total water footprint. It turns out everything has a hidden water cost, from the meat and produce we consume to every product we purchase. For instance, a pair of leather shoes takes 4,400 gallons of water to make—yet another reason to go barefoot! Along with tossing the shoes, eating meat is out, because it uses up to two hundred times more water than vegetables and in most cases destroys forests, pollutes groundwater, poisons the soil, and increases greenhouse gases. Refined sugar and nonorganic fruits and vegetables are out for the same reasons—polluted water, air, and soil. And it just so happens that cutting these way back is much better for your health.

As for home water usage, we don't use the washer or dishwasher without a full load. We take shorter showers too, which again happens to be healthier because we minimize the chlorine and fluoride absorbed through our skin.

Eighth, we conserve fuel whenever possible. We zip around on a 150 cc scooter, which, even carrying the two of us plus groceries, still gets an impressive 75 to 90 mpg. And when we need more storage capacity or in times of inclement weather, we drive a used Prius, and like Grandma and Grandpa, we try to keep it under sixty in the slow lane. To our surprise, we've found slower driving more relaxing and even enjoyable.

Ninth, we avoid buying new precious metals and stones. These often require strip mining, which destroys the land. For our wedding we purchased used rings. In general we prefer jewelry and art that are made from seeds, shells, and other found or reclaimed natural materials.

Last, we volunteer. We volunteer with groups that help replant trees, save forests, restore wildlife, conserve nature, organize local cleanups, build trails, and educate others about what we all can do. And we've joined global communities online that work to protect the land.

We're far from perfect, and there's a lot we can do to improve. But these little steps add up; everything does matter, and each action helps. You can takes steps too. By doing so, you lead by example, showing others the simple changes they can make. Each one of us can make a difference.

When we take care of Mother Earth and the health of our soil, we're taking care of our own health and the health of generations to come.

ONLY THE BEGINNING

Barefoot Walking is really about reconnecting with the earth and rediscovering who we are, who we were, and who we are meant to be. It's about waking up our bodies and discovering what we're capable of—at any age.

It's about seeing the world in a new light. When you feel the earth beneath your feet, you can't help but change the way you think.

Change isn't easy. It often requires an uncomfortable paradigm shift. Yet changes such as shedding your shoes are often for the best. In the beginning, your bare feet may feel weak and unsteady. Know that this temporary awkwardness will be well worth the gains you'll reap, for your feet will grow strong and you will become empowered to take the next step—to hike, to run, to be a steward of the earth, or simply to lead by example.

Thank you for reading this book. Baby-step your way in, listen on the inside, and have fun. You are now a designated change maker in society. With your enlightened footprint, you have the ability to make big changes through your graceful steps.

Nurture your own earth connection. Be well, and bless the soil with your bare feet. Give thanks for the earth and your newfound health and happiness. Congratulations, you're now an official barefoot walker. Stand tall, smile, and walk free!

Acknowledgments

Maui is a very special place, a real microcosm of the rest of the world. Everywhere we've gone we've run into the right helpful person at the right time. We call it "Maui magic."

But Maui magic isn't limited to the island. We find the more we align ourselves with our spiritual path, the more we experience magic everywhere we go.

If we were to thank everyone who's touched our lives, it'd be its own book, for we are extremely grateful for everyone on our path.

It's been a challenging few years. Though we went broke three times before getting out *Barefoot Running*, we never gave up. Our path turned us into temporary vagabonds: after a five-month book tour, we bounced from Colorado to New Mexico to New Jersey and then finally on to Maui.

It seems everything's always worked out. We always had just enough to survive. It was sometimes scary, but even when we mailed our last dollar to the printers for our self-published edition of *Barefoot Running*, we knew we'd be all right. As our documentary filmmaker puts it, we've been operating on bare faith.

And though sometimes uncomfortable, this amazing journey has exceeded all expectations.

This has been a path of knowing, and a path of faith. It's been a true test of letting go and letting God.

And so we place all of our thanks and gratitude where it belongs, with the Big Guy (or Gal) upstairs. We know we didn't choose this path, or really write the words you see here. We're just an instrument, dictating what comes to us. We do our best to flow like water and get the heck out of the way. This is how

Michael survived his accident, how Jessica found her path toward helping others, and how we both came together after a meditation one fateful evening at the Shambhala Meditation Center in Boulder. In Michael's words, "I just knew."

Our ideas, thoughts, and direction come through prayer, meditation, and connecting with the earth. And they come from connecting with people.

Our journey would not have been possible without the help of countless others. First off, to Jack Burden, our "pain in the butt" best man, who at ninety years young still gives us a good kick in the pants when we need it. To serial entrepreneur Mike Stemple, whose guidance helped convince us to "make the impossible possible." To our editor, Sandra Wendel, who could find time where there was none and always told it like it is. To our agent, Stephanie Tade—you were right, we had to go with you! Thank you for your persistence, for believing in us and our message, and for the whirlwind day in New York. To Three Rivers Press, Crown Publishing, Random House, Sydny Miner, and Stephanie Knapp for believing in us and helping us put together a beautiful book. To our publicist Beth Grossman for her manifestation in helping us get the word out and getting us "out of the vacuum." To Laurie Huseby at Miami Footworks, whose support was fundamental for keeping us going when we needed it most. To Danny Dreyer, cofounder of Chi Running and Chi Living, our friend and mentor, thank you so much for your *chi* guidance in building our business! To Barefoot Ted for your Zen monkey guidance. And to the late Micah True, aka Caballo Blanco: you touched us more than you may ever know, and your example of integrity gives us the courage to stay true to our message.

In Colorado, to Lhoppon Rechung, our Tibetan Buddhist teacher at Mipham Shedra, for your invaluable lessons on love, patience, and compassion. All good things happen "slowly, slowly."

To Bill Weber for helping us see the beauty and wonder of nature and the earth as nature intended, and of what's truly native, from the lichen on up. To Paul Weppler, aka St. Paul, a true superman of a friend, who knows no limits to giving. To Scott McLean, without whose incredible energy, enthusiasm, and assistance we'd never have gotten out of Boulder. We hope your journey brings you back to Boulder, or wherever your heart takes you. To Benji Covington for dragging us away from our computers to feed us with food made with love. To Don Spence, whose Pilates and tennis ball work performed miracles and helped turn Michael into a "superstar." He will always think "one gear harder"! To Tevis Morrow and Deb Conley for opening your doors and hearts, to Michael Sandrock for sharing your childlike enthusiasm and letting us know we're on the right path, to RL Smith and Tricia Vieth of In-Step for believing in us and spurring Michael to strip off his shoes, to Erwan Le Corre of Movnat .com for challenging us to be true to our nature, to Gina Kremer for support and friendship that go way beyond the call of duty. And to Dennis Shaver for reminding us to prioritize and manifest in the now. To Valeria Solheim for pointing us back to Source. To Vincent Gerbino, our mobile yogi friend, for helping people understand the connection between yoga and barefoot movement. To Josephine Pham for your fantastic photography, patience, and humor. You helped us smile.

In Taos, New Mexico, to Robert Mirabal for sharing your magical world, miracle moccasins, and work to help the Taos Pueblo, the "people of the corn." To Bruce Marshall for saving us from a sinking ship with your courage and honesty. To Chris and Corina, who offered a Moroccan palace in the middle of the desert when there weren't many places to turn to. To Elizabeth Burgess for lending a compassionate ear and providing Jessica the best massage of her life when she needed it most. To Susan Marie Frozneck and Tripp Hammond, who provided the basic necessities of food and water before our flight from Taos. To our moving angel, Ted Remillard, who swooped in from the north, helped, and then disappeared. Godspeed on your journey!

While on Maui, to David Meredith, who helped us see the magic on Maui and to "be the mountain goat." Thank you for sharing the trails and opening doors. To Auntie Puanani Mahoe, who embodies aloha and continues to teach us how to do the same. We love you, Auntie Pua! To Auntie Maile Shaw, a living example of living life to the fullest. To Uncle Jim Canonn for your lessons on connecting with the dirt. To Shaun Simmons, thank you for reminding us that when you give love, you receive love. Your optimism and perma-grin are infectious. To "Brother Philip" Oje for helping us stay connected to the creative energy of the earth. To Darshan Zenith for reminding us to breathe deeply in order to live deeply. To the Honey Badgers: Adam Brix for helping us get down to the essence and realize it all comes back to the earth, and Thomas Scavenius for your patience and willingness to flow rock-and-roll style. *Barefoot Running—The Movie* turned out great! See you both on Hah-lee-ah-ka-la.

To Lion for sharing your incredible inner peace and helping us to "see" we're just where we're supposed to be. To Ruthie Goodfellow for reminding us that the Love is always there, that we need only to walk through the door. To Jim Henry, a true servant to humankind: we are honored to be in your fellowship, and we can't wait to sleep in the teepee! To Kamana for sharing knowledge and wisdom of the Aina and for speaking the truth about Hawaii's past and present. To Maui Nui Farm for keeping us well fueled with fresh local produce, and to Kit, who's taught us so much about every fruit and vegetable under the sun. And to Mark and Leah Damon for teaching us the importance of "raising soil," not just plants, with loving energy.

The best doctors we know don't just treat symptoms but help heal. To Dr. Marc Silberman for being bold, shedding your shoes, and going against conventional wisdom. To Dr. Ray McClanahan, a long-lost brother—keep up the great fight; you're changing lives! To Doc Gurney and everyone at Aspen Park Medical Center—if you have a pet with cancer or in need, these guys are miracle workers! To Nashalla Gwinda for using traditional Tibetan medicine to return Michael to health antibiotic-free after a difficult year with walking pneumonia. To Dr. Warren Grossman for helping us connect and heal through the earth. To Dr. Maureen Traub for helping us tap into the "intranet" aka the message center that is your heart. And to the Barefoot Professor, Dr. Daniel Howell, for pushing past social norms and into what's natural.

To the doctors and researchers who are doing the research that is the backbone of what we teach. To Clint Ober, the father of Earthing—thank you for helping people see why grounding is so necessary, and helping thousands to overcome their challenges and heal. To Dale Teplitz for being the first to get us grounded while explaining the physics behind it all. To Martin Zucker for your continued mission to share the message and help everyone discover the benefits of Earthing. Thank you too for getting us grounded in our home. To Dr. Daniel Lieberman for your pioneering work into why going barefoot is so great, and why we are the way we are. To Dr. Michael Merzenich, thank you for helping people understand how to work with their minds and grow their brains stronger. To Adrienne Samuels for helping set us and the world straight about free glutamic acid at truthinlabeling.org.

And to our inspiring raw foodies. First to Dave Smith, who introduced us to the concept of a raw diet with awesome homemade squash spaghetti. Know that anything you touch turns to gold. To Glen Collelo of Catch a Healthy Habit, our second raw foodie instigator, whose skin shines so bright we have to wear shades. To Tarah Michelle Cech, a kindred spirit, thank you for your spiritual nutritional guidance and your infectious enthusiasm. And to our new friend Ceci, for sharing your story and your guidance, and for giving us hope and inspiration as we embark further down the raw road.

To Jessica's parents, William and Esther Lee, for your support and for taking us in when we needed a little shelter. To Michael's sister, Elisa, for your love and guidance. Keep up your amazing work healing through nutrition and helping others overcome lupus. Your inspirational song www.tinyurl.com/fly-free-butterfly helps people to soar! To Michael's parents, Marc and Sydelle Sandler, for cheering us on. To Amy Silberman and her daughters, Rebecca and Jackie, for demonstrating what it really means to be a kid. To Karl Sandler for your website troubleshooting assistance. And to What About Bob—you've always been there for us, like Houston to Apollo; now it's our turn to say, "Ground Control to Major Bob, you're clear for takeoff!" To Zachary Bergen, a modern-day Renaissance man, for presiding over our wedding and blessing our marriage. Thank you for being a bright beacon of light and for sharing your loving vibration through music. Thank you for your infinite friendship, mentorship, and unofficial couples counseling.

To Lou Paradise, a beautiful human being and founder of Topricin: Please consider motivational speaking. Your talks are inspirational. To Bob's Red Mill, for wholesome organic grains, and to Nutiva, for your hemp, chia seed, and coconut superfoods. You were both instrumental in keeping us well fueled on the road. And to Primal Spirit Foods for your vegan Primal Strip "emergency food" that helped stabilize Michael's blood sugar before we went raw. To Prana for providing beautiful organic cotton clothing for Jessica's photos in this book. To Amphipod for keeping us hydrated with smart ergonomics in mind. To Golden Harper of Altra, another long-lost brother, for being our confidant in challenging times. We love your vision. To Lena Phoenix and Steven Sashen of Xero Shoes for keeping your fingers on the pulse of the barefoot movement.

And to our new four-legged feline friend and hiking companion, Bam Bam, a pedigree specimen of a Japanese bobtail with a full-on corkscrew tail, who bamboozled his way into our hearts. Thanks for bamming us awake at four every morning to get to work, and for keeping our laps warm during late nights in front of the computer . . . Bambaroooo! And last but not least to our somewhat bipolar kitty Meow Meow, aka Joe Black, aka Bubbles, who meditates with Michael and weaseled her . . . errr, his way in, using sweetness, when we thought one cat was enough. Honk!

For all of those who have touched our lives in one way or another, we send light and love to each and every one of you.

Blessings and Aloha!

Notes

As of this printing, all URLs are accurate, but of course Internet links may change or disappear with time.

Introduction

Richard Louv, *Last Child in the Woods: Saving Our Children from Nature-Deficit Disorder* (Algonquin Books, 2011).

Chapter 2: Why Barefoot Is Best

Philip Hoffmann, "Conclusions Drawn from a Comparative Study of the Feet of Barefooted and Shoe-Wearing Peoples," *Journal of Bone and Joint Surgery* s2–3(2) (1905): 105–136.

Danielle Barkema et al., "ISU Study Finds High Heels May Lead to Joint Degeneration and Knee Osteoarthritis," paper presented at the American Society of Biomechanics, August 2010 (Iowa State University press release).

U. B. Rao and B. Joseph, "The Influence of Footwear on the Prevalence of Flat Foot, a Survey of 2300 Children," *Journal of Bone and Joint Surgery* 74(4) (July 1992): 525–527.

Greg Downey, "Lose Your Shoes: Is Barefoot Better," 2009, http://neuroanthropology .net/2009/07/26/lose-your-shoes-is-barefoot-better.

B. Zipfel and L. R. Berger, "Shod Versus Unshod: The Emergence of Forefoot Pathology in Modern Humans?" *The Foot* 17(4) (December 2007): 205–213.

N. D. Carter, P. Kannus, and K. M. Khan, "Exercise in the Prevention of Falls in Older People," *Sports Medicine* 31(6) (2001): 427–438.

S. Robbins, E. Waked, and J. McClaran, "Proprioception and Stability: Foot Position Awareness as a Function of Age and Footwear," *Age and Ageing* 24(1) (January 1995): 67–72.

Joseph Froncioni, "Athletic Footwear and Running Injuries," originally published in the German magazine *Spiridon* in 2006, also at http://www.quickswood.com/my_weblog/2006/08/ athletic_footwe.html#more.

Chapter 3: Barefoot Walking: The New Fountain of Youth

Marianne David-Jürgens, "Differential Effects of Aging on Fore- and Hindpaw Maps of Rat Somatosensory Cortex," *Plos One* 3(10) (2008): e3399.

Chapter 4: Vitamin G: The Lost Supplement

C. Ober, S. T. Sinatra, and M. Zucker, *Earthing: The Most Important Discovery Ever?* (Basic Health Publications, 2010).

M. Ghaly and D. Teplitz, "The Biological Effects of Grounding the Human Body During Sleep, as Measured by Cortisol Levels and Subjective Reporting of Sleep, Pain, and Stress," *Journal of Alternative and Complementary Medicine,* 10 (2004): 767–776.

G. Chevalier, K. Mori, and J. L. Oschman. "The Effect of Earthing [Grounding] on Human Physiology," *European Biology and Bioelectromagnetics,* January 31, 2006, 600–621.

J. L. Oschman, "Charge Transfer in the Living Matrix," *Journal of Bodywork and Movement Therapies* 13 (2009): 215–228.

Gerald Draper et al., "Childhood Cancer in Relation to Distance from High Voltage Power Lines in England and Wales: A Case-Control Study," *British Medical Journal* 330 (June 2005): 1290.

World Health Organization, International Agency for Research on Cancer, "Non-ionizing Radiation, Part 1, Static and Extremely Low-Frequency (ELF) Electric and Magnetic Fields," *IARC Working Group on the Evaluation of Carcinogenic Risks to Humans* (80) 2002.

N. P. Dharmadhikari et al., "Geopathic Stress: A Study to Understand Its Nature Using Light Interference Technique," *Current Science* 98(5) (March 10, 2010): 695–697.

M. A. Persinger, "Possible Cardiac Driving by an External Rotating Magnetic Field," *International Journal of Biometeorology* 17 (1973): 263–266.

M. A. Persinger et al., "Psychophysiological Effects of Extremely Low Frequency Electromagnetic Fields: A Review," *Perceptual and Motor Skills* 36(3) (June 1973): 1139–1151.

"The Schumann's Resonances and Human Psychobiology," *Nexus Magazine,* April-May 2003.

N. J. Cherry, "Human Intelligence: The Brain, an Electromagnetic System Synchronised by the Schumann Resonance Signal," *Medical Hypotheses* 60(6) (June 2003): 843–844.

A. C. Ober, "Grounding the Human Body to Earth Reduces Chronic Inflammation and Related Chronic Pain," *ESD Journal,* July 2003.

A. C. Ober, "Grounding the Human Body to Neutralize Bioelectrical Stress from Static Electricity and EMFs," *ESD Journal,* February 22, 2004.

A. C. Ober and R. W. Coghill, "Does Grounding the Human Body to Earth Reduce Chronic Inflammation and Related Chronic Pain?" paper presented at the European Bioelectromagnetics Association annual meeting, November 12, 2003, Budapest, Hungary.

J. L. Oschman and J. Kosovich, "Energy Medicine and Matrix Regeneration," *Anti-Aging Therapeutics* 10 (2004): 203–210.

R. Applewhite, "Effectiveness of a Conductive Patch and a Conductive Bed Pad in Reducing Induced Human Body Voltage via the Application of Earth Ground," *European Biology and Bioelectromagnetics*, November 2005, 23–40.

G. Chevalier, K. Mori, and J. L. Oschman, "The Effect of Earthing (Grounding) on Human Physiology," *European Biology and Bioelectromagnetics*, January 31, 2006, 600–621.

G. Chevalier and K. Mori, "The Effect of Earthing on Human Physiology, Part 2: Electrodermal Measurements," *Subtle Energies and Energy Medicine* 18 (2006): 11–34.

M. Ghaly and D. Teplitz, "The Biological Effects of Grounding the Human Body During Sleep, as Measured by Cortisol Levels and Subjective Reporting of Sleep, Pain and Stress," *Journal of Alternative and Complementary Medicine* 10 (2004): 767–776.

D. Brown et al., "Pilot Study on the Effect of Grounding on Delayed-Onset Muscle Soreness," *Journal of Alternative and Complementary Medicine* 16(1) (2010): 1–9.

G. Chevalier, "Changes in Pulse Rate, Respiratory Rate, Blood Oxygenation, Perfusion Index, Skin Conductance and Their Variability Induced During and After Grounding Human Subjects for Forty Minutes," *Journal of Alternative and Complementary Medicine* 16(1) (2010): 81–87.

D. D. Sentman and B. J. Fraser, "Simultaneous Observations of Schumann Resonances in California and Australia—Evidence for Intensity Modulation," *Journal of Geophysical Research* 96 (1991): 15973–15984.

L. Assersohn et al., "A Randomized Pilot Study of SRL172 (*Mycobacterium vaccae*) in Patients with Small Cell Lung Cancer (SCLC) Treated with Chemotherapy," *Clinical Oncology* 14(1) (February 2002): 23–27.

C. A. Lowry et al., "Identification of an Immune-Responsive Mesolimbocortical Serotonergic System: Potential Role in Regulation of Emotional Behavior," *Neuroscience* 145(2–5) (May 2007): 756–772.

Chapter 5: Discover Your True Nature

Joshua W. Brown and Todd S. Braver, "Learned Predictions of Error Likelihood in the Anterior Cingulate Cortex," *Science* 307 (February 18, 2005): 1118–1121.

Ronald A. Rensink, "Change Detection," *Annual Review of Psychology* 53 (February 2002): 245–277.

Tony Perry, "Some Troops Have a Sixth Sense for Bombs," *Los Angeles Times*, October 28, 2009.

Chapter 10: Turn Your Feet into Living Shoes

American Academy of Orthopaedic Surgeons, "If the Shoe Fits, Wear It," http://orthoinfo.aaos .org/topic.cfm?topic=A00146.

Arthritis Guide, http://arthritis-guide.com/arthritis-glossary.htm.

"Exercise Adaptation/Injury Prevention Tidbits," Exercise Prescription, http://exrx.net/ExInfo/ InjuryTidbits.html.

L. Klenerman and B. Wood, *The Human Foot: A Companion to Clinical Studies* (Springer, 2006), 45–48, 95–96.

Peter Nabakov, *Indian Running: Native American History and Tradition* (Ancient City Press, 1987).

Chapter 13: On the Right Path with Nutrition

Ronald A. Hites et al., "Global Assessment of Organic Contaminants in Farmed Salmon," *Science* 303 (January 9, 2004): 226–229.

Deepak Chopra, *Magical Mind, Magical Body* [audiobook], (Nightingale Conant Corporation, 1994).

"Infant Formula Contains MSG," Truth in Labeling, www.truthinlabeling.org/formulacopy .html.

Gabriel Cousens, *There Is a Cure for Diabetes: The Tree of Life 21-Day+ Program* (North Atlantic Books, 2008).

Robert H. Lustig, Laura A. Schmidt, and Claire D. Brindis, "Public Health: The Toxic Truth About Sugar," *Nature*, February 2009.

World Wildlife Foundation, "Sugar and the Environment: Encouraging Better Management Practices in Sugar Production," 2004, assets.panda.org/downloads/sugarandtheenvironment _fidq.pdf.

Haibo Liu et al., "Fructose Induces Transketolase Flux to Promote Pancreatic Cancer Growth," *Cancer Research* 70 (August 1, 2010): 6368–6376.

Christopher R. Mohr, "The Dangers of High Fructose Corn Syrup: Is This Disguised Sugar Affecting Your Diabetes?" *Diabetes Health*, May 2005.

Emily Ventura et al., "Sugar Content of Popular Sweetened Beverages Based on Objective Laboratory Analysis: Focus on Fructose Content," *Obesity*, 2010.

V. S. Malik et al., "Intake of Sugar-Sweetened Beverages and Weight Gain: A Systematic Review," *American Journal of Clinical Nutrition* 84(2) (2006): 274–288.

L. R. Vartanian et al., "Effects of Soft Drink Consumption on Nutrition and Health? A Systematic Review and Meta-analysis," *American Journal of Public Health* 97(4) (2007): 667–675.

G. A. Bray, "How Bad Is Fructose?" *American Journal of Clinical Nutrition* 86(4) (2007): 895–896.

Aziz Aris and Samuel Leblanc, "Maternal and Fetal Exposure to Pesticides Associated to Genetically Modified Foods in Eastern Townships of Quebec, Canada," *Reproductive Toxicology* 31(4) (2011): 528–533.

Joël Spiroux de Vendômois, François Roullier, Dominique Cellier, and Gilles-Eric Séralini, "A Comparison of the Effects of Three GM Corn Varieties on Mammalian Health," *International Journal of Biological Sciences* 5(7) (2009): 706–726.

A. K. Susheelal et al., "Effective Interventional Approach to Control Anaemia in Pregnant Women," *Current Science* 98(10) (May 25, 2010).

M. Diesendorf et al., "New Evidence on Fluoridation," *Australian and New Zealand Journal of Public Health* 21(2) (1997).

D. H. Gutteridge et al., "Spontaneous Hip Fractures in Fluoride-Treated Patients: Potential Causative Factors," *Journal of Bone Mineral Research* 5, suppl. (March 1990): S205–215.

Y. Li et al., "Effect of Long-Term Exposure to Fluoride in Drinking Water on Risks of Bone Fractures," *Journal of Bone Mineral Research* 16(5) (May 2001): 932–939.

"EPA to Bar Fluoride-Based Pesticide; Decision Aims to Protect Children's Health," Environmental Working Group news release, January 10, 2011, http://ewg.org/release/epa-bar -fluoride-based-pesticide.

"Study Proves Benefits of Korean Fermented Paste," *Chosunilbo*, October 24, 2009, at http://english.chosun.com/site/data/html_dir/2009/10/24/2009102400127.html.

F. Batmanghelijd, M.D., *Your Body's Many Cries for Water* (Global Health Solutions, Inc., 2008).

Chapter 14: Barefoot Children

William A. Rossi, "Children's Footwear: Launching Site for Adult Foot Ills," *Podiatry Management*, October 2002, 83–100.

Michael Nirenberg, "Footnotes," *NWI Parent*, July/August 2008, 20.

U. B. Rao and B. Joseph, "The Influence of Footwear on the Prevalence of Flat Foot, a Survey of 2300 Children," *Journal of Bone and Joint Surgery* 74(4) (July 1992): 525–527.

Michael Nirenberg, "What Are the Best Shoes for Children? The Answer May Surprise You," America's Podiatrist, http://americaspodiatrist.com/2009/12/what-are-the-best-shoes-for-children-the-answer-may-surprise-you.

Shin-Jung Park et al., "Effects of Barefoot Habituation in Winter or Thermal and Hormonal Responses in Young Children—A Preliminary Study," *Journal of Human Ergology* 33 (2004): 61–67.

Sebastian Wolf et al., "Foot Motion in Children's Shoes: A Comparison of Barefoot Walking with Shod Walking in Conventional and Flexible Shoes," *Gait and Posture* 27 (2008): 51–59.

M. Walther et al., "Children's Sport Shoes—A Systematic Review of Current Literature," *Journal of Foot and Ankle Surgery* 14 (2008): 180–189.

Canadian Pediatrics Society statement, *Pediatrics and Child Health* 3(5) (1998): 373.

Anton Tudor et al., "Flat-Footedness Is Not a Disadvantage for Athletic Performance in Children Aged 11 to 15 Years," *Pediatrics* 123 (2009): 386–392.

William A. Rossi, "Fashion and Foot Deformation," *Podiatry Management*, October 2001, 103–118.

Chapter 15: Barefoot Seniors Turn Back the Clock

Norman Doidge, *The Brain That Changes Itself: Stories of Personal Triumph from the Frontiers of Brain Science* (Penguin, 2007).

Tobias Kalisch, et al., "Improvement of Sensorimotor Functions in Old Age by Passive Sensory Stimulation," *Clinical Interventions in Aging* 3(4) (2008): 673–690.

Gary Null and Amy McDonald, *Be a Healthy Woman!* (Seven Stories Press, 2009).

R. S. Rector et al., "Participation in Road Cycling vs. Running Is Associated with Lower Bone Mineral Density in Men," *Metabolism* 57 (2008): 226–232.

Joseph A. Buckwalter, "Decreased Mobility in the Elderly: The Exercise Antidote," *Physician and Sportsmedicine* 25(9) (1997): 126–133.

F. Li et al., "Health Benefits from a Cobblestone-Mat Walking Activity: Findings from a Pilot Study," *Medicine and Science in Sports and Exercise* 35 (May 2003): S375.

Najia Shakoor et al., "Effects of Specialized Footwear on Joint Loads in Osteoarthritis of the Knee," *Arthritis and Rheumatism* 59 (September 15, 2008): 1214–1220.

Chapter 17: Exploring Terrain

Ethan Todras-Whitehill, "Footloose and Boot Free: Barefoot Hiking," *New York Times,* September 22, 2006.

Chapter 18: Overcoming the Agony of the Feet

J. Li and C. Muehleman, "Anatomic Relationship of Heel Spur to Surrounding Soft Tissue: Greater Variability than Previously Reported," *Clinical Anatomy* 20 (2007): 950–955.

P. Jonsson et al., "New Regimen for Eccentric Calf-Muscle Training in Patients with Chronic Insertional Achilles Tendinopathy: Results of a Pilot Study," *British Journal of Sports Medicine* 42 (2008): 746–749.

Chapter 19: Minimalist Footwear—Uncensored

William A. Rossi, "Why Shoes Make 'Normal' Gait Impossible," *Podiatry Management*, March 1999.

Michael Nirenberg, "Can the Color of Your Shoes Affect Your Feet?" America's Podiatrist, http://americaspodiatrist.com/2009/09/can-the-color-of-your-shoes-affect-your-feet.

Chapter 20: Leading by Your Footprints

Thomas M. Kostigen, "Everything You Know About Water Conservation Is Wrong," *Discover*, June 2008.

Resources

Books

Ali, Majid. *The Ghoraa and Limbic Exercise.* Life Span Books, 1993.

Bragg, Patricia, and Paul C. Bragg. *Apple Cider Vinegar: Miracle Health System (Bragg Apple Cider Vinegar Miracle Health System: With the Bragg Healthy Lifestyle).* Bragg Health Sciences, 2008.

Brennan, J. H. *Tibetan Magic and Mysticism.* Llewellyn, 2006.

Campbell, T. Colin, and Thomas M. Campbell II. *The China Study.* BenBella Books, 2006.

Chopra, Deepak. *Magical Mind, Magical Body* (audiobook). Nightingale Conant Corporation, 1994.

Cousens, Gabriel. *There Is a Cure for Diabetes: The Tree of Life 21-Day+ Program.* North Atlantic Books, 2008.

Crowley, Chris, and Henry Lodge. *Younger Next Year: Live Strong, Fit, and Sexy—Until You're 80 and Beyond.* Workman, 2007.

Dispenza, Joe. *Evolve Your Brain: The Science of Changing Your Mind.* HCI, 2008.

Doidge, Norman. *The Brain That Changes Itself: Stories of Personal Triumph from the Frontiers of Brain Science.* Penguin, 2007.

Dreyer, Danny, and Katherine Dreyer. *ChiRunning: A Revolutionary Approach to Effortless, Injury-Free Running.* Fireside, 2009.

Emoto, Masaru. *The Hidden Messages in Water.* Atria, 2005.

Grossman, Warren. *To Be Healed by the Earth.* Seven Stories Press, 1999.

Howell, L. Daniel. *The Barefoot Book: 50 Great Reasons to Kick Off Your Shoes.* Hunter House, 2010.

Klenerman, L., and B. Wood. *The Human Foot: A Companion to Clinical Studies.* Springer, 2006.

Logan, William Bryant. *Dirt: The Ecstatic Skin of the Earth.* Norton, 2007.

Louv, Richard. *The Nature Principle: Human Restoration and the End of Nature-Deficit Disorder.* Algonquin Books, 2011.

———. *Last Child in the Woods: Saving Our Children from Nature-Deficit Disorder.* Algonquin Books, 2008.

McDougall, Christopher. *Born to Run: A Hidden Tribe, Superathletes, and the Greatest Race the World Has Never Seen.* Knopf, 2009.

Mipham, Sakyong. *Running with the Mind of Meditation.* Harmony Books, 2012.

Nabakov, Peter. *Indian Running: Native American History and Tradition.* Ancient City Press, 1987.

Nhat Hanh, Thich. *The Miracle of Mindfulness.* Beacon Press, 1999.

————. *Peace Is Every Step: The Path of Mindfulness in Everyday Life.* Bantam, 1992.

Null, Gary, and Amy McDonald. *Be a Healthy Woman!* Seven Stories Press, 2009.

Ober, Clinton, Stephen T. Sinatra, and Martin Zucker. *Earthing: The Most Important Health Discovery Ever?* Basic Health Publications, 2010.

Rossi, William. *The Complete Footwear Dictionary.* Krieger, 2000.

————. *The Sex Life of the Foot and Shoe.* Krieger, 1993.

Ruebush, Mary. *Why Dirt Is Good: 5 Ways to Make Germs Your Friends.* Kaplan Publishing, 2009.

Sandler, Michael and Jessica Lee. *Barefoot Running: How to Run Light and Free by Getting in Touch with the Earth.* Three Rivers Press, 2011.

Schaefer, Monika. *Reflexology Massage.* Sterling, 2008.

Schenck, Susan E., and Victoria Bidwell. *The Live Food Factor: The Comprehensive Guide to the Ultimate Diet for Body, Mind, Spirit and Planet.* Awakenings Publications, 2009.

Stevens, John. *The Marathon Monks of Mount Hiei.* Shambhala, 1988.

Wolfe, David. *Superfoods: The Food and Medicine of the Future.* North Atlantic Books, 2009.

Videos

The Art of Aging: The Limitless Potential of the Brain. Dir. Nicholas Blair. Documentary for PBS television. Old Dog Productions, 1999.

Barefoot Running—The How-To Movie. Dir. Adam Brix. DVD. RunBare Company, 2012.

The Beautiful Truth. Dir. Steve Kroschel. DVD. Kroschel Films, 2008.

Dirt! The Movie. Dir. Bill Logan, Gene Rosow, and Eleonore Dailly. DVD. Docurama, 2010.

Fat, Sick, and Nearly Dead. Dir. Joe Cross and Kirt Engfehr. DVD. Warner Bros., 2010.

Food Inc. Dir. Robert Kenner. DVD. Magnolia Home Entertainment, 2009.

Food Matters. Dir. James Colquhoun and Carlo Ledesma. DVD. Passion River Films, 2009.

Forks over Knives. Dir. Lee Fulkerson. DVD. Virgil Films and Entertainment, 2011.

Fresh. Dir. Ana Sofia Joanes. DVD. Docurama, 2009.

GasLand. Dir. Josh Fox. DVD. Docurama, 2010.

King Corn. Dir. Aaron Woolf. DVD. New Video Group, 2008.

Marathon Monks of Mount Hiei. Dir. Christopher J. Hayden. DVD. Documentary Educational Resources, 2002.

No Impact Man. Dir. Laura Gabbert and Justin Schein. DVD. Oscilloscope Laboratories, 2010.

The Meatrix. www.themeatrix.com.

Peaceful Warrior. Dir. Victor Salva. DVD. Universal Studios, 2007.

Simply Raw: Reversing Diabetes in 30 Days. Dir. Aaron Butler, DVD. Raw for Thirty, LLC, 2009.

What the Bleep Do We Know? Dir. Betsy Chasse, Mark Vicente, and William Arntz. DVD. 20th Century Fox, 2004.

What the Bleep? Down the Rabbit Hole. Dir. Betsy Chasse, Mark Vicente, and William Arntz. DVD. 20th Century Fox, 2006.

Yoga/Feet: Strong, Pain-free Feet. Dir. Warren Grossman, Sherri Mills, and Jimmy Maguire. DVD. 2012.

Websites

Barefoot Resources

www.RunBare.com Our barefoot wellness center devoted to helping people experience the spiritual, healing, and antiaging benefits of reconnecting with Mother Earth. We apply natural movement, conscious living practices, and delicious raw foods to help awaken and enliven your true nature. RunBare.com also includes tips, videos, and upcoming events.

Follow a thoughtful and insightful blog on barefoot living, the barefoot lifestyle, your barefoot rights, and more at Dr. Daniel Howell's site **www.BarefootProf.blogspot.com**.

www.Barefooters.org is home of the Society for Barefoot Living, dedicated to the barefoot movement since 1994.

PrimalFootalliance.org is an organization dedicated to the support and advocacy of those who choose to bare their feet.

Aids for Relaxation and Getting Grounded

Learn everything there is to know about how and why Earthing works to help you live more vibrantly at **www.Earthing.com**.

Michael Sandler shares the nature photography that helped quiet his mind and heal his spirit at **www.RunBare.com/Photography**.

Earth Songs: Mountain, Water, and the Healing Power of Nature, a documentary produced by stress expert Brian Luke Seaward, narrated by actor Michael York, with music composed by Academy Award–winning composer Brian Keane, is a breathtaking symphony of life that invites us all to renew our relationship with nature. *Earth Songs* was made as a relaxation DVD. Visit **www.BrianLukeSeaward.net**. Preview on YouTube at **www.youtube.com/watch?v=swE5aYurZcg**.

Foot Aids and Footwear Sources

Originator of the "zero drop" concept, Altra founder Golden Harper spent years cutting the heels off running shoes at his father's running shoe store (where he grew up and worked with co-designer Brian Beckstead), hoping to make a more biomechanically correct shoe. Years later, along with partner Jeremy Howlett, they designed Altras. **www.AltraZeroDrop.com**.

In 1993 the Pulka family had a vision to provide products for healthier feet. Mate a socklike upper with a 1-mm Kevlar bottom, and you've got the makings of a Feelmax. Their shoes are some of the thinnest and lightest out there, allowing full natural mobility of the foot. **www.Feelmax.fi/en** and **www.GiftsfromFinland.com**.

www.LemsShoes.com Originally called Stem Footwear, Lems were inspired by creator and CEO Andrew Rademacher after years of injuries on the track. Going barefoot, he sought to deconstruct the shoe and come up with something better. His company seeks to follow the 50 percent eco rule: 50 percent less consumption (smaller carbon footprint), 50 percent less shoe (more natural movement), 50 percent less material, 50 percent less of everything.

Inspired by Manuel Luna, Barefoot Ted began creating his own huaraches. His idea caught on and grew into a forward looking, eco-friendly company, **www.LunaSandals.com**. They seek to design sandals that are "made out of natural, sustainable materials that are easy to make by hand with simple tools."

Two-time Grammy Award winner and Native American "Renaissance man" Robert Mirabal "talks story" about how he began re-creating Taos Pueblo moccasins based on traditional designs handed down from his grandmother at **www.redwillowvoices.blogspot.com/ search?q=moccasins**. Pick up your own pair at **www.RobertMirabal.com**.

The **www.SoftStarShoes.com** elves are busy at work in Corvallis, Oregon, hand-crafting moccasins made with eco-friendly leathers, sheepskin, and Vibram soles, for every occasion, season, and age, from baby to adult.

From the Maori to the Incans to the gladiators, Tread Light Gear showcases a wide variety of handmade ancestral-inspired footwear at **www.etsy.com/shop/TreadLightGear**.

For a modern take on huaraches, the traditional Mexican running sandals of the Tarahumara and a "barefoot-plus protection feel," check out Xero Shoes, at **www.XeroShoes.com**.

Designed as "performance protection for bare feet," **www.ZEMGear.com** offers protection for the sole without much else. If your feet need mittens, check out the split-toe designs.

Start your feet and ankles on the path to recovery with Correct Toes at **www.NWfootankle .com**. Realigning your toes as nature intended realigns your body for better balance and stride.

Check out **www.Topricin.com** for a homeopathic solution to your aches, pains, and inflammation. Invented by Vietnam veteran Lou Paradise to overcome his postwar challenges, this revolutionary nonpharmaceutical product has no parabens, no petroleum derivatives, or any other harmful ingredients.

If you're in Boulder, Colorado, stop in at In-Step, a minimalist-friendly footwear shop and a great place to hang out. Be sure to check out Spencer's train set. Or visit online at **www.InStepBldr.com**.

Resources for Eating and Drinking Well

For the latest health news, articles, and information on diet, nutrition, and natural health, check out **www.Mercola.com**.

To ensure healthy living for future generations, strive to bring only sustainable food to your dinner table with the help of Sustainable Table at **www.sustainabletable.org/home.php**.

An indispensable resource for all families that desire to eat well: Encyclopedia of Macrobiotic and Nutrition Info at **www.macrobiotics.nl/encyclopedia/encyclopedia_a.html**.

You can't go wrong with **www.Nutiva.com**, a company that strives to change the world, promoting health and sustainability while offering high-quality, organic superfoods.

For an incredible selection of superfoods, visit David Wolfe's **www.LongevityWarehouse.com** and for delicious organic, vegan, raw chocolate, **www.sacredchocolate.com**.

This raw family offers delicious green smoothie recipes. Follow the Boutenko family's remarkable healing journey through raw food eating at **www.RawFamily.com**.

From seeds to sprouters, **www.SproutPeople.org** offers everything you could possibly need to get started on your sprouting journey.

A true employee-owned, family-started business, **www.BobsRedMill.com** strives to make grains the old-fashioned way, stone ground, with a huge selection of gluten-free grains and foods.

Remember to bless your water. See with your own eyes how our thoughts affect water crystals when you use Dr. Masaru Emoto's iPhone app: **www.MyHado.com**.

Footprint Calculators

Measure the walkability of any address at **www.WalkScore.com** and make better living choices.

In addition to consuming water directly, water is used to produce the goods and services you consume. Calculate your water footprint at **www.WaterFootprint.org**, by considering both your direct and indirect use of water.

Get *Rippl*. Learn how to make simple, sustainable choices and form life-changing habits with this fantastic app from **http://www.oceanconservancy.org/do-your-part/rippl.html**.

Take an ecological footprint quiz at **www.Earthday.org/footprint-calculator** and explore simple actions to minimize your family's footprint.

For the next step on your barefoot journey, check out our how-to book, *Barefoot Running: How to Run Light and Free by Getting in Touch with the Earth*.

Take the Next Step

www.richardlouv.com/blog Follow author of *Last Child in the Woods* Richard Louv's commentary on society and what choices we can make to coexist and reconnect with nature.

Looking for a barefoot walking or running club? Check out **meetup.com** and the Barefoot Runner's Society, an international barefoot running club and forum with chapters and events in nearly every state and many countries around the world. **http://www.thebare footrunners.org**.

Read up on Dr. Daniel Lieberman's latest studies on the biomechanics of running shod versus running barefoot at **www.barefootrunning.fas.harvard.edu**.

www.barefootrunning.com, the "original barefoot running website, since 1997"—site of Ken Bob Saxton, an early guru of the barefoot movement.

Meet up with the original Barefoot Running Club for a barefoot run, walk, or hike in Boulder, Colorado. **www.meetup.com/Barefoot-Running-Club**.

Danny and Katherine Dreyer's revolutionary approach to effortless and injury-free running is spelled out in their best-selling book *ChiRunning* and in their clinics. Find out more at **www.ChiRunning.com**.

Follow Don Spence, the Pilates and health guru in Fort Collins, Colorado, who saved Michael's back after an injury, at **www.MYBQA.com**.

Now that your time out in nature has made you smarter, keep the brain stimulation going by visiting **www.PositScience.com**, Dr. Michael Merzenich's brainpower site.

Photos

Take a deep breath, relax, and enjoy our sunrise and sunset photos from nature at **www.RunBare.com/photography**.

Retreats

Come walk and dine with us. For rejuvenating healing retreats and delicious raw foods at exotic eco-friendly locations around the world, visit **www.RunBare.com/Retreats**.

The Movie

For the most beautiful and inspiring how-to movie on barefoot running and playing in nature, starring the authors of this book, visit **www.RunBare.com/TheMovie**.

Social Media

Follow us and get the latest advice and information on **www.Facebook.com/RunBare**.

Get the skinny with quick tips and updates at **www.twitter.com/RunBareCompany**.

Watch our cool videos at **www.youtube.com/RunBareCompany**.

Check out the latest eco-adventures, inspirational posts, and photos by Michael at **www.Facebook.com/RunsWithSpirit**.

Visit Jessica's page for her latest stories and adventures in nature, with a lighthearted take on life's lessons: **www.Facebook.com/Jessica.Lee.Sandler**.

Photo Credits

Index

Hills, 154–155, 329–330
Hindfoot, 173, 175, 178–179
Hinduism, 6
Hippocampus, 55
Hippocrates, 242
Hips, 21, 22, 32, 351
Honey, 110, 266
Hot Potato game, 211
Hot tubs, 201, 231, 233
Hot-weather walking, 99, 100, 197, 279,
    306–311
Hundreds exercise, 213–214
Hydration belt/pack, 311
Hygiene hypothesis, 75, 76
Hypoglycemia, 241, 251
Hypothalamus, 252

Icing feet, 199, 339, 345
Iliotibial (IT) bands, 122, 234
IllumiNite, 321
Immune system, 4, 41–43, 65, 75, 109, 226,
    241, 244, 265, 298, 299, 312
Impact fractures, 343
Impact transient, 137
Inch Worm exercise, 184
Indian Ocean tsunami (2004), 83
Indian Running (Nabokov),
    278
Infections, 335, 362
Inflammation, 4, 42, 65–66, 77, 78, 200,
    257, 299, 337–340, 345
Inflare, 368, 369
Inflate the Balloon exercise, 127
Information overload, 52, 53
Ingrown toenails, 344
Injuries, 331–355
Inmon, Raymond, 169
Inov-8, 216
Insoles, 171, 371
Insulin resistance, 252
Insulin response, 61
Integration, 52, 53
International Mud Day, 76
Intuition, 83
Iron, 266

Jarawa tribe, 83
Jazzercise, 227

Jesus, 6, 61
Jet lag, 67
Jumping Jacks, 213

Kale, 265
Katz, Sandor Ellix, 262
Keller, Helen, 316
Kelp, 265
Knee Kick exercise, 214
Knees, 20–23, 32, 123, 348–349
Koran, 6

Labyrinths, 5, 168–169, 287
Lactic acid, 200
LaLanne, Jack, 298
Lamisil, 334
Lao Tsu, 115
Last Child in the Woods (Louv), 84,
    276
Laughter, 133
Lauric acid, 264
Lava rock, 327
Left hemisphere of brain, 53
Leg length discrepancy (LLD), 3, 139, 236,
    350
Legs, stress on, 21
Lems, 149, 360
Leonardo da Vinci, 173
Lhoppon Rechung, 144
Libido, 58
Lieberman, Dan, 137
Lifting Your Arch exercise, 184
Ligaments, 174, 220, 224
Lightning, 68
Lignans, 266
Live Food Factor, The (Cousins), 263
Live foods, 262–263
Local foods, 244
Lodge, Henry S., 289–290, 297
Log Roll exercise, 192
Louv, Richard, 83, 84, 276
Lowry, Chris, 77
Luna Sandals, 360, 370
Lung-gom-pa runners, 7
Lunges, 220
Lymphatic fluid, 200, 288
Lymphatic system, 42, 225–226
Lyons, Oren, 373

About the Authors

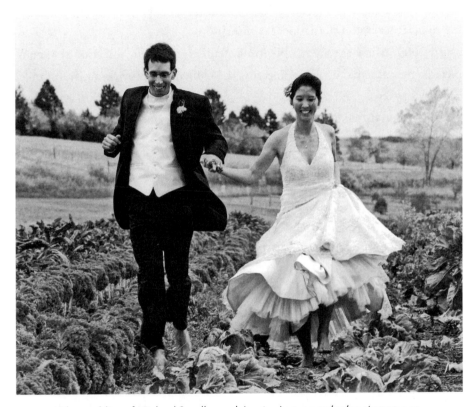

The wedding of Michael Sandler and Jessica Lee, on 10/10/10 at 10:10 a.m.

MICHAEL SANDLER, the co-author of *Barefoot Running: How to Run Light and Free by Getting in Touch with the Earth*, is an internationally recognized barefoot running and walking coach, teaching thousands of runners, walkers, and hikers of all abilities. He has coached athletes professionally for nearly twenty years.

After a near-fatal in-line skating accident in 2006, he was told he was lucky to keep his leg, but that he might never walk again. With a titanium femur and hip, he found that it was only through barefoot walking and running and the lessons learned on the trails that he was able to heal. He now walks and runs barefoot ten to twenty miles a day.

Among Michael's other personal athletic achievements are training for the 1992 and 1996 Olympics in both cycling and speed skating at the Olympic Training Center in Colorado Springs. While racing in Europe aiming for the Tour de France, an unexpected vehicle collision on a closed race course dashed his chances for both international competitions.

In 2004, Michael rode his bike in an entirely different direction. He completed a monumental bicycle trip across the United States by riding 5,000 miles in forty days, solo and unsupported, to raise awareness for children and adults with attention deficit disorder (ADD). He ended the ride in Washington, D.C., where he was invited to speak before members of the U.S. House and Senate on the Mental Health Parity Act, urging equal health coverage for psychological as well as physical health.

Michael is also an accomplished professional photographer. He began taking sunrise and sunset photos while healing from his near-fatal accident. He now takes photographs on his barefoot walks and hikes daily. His works are featured in select galleries around the world.

Michael has been featured on NPR, the BBC, ABC News, CBS News, NBC News, and Fox News, and in *Men's Health Asia*, *Shape Magazine Asia*, *Asian Geographic*, and elsewhere.

JESSICA LEE holds a bachelor's of science degree in learning and organizational change from Northwestern University's School of Education and Social Policy. Following graduation, she served two years with the U.S. Peace Corps working on sustainable youth and community development projects in St. Vincent and the Grenadines.

Envisioning a world with more eco-friendly practices, she then went on to work in the renewable energy industry, marketing and promoting green projects in both the solar and geothermal energy fields.

Meanwhile in 2007, she ran the Bolder Boulder 10K and felt crippled with knee pain after the first 3K. Following the race, she decided to give up the sport and focus her athletic efforts on cycling. This lasted until she met Michael and became inspired to run again, discovering a pain-free joyous experience in barefoot movement. So inspired by this newfound freedom, she convinced Michael that they should quit their jobs, start writing *Barefoot Running*, and launch RunBare Company as a team.

Today RunBare is a thriving barefoot wellness center devoted to helping people experience the spiritual and antiaging benefits of reconnecting with Mother Earth and with one's true nature through natural movement and conscious living practices. Jessica designs, coordinates, and co-instructs multiday retreats and weekend workshops nationwide and at exotic eco-friendly locations around the world for destination travel adventurists. Now married, Michael and Jessica enjoy starting each day with a grounded meditation and a barefoot sunrise hike before embracing the joyous work that lies ahead.